Contents

D1332715

Child and Adolescent Mental Health Nursing

Edited by Tim McDougall

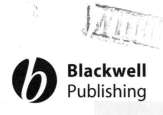

Blackwell
Publishing

Editorial offices:
Blackwell Publishing Ltd, 9600 Garsington Road, Oxford OX4 2DQ, UK
   Tel: +44 (0)1865 776868
Blackwell Publishing Inc., 350 Main Street, Malden, MA 02148-5020, USA
   Tel: +1 781 388 8250
Blackwell Publishing Asia Pty Ltd, 550 Swanston Street, Carlton, Victoria 3053, Australia
   Tel: +61 (0)3 8359 1011

First published 2006 by Blackwell Publishing Ltd

ISBN-10: 1-4051-2801-1
ISBN-13: 978-1-4051-2801-8

Library of Congress Cataloging-in-Publication Data

Child and adolescent mental health nursing / edited by Tim McDougall.
     p. ; cm.
   Includes bibliographical references and index.
   ISBN-13: 978-1-4051-2801-8 (pbk. : alk. paper)
   ISBN-10: 1-4051-2801-1 (pbk. : alk. paper)   1. Child psychiatric nursing.   2. Adolescent psychiatric nursing.
   [DNLM: 1. Child.   2. Mental Disorders–nursing.   3. Adolescent.   4. Psychiatric Nursing–education.   5. Psychiatric Nursing–legislation & jurisprudence.   WY 160 C5357 2006]   I. McDougall, Tim.
   RJ502.3.C48 2006
   618.92′89–dc22
                                        2005036417

A catalogue record for this title is available from the British Library

Set in 10/12.5 pt Palatino
by Graphicraft Limited, Hong Kong, China
Printed and bound in India by Replika Press Pvt. Ltd, Kundli

The publisher's policy is to use permanent paper from mills that operate a sustainable forestry policy, and which has been manufactured from pulp processed using acid-free and elementary chlorine-free practices. Furthermore, the publisher ensures that the text paper and cover board used have met acceptable environmental accreditation standards.

For further information on Blackwell Publishing, visit our website:
www.blackwellnursing.com

Contributing authors

Marie Armstrong is a Nurse Consultant leading the child and adolescent mental health self-harm service in Nottingham. Having worked in CAMHS for 18 years, she has vast experience in a variety of settings, including adolescent in-patient, children's day service, community mental health teams, and primary care liaison nursing. Marie has been a nurse consultant since 2000. Her current post involves 50% direct clinical practice, as well as leadership and consultancy, teaching, research and service development. Marie has developed and implemented good practice guidelines for the management of young people who self harm and has helped develop the National Institute for Clinical Excellence (NICE) guidelines on selfharm. Marie has provided training workshops and spoken at conferences. As well as being trained in child and adolescent mental health nursing, Marie is a qualified and United Kingdom Council for Psychotherapy (UKCP) registered systemic psychotherapist.

Moira Davren, RMN, MSc, BSc (Hons), a Registered Systemic Therapist, is Senior Practice Development Fellow at the RCN Institute, Northern Ireland. Moira's experience has been in child and adolescent mental health services as a nurse specialist and registered family therapist. She joined the RCN in 2000. Moira has been, and continues to be, involved in an array of research and development activities, locally, nationally and internationally and has worked as the acting head of professional development at the RCN in Northern Ireland for the last two years. Moira is currently acting as Convenor of the expert Child & Adolescent Mental Health Committee within the Review of Mental Health and Learning Disability in Northern Ireland and is a member of the Children's Legal Issues Committee, the main review-steering committee, and the Convenors Expert Reference Committee. Moira has held several consultative and advisory roles at a regional, national and international level and has extensive experience in practice development, policy development, work-based learning programmes, lifelong learning programmes and project management. Moira also contributes to community and public health initiatives by acting as a consultant to DELTA, an early learning project for families in the Southern Health and Social Services Area Board in Northern Ireland, and contributes in a voluntary capacity to her local community and to Barnardo's as a family therapist.

Fiona Gale, RMN, BSc, PG Dip, MA, PhD, ENB 603 (higher award) is Associate Director and the CAMHS programme leader for the East Midlands, National CAMHS Support Service within the Care Services Improvement Partnership (CSIP). Her role is to support CAMHS in developing their services to a sustainable and comprehensive level. Within her portfolio, Fiona is also the national lead on the development of the primary mental health worker role, and the advanced CAMHS training programme for England. She has 18 years' experience in CAMHS as a mental health nurse, primary mental health worker, service manager and joint commissioning and strategy manager for CAMHS. She has substantial clinical and managerial experience in all tiers of CAMHS. In the last few years, Fiona has undertaken much work on a local and national basis in relation to the role of the primary mental health worker in CAMHS, and has published widely on the subject. Fiona's PhD thesis is a research study of children's and families' perceptions of mental health and stigma. She is also an honorary lecturer on the CAMHS MSc at University College Northampton.

Ian Higgins, RMN, RSCN, RGN, MBA, is Nurse Consultant in Tier 4 Services, South West London & St George's NHS Trust. Ian has 20 years' experience most of which has been in specialist CAMHS. He is one of the founding members of the Children's In-patient Special Interest Group (CHIPSIG) and is currently Chair of the National Nurse Consultants in CAMHS Forum. Ian is particularly interested in highlighting the complex and multiskilled role of the nurse in CAMHS and health services in general. Ian's clinical interests include the role of fathers in CAMHS and also the impact of parental mental health on children and young people.

Sharon Leighton, RMN, PG Dip, MSc, is a Nurse Consultant in Stafford and has worked in child and adolescent services for 15 years. Sharon has close links with Staffordshire University where she has been involved in setting up CAMHS training for practitioners in primary settings. This work has been evaluated and recently published. Sharon has also been working on implementing school-based mental health services for children. Sharon has helped develop the National Institute for Clinical Excellence (NICE) guidelines for depression in children and is a member of the National Nurse Consultants in CAMHS Forum. Sharon has a clinical interest working with children who have suffered bereavement or loss; and particularly adolescents who present with delayed symptoms of complicated grief.

Lisa Lewer is Nurse Consultant at the Ellern Mede Centre for Eating Disorders in north London. Lisa has worked in CAMHS in-patient settings for the past 12 years. Throughout this time, she has maintained a keen interest in the therapeutic milieu, and organisational dynamics. She has recently begun to develop the concepts of 'affect regulation' and 'mentalisation' within the in-patient setting with her colleagues at the Ellern Mede Centre.

Tim McDougall, RMN, BSc (Hons), PG Dip, Specialist Practitioner (Mental Health), ENB 603 (higher award) is a Nurse Consultant in Tier 4 CAMHS. Tim has worked in a range of CAMHS settings, including community child mental health teams, adolescent in-patient services and secure adolescent forensic services. Tim has a national profile in CAMHS and, with over 50 publications, has spoken at national and European conferences about the mental health of children and adolescents. Whilst Tim is primarily interested with the strategic development and leadership of CAMHS and nursing, clinical interests include working with violent young people, early onset psychosis and adolescent bipolar disorder. Tim help found the National Nurse Consultants in CAMHS Forum and has helped develop the NICE guidelines for bipolar disorders and the Chief Nursing Officer's review of mental health nursing.

Ray McMorrow is Nurse Consultant for Community CAMHS at Birmingham Children's Hospital. Ray has worked in mental health settings in East London, Northampton, Bermuda and the east and west Midlands. His interest in the cultural competency of services started early in his nursing career as he observed the over-representation of some groups in secure hospital settings and the paucity of cultural competence in service provision. During his 15-year nursing career Ray has become passionate about service equity and community needs. He has published articles on the role of nursing in CAMHS and presented at conferences on service development and cultural impacts on mental health. Ray is Treasurer of the Association of Nurses in CAMHS, a council member of YoungMinds and a CAMHS nurse representative to the NIMHE (National Institute for Mental Health in England) Nursing Advisory Group.

Paul Mitchell is Clinical Nurse Specialist in the Forensic Adolescent Consultation and Treatment Service, Manchester. Paul has over 15 years' experience in community and in-patient CAMHS and worked in one of the first pilot Youth Offending Teams (YOT) as a mental health worker. Paul has always had a keen interest in the interface between CAMHS and the youth justice system. Paul has previously undertaken research with service users regarding their views of forensic services and was one of the founding members of the Adolescent Forensic Professional Network. On behalf of the Youth Justice Board (YJB) Paul has delivered mental health training to YOT workers, and is currently working on a pilot project providing CBT (cognitive behaviour therapy) interventions to young offenders with mental health problems. Paul is currently working towards his doctorate.

Barry Nixon currently combines two roles, being the National Workforce Lead for CAMHS and the Northwest Regional CAMHS Workforce Project Director based with the Greater Manchester Strategic Health Authority. Barry has worked in a variety of learning disability and CAMHS settings across a range of services including the health, education, social services and voluntary sectors. Having now moved away from clinical practice Barry has been instrumental in the development of education programmes in child and adolescent mental health practice and more recently in supporting the development of the National Workforce Strategy for CAMHS.

Ian Roberts is a Service Manager in the Central Cheshire Child and Adolescent Mental Health Service. After completing his initial RMN (Registered Mental Health Nurse) training in Chester, Ian worked in both Bolton and Liverpool before moving back to Cheshire. Ian has been working within CAMHS for 15 years in Tier 4 and community settings, as well as in the independent sector. Ian has developed a clinical interest in therapeutic fostering, systemic consultation and systemic approaches and interventions. Ian has completed training in several therapeutic modalities and is registered with the UKCP as a systemic therapist. Ian's current role delivers both a clinical specialist therapeutic function and a management role to CAMHS services in Cheshire.

Noreen Ryan, RGN, RMN, ENB 603, ENB 998, BA (Hons), MSc is Nurse Consultant at Bolton CAMHS. Noreen's areas of expertise are attention deficit hyperactivity disorder (AD/HD) and neurodevelopmental disorder. As lead of the ADHD service in Bolton, Noreen is responsible for the strategic and clinical development of the service. As part of her consultation role Noreen helps other professionals develop skills and competencies and provides expert opinions in relation to ADHD. After training as a general nurse, Noreen worked as a staff nurse on a neurosurgical unit. On completing post-registration mental health nurse training, Noreen worked on a psychogeriatric ward before starting her career as a CAMHS nurse. Noreen has worked in both in-patient and community settings and has developed skills in assessment, parenting and groupwork, as well as in providing liaison and consultation to colleagues in statutory and voluntary services in primary care, education and social services.

Augustine Sagoe is a Nurse Consultant in the Child, Adolescent and Family Mental Health, South Essex Partnership NHS Trust. He has several years' experience in CAMHS and has worked in both in-patient and community settings in the NHS, independent services and voluntary sector. Augustine specialises in consultation and provides training, supervision and group facilitation to nurses, multidisciplinary teams and organisations. Augustine is passionate about mental health promotion and the prevention of mental ill-health in children.

Sally Sanderson is the Team Manager for a newly established early onset psychosis service in the Cheshire & Wirral NHS Partnership Trust. Sally has worked in adult mental health for over 20 years, primarily with people who have severe mental health problems. Due to a belief that there must be more to treatment than the traditional medical models and high levels of medication, Sally became attracted to the growing body of evidence supporting the use of psychosocial approaches to treatment. Having completed her BSc (Hons) course, Sally developed a specific interest in the emergent early psychosis services, becoming involved in the planning and implementation process. Sally is involved with a wide range of training programmes focusing on psychosocial approaches to the management of severe mental health problems.

Eileen Woolley is a Nurse Consultant for CAMHS in the Cambridge and Peterborough Partnership NHS Trust. Eileen trained as a psychiatric nurse and began her career in CAMHS after helping to develop and open an adolescent unit in the Midlands. Eileen obtained her first degree from the University of Armidale in Australia via distance learning and obtained an MSc from Cambridge University in 1999. Eileen is an honorary lecturer at Homerton College in Cambridge and is about to begin a doctorate at Cambridge University.

Tina Hatton and **Debra McKay** are both Clinical Nurse Specialists in substance misuse (young people and their carers) working for CAMHS at South West London and St George's NHS Trust. Tina and Debra have backgrounds in adult addiction and CAMHS in the statutory and voluntary sectors. Between them they have developed expertise in the area of substance misuse and have worked in London, Surrey, Sheffield and Brazil.

Preface

Readers will note that this is a book written by nurses for nurses. However, this does not mean that nurses work in isolation and they have nothing to learn from other professions. On the contrary, nurses who work with children with mental health problems do so in a multiprofessional and interagency context, and have much to learn from, and to share with their colleagues. There exists a wealth of knowledge, skills and competencies across the specialist CAMHS workforce. Just as professionals in health, social care, education and youth justice provide complimentary services to children and young people, so too the roles and responsibilities of professionals should interact to produce the best possible outcome for children. Specialist CAMHS form a workforce which includes all disciplines and talents: psychiatrists, psychologists, paediatricians and nurses all have a different education and training, different philosophies and objectives as well as different roles and functions. Together they all form part of the rich tapestry of specialist CAMHS which should be celebrated and embraced by nurses.

Foreword

by Professor Susan Bailey

Child and Adolescent Mental Health Nursing represents a landmark event at many different levels. During a period of unprecedented change and development in child and adolescent mental health services across the jurisdictions of the UK, a real opportunity has been given to all professionals working with children and adolescents to meet their mental health needs, whatever the nature and degree of their difficulty and circumstance.

Through this book, the editor and individual authors have brought together a unique blend of clinical knowledge, evidence-based practice and practical pragmatics of working day to day, out in the field, managing and steering a complex variety of service provision across community settings and specialist community and child and adolescent inpatient provision.

This book is a realisation of the pivotal role of nurses in research, management, leadership and innovative practice across child and adolescent mental health.

Each chapter addresses the key child and adolescent mental health problems and distils down the science and complexity of the subject into a framework that will better enable all practitioners of whatever discipline to understand and carry out their role as part of multiagency, multidisciplinary teams.

In essence, what follows represents far more than the sum of its constituent parts. Mental health nurses have come together at a time when it seemed there was little outside incentive to move on and develop this important speciality. Child and adolescent mental health nursing has come of age and in doing so has delivered a thoroughly informed, clear, helpful text, providing a platform from which to develop the vitally important role of the nursing profession in what is at least for me and clearly the authors is a most exciting area of work, providing resilience and restoring wellbeing to children and adolescents.

Dedication

For my wonderful children: Amy, Sam and Jack.

Acknowledgements

As well as each contributing author, I would like to thank the following people for their advice, guidance, support and patience during the development of this book:

Professor Susan Bailey (University of Central Lancashire); Professor Simon Gowers (University of Liverpool); Mervyn Townley (Gwent Healthcare NHS Trust); Keith Escott (Department of Health); Richard Wistow (University of Durham); Tim Docking (Northgate & Prudhoe NHS Trust); Sarah Corcoran (Scottish Executive Government); Helen Scott (Cheshire & Merseyside Adolescent Eating Disorders Service); Alison Tingle (Department of Health); Susan Aitkenhead (Nursing & Midwifery Council); Bev Reid (North Tyne Commissioning Group); Carys Jones (Cheshire & Wirral Partnership NHS Trust); Andrew Cresswell (Gwent Healthcare NHS Trust).

Note

All the case studies used in this book are real. However, the names of the young people concerned and some of their details have been changed. This is to protect their identity and respect their confidentiality.

List of abbreviations and glossary of useful terms

Term	Meaning	Applicable
ADD	Attention deficit disorder	
ADHD	Attention deficit hyperactivity disorder	
AHPs	Allied health professionals	
AN	Anorexia nervosa	
ASEBA	Achenbach system of empirically based assessment	
BAVQ	Beliefs about voices questionnaire	
BDI	Beck's depression inventory	
BME	Black and minority ethnic	
BMI	Body mass index	
BN	Bulimia nervosa	
BSFT	Brief solution-focused therapy	
CAMHS	Child and adolescent mental health services	
CAS	Cognitive assessment schedule	
CASR	Connors adolescent self report	
CBC	Child behaviour checklist	
CBGT	Cognitive behavioural group treatment	
CBT	Cognitive behavioural therapy	
CGAS	Children's global assessment of functioning	
CGWT	Care group workforce team	[England only]
Childline	Free telephone helpline for children and young people	
CHIPSIG	Children's in-patient special interest group	
CHSG	Scottish Executive's Child Health Support Group	[Scotland only]
Connexions	Information, advice and support service for young people aged 13–19	[England only]
CORC	CAMHS Outcome Research Consortium	
CMP	Clinical management plan	
CNO	Chief Nursing Officer	
CPA	Care programme approach	
CPD	Continuing professional development	

CPRS	Connors parent rating scale	
CSE	Coping strategy enhancement	
CTRS	Connors teachers rating scale	
CSIP	Care Services Improvement Partnership	*[England only]*
CYPU	Children and Young People's Unit	*[England only]*
DAMP	Deficits in attention, motor function and perception	
DAAT	Drug and alcohol team	
DAT	Drug action team	
DBT	Dialectical behavioural therapy	
DfES	Department for Education and Skills	*[England only]*
DoH	Department of Health	*[England only]*
DHSSPS	Department of Health, Social Services and Public Safety	*[Northern Ireland only]*
DNA	Did not attend	
DRE	Delivering race equality	
DSH	Deliberate self-harm	
DSM	Diagnostic and Statistical Manual of Mental Disorders	
EBD	Emotional and behavioural difficulties	
ECBI	Eyberg child behaviour inventory	
ECHR	European Convention on Human Rights	
ECT	Electroconvulsive therapy	
EDNOS	Eating disorder not otherwise specified	
ENB	English National Board	
EPPIC	Early Psychosis Prevention and Intervention Centre	*[Australia only]*
FPLD	Foundation for People with Learning Disabilities	
GCSE	General Certificate of Secondary Education	*[England, Wales & Northern Ireland only]*
HAS	Health Advisory Service	*[England and Wales only]*
HMSO	Her Majesty's Stationary Office	
HoNOSCA	Health of the nation outcome scale for children and adolescents	
HoNOSCA-SR	Health of the nation outcome scale for children and adolescents – self-rated	
GAS	Severe Group A streptococcus	
GHQ	General health questionnaire	
GP	General practitioner	
Heads Up Scotland	National project for child and adolescent mental health	*[Scotland only]*

HCW	Health Commission Wales	*[Wales only]*
HKD	Hyperkinetic disorder	
HPA	Health Protection Agency	
HRA	Human Rights Act	
ICD	International classification of diseases	
IP	Independent prescriber	
IQ	Intelligence quotient	
IRIS	Initiative to Reduce the Impact of Schizophrenia	
ISSP	Intensive supervision and surveillance programmes	
KIDDIE-SADS	Kiddie schedule for affective disorders and schizophrenia	
LAC	Looked-after children	
LASCH	Local authority secure children's home	
LDP	Local delivery plan	
LHB	Local health board	*[Wales only]*
LSCB	Local safeguarding children's boards	*[England and Wales only]*
MHA	Mental Health Act	*[England and Wales only]*
MHAC	Mental Health Act Commission	*[England and Wales only]*
MHF	Mental Health Foundation	
MRSA	Methicillin-resistant staphylococcus aureaus	
MST	Multisystemic therapy	
NACRO	National Association for the Care and Rehabilitation of Offenders	
NCH	National Children's Home	
NCSS	National CAMHS Support Service	*[England only]*
NHS	National Health Service	
NICE	National Institute for Health and Clinical Excellence	*[England and Wales only]*
NIMHE	National Institute for Mental Health in England	*[England only]*
NSF	National Service Framework	
NSPCC	National Society for the Prevention of Cruelty to Children	
NTA	National Treatment Agency	
NVLD	Nonverbal learning difficulties	
OCD	Obsessive compulsive disorder	
ONS	Office for National Statistics	
PCT	Primary care trust	*[England only]*
PHIS	Public Health Institute for Scotland	*[Scotland only]*
PHSE	Personal Health and Social Education	
PMHW	Primary mental health worker	

PSA	Public service agreement	
PSI	Psychosocial interventions	
PTSD	Post-traumatic stress disorder	
RCN	Royal College of Nursing	
RCP	Royal College of Psychiatrists	
RCT	Randomised controlled trial	
RDW	Regional development worker	*[England only]*
RMN	Registered Nurse – mental health	
RNLD	Registered Nurse – learning disabilities	
RSCN	Registered Nurse – children	
SAAT	Self-assessment audit tool	*[Wales only]*
SBHC	School-based health clinic	
SAVRY	Structured assessment of violence risk in youth	
SBMHS	School-based mental health services	
SCMH	Sainsbury Centre for Mental Health	
SDQ	Strengths and difficulties questionnaire	
SEN	Special educational needs	
SENCO	Special educational needs coordinator	
SHA	Strategic health authority	*[England only]*
SIFA	Mental health screening interview for adolescents	
SIS	Suicidal intent scale	
SNAP	Scottish Needs Assessment Programme	*[Scotland only]*
S-NASA	Salford needs assessment schedule for adolescents	
SP	Supplementary prescriber	
SQUIFA	Screening questionnaire interview for adolescents	
SSRI	Selective serotonin reuptake inhibitor	
TVRS	Topography of voices rating scale	
STC	Secure training centre	*[England only]*
UKCC	United Kingdom Central Council	
UKCP	United Kingdom Council for Psychotherapy	
UNCRC	United Nations Convention on the Rights of the Child	
WHO	World Health Organization	
YJB	Youth Justice Board	*[England and Wales only]*
YOI	Young offender institution	
YOT	Youth offending team	*[England and Wales only]*
YoungMinds	National charity committed to improving the mental health of all babies, children and young people.	

Chapter 1

Defining the Terms

Tim McDougall

Key points

- All nurses and other professionals who work with children share a responsibility to ensure that every child is given every opportunity to reach their fullest potential and to enjoy good mental health. Good mental health involves the ability to develop emotional resilience, good self-esteem and the skills to cope in the face of stress and adversity.

- In addition to the 2500 nurses in specialist child and adolescent mental health services, there are an estimated 15 000 children's nurses, 13 000 health visitors and 2500 school nurses who work in primary CAMHS (child and adolescent mental health services) and also have a role in meeting the mental health needs of children and adolescents.

- Primary mental health workers work in a range of settings and in a variety of ways. They have been successful in reducing inappropriate referrals to specialist CAMHS and in developing the mental health skills of staff whose core business is not child and adolescent mental health.

- Since the large majority of nurses in specialist CAMHS are mental health nurses, the reviews underway in England and Scotland will impact directly on their future roles and responsibilities.

- CAMHS in all four countries of the UK are facing workforce pressures. There are significant challenges in the recruitment and retention of mental health nurses across England, Northern Ireland, Scotland and Wales, and a substantial proportion of the exiting nursing workforce is approaching retirement.

Introduction

Contrary to popular belief, mental health problems and mental health needs are not the same thing. Whilst all children have mental health needs, one in five have mental health problems (Mental Health Foundation 1999) and as many as one in ten children and young people aged 5–15 years in England, Scotland and Wales will have a diagnosable mental disorder (Meltzer et al. 2000; Green et al. 2005). This means that in an average secondary school with 1000 pupils, as many as 50 will be depressed, between 10 and 20 will be anxious, and between 5 and 10 will have an eating disorder (YoungMinds 1999). It is widely agreed that rates of substance misuse, antisocial behaviour and crime by children and young people are on the increase and that these psychosocial problems are strongly associated with poor mental health (Rutter & Smith 1995; Rutter et al. 1998).

The mental health of children and young people is now widely recognised as everyone's business in all four areas of the UK. Government departments are increasingly aware that there are many reasons to invest early in order to save later. Untreated mental health problems are linked to educational failure, family and social problems, crime and antisocial behaviour. As well as placing demands on specialist mental health services, there are also costs to social services, schools and the youth justice system. Many unresolved mental health problems during childhood continue into adulthood, disrupting personal and social functioning. All nurses and other children's professionals share a responsibility to ensure that every child is given every opportunity to reach their fullest potential and to enjoy good mental health. This is to give them the best start in life. Good mental health involves the ability to enter into and sustain mutually satisfying personal relationships. It is about having emotional resilience, good self-esteem and the skills to cope in the face of stress and adversity.

Mental health problems and disorders manifest in children's behaviour, in how they feel and in what they tell us. Whilst mental health problems can interfere with a child's development and functioning, they are distinguished from mental disorders as being less severe, less complex or less persistent in nature. There is growing interest in creating prevention programmes and setting developmental trajectories for mental health problems and disorders. This is illustrated by the rapidly expanding evidence base showing that strategies to promote, prevent and intervene early can offset the development of mental health problems and disorders in children and young people. All nurses and other children's professionals also share a responsibility for promoting mental health by strengthening communities, improving social inclusion and reducing the stigma associated with mental health. This is to help prevent mental disorder and involves universal public mental health promotion, targeted and selective intervention and treatment for mental disorder with the aim of reducing severity, complexity and persistence. Primary mental health prevention refers to those interventions that are aimed at the general population and are intended to preclude the possibility of mental health problems occurring in the first place. Secondary prevention, otherwise called early intervention, is intended to prevent mental health problems evolving into mental disorders. Nurses across all settings must weave mental health prevention strategies into their everyday work with children and young people.

What do we mean by child and adolescent mental health services (CAMHS)?

CAMHS refers to services that are designed to meet the mental health needs of children and young people. However, the term CAMHS is used in a variety of different ways and this can often cause confusion. This includes confusion not only among those who commission, provide and evaluate mental health services for children; but also in the minds of nurses, other professionals and the general public. Although various attempts have been made to clarify what CAMHS means in practice, consensus has not yet been achieved (Wolpert & Wilson 2003). The National Service Frameworks for Children, Young People and Maternity Services (Department of Health 2004a; National Assembly for Wales 2005) provide some guidance on providing comprehensive CAMHS, and the Royal College of Psychiatrists has attempted to define specialist CAMHS in their consultation paper on the workforce, capacity and functions of CAMHS at Tiers 2, 3 and 4 (Royal College of Psychiatrists 2005). For the purposes of this book, CAMHS is used in two ways. First, it refers to all provision that aims to meet the mental health needs of children and young people, whether provided by specialist teams or by professionals whose responsibility for the mental health of children and young people is only one part of their role. Here, the terms 'primary', 'universal', 'mainstream' and 'Tier 1' CAMHS are also used to refer to a comprehensive range of mental health services for children and young people in health, education, social services, youth justice and voluntary sector agencies. Second, where the term 'specialist CAMHS' is used, this refers to individuals or teams whose primary function is to work with children and young people with complex, severe or persistent mental disorders.

The most important strategic document to set the context in which CAMHS in the UK have evolved was the NHS (National Health Service) Health Advisory Service (HAS) report, *Together We Stand* (NHS HAS 1995). This report introduced the now widely applied tiered model of service delivery, explored the commissioning, role and management of CAMHS and recommended a coordinated, tiered approach to service delivery. Within this framework, mental health services for children and young people are described according to a four-tier framework, with each tier characterised by increasingly specialised service provision (see Figure 1.1). Whilst the tiered model has now been widely adopted by CAMHS across the UK, it is increasingly recognised that neither children/young people nor services meeting local need fit neatly into a structural interpretation of the tiers (Royal College of Psychiatrists 2005).

Primary services at Tier 1 are usually the first point of contact for children and young people with mental health problems (McDougall & Crocker 2001). Here, non-specialists such as GPs (general practitioners), school nurses and health visitors promote mental health and emotional well-being, prevent mental health problems and disorders, and offer support for less complex

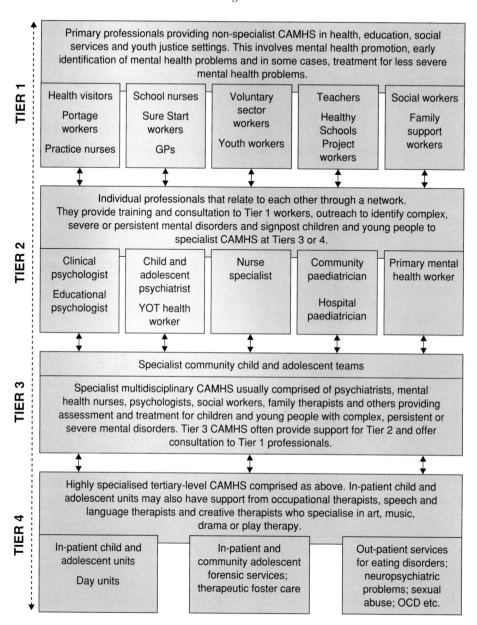

Figure 1.1 CAMHS tiered model of service delivery.
Source: NHS Health Advisory Service (1995). *Together We Stand: the commissioning, role and management of child and adolescent mental health services.* London: HMSO.

mental health problems. CAMHS professionals working at Tier 2 provide training and consultation for Tier 1 workers and usually practice as part of a multiprofessional network rather than a multidisciplinary team. Professionals working in services at Tiers 1 and 2 must be able to access specialist CAMHS. Tiers 3 and 4 CAMHS provide assessment and treatment interventions for children and young people with complex, persistent or severe mental health needs and disorders. These CAMHS are usually multidisciplinary teams that include nurses, psychiatrists, psychologists, family therapists, social workers and creative therapists. Sometimes young people have very complex or debilitating mental disorders and Tier 4 CAMHS are highly specialised CAMHS and may include in-patient child and adolescent units, specialised eating disorders services and forensic CAMHS, as well as multiagency services such as home treatment services, community support teams and crisis teams (see Figure 1.1).

What is CAMHS nursing?

Like all professionals charged with the care and welfare of children, nurses share joint responsibility for safeguarding and promoting their mental health. School nurses, health visitors or nurses on paediatric wards may be the first point of professional contact for children and young people with mental health problems. This group are not usually referred to as CAMHS nurses. They may encounter children and young people who have been traumatised, abused or bereaved, those who harm themselves or others and those with emotional and behaviour problems. Many such nurses will be involved in helping children to develop self-esteem, emotional literacy and the skills to resolve conflict in non-destructive and prosocial ways. A substantial number of nurses in CAMHS are practising as primary mental health workers (PMHWs) within all four regions of the UK (Gale et al. 2005). Sometimes known as CAMHS link workers, their role is to act as an interface or conduit between universal first-contact services for children and families and specialist CAMHS, with the aims of:

(1) Supporting and strengthening Tier 1 CAMHS through the building of capacity and capability within community and primary care workers, in relation to the recognition and early identification of mental health problems in children and young people.
(2) Promoting the mental health and psychological wellbeing of children and young people, their families and carers, in line with policy, strategy and good practice guidance.
(3) Enhancing accessibility and equity for CAMHS service users, especially those who may experience difficulties with access, such as black and minority ethnic communities, asylum seekers or refugees and homeless families.
(4) Working across professional, service and agency boundaries to develop a coordinated response to the mental health needs of children and young people.
(5) Facilitating appropriate access to specialist CAMHS and other relevant provision according to the level and nature of the need.
(6) Providing a direct service to children and young people, their families and carers, in an accessible and least stigmatising environment.

Primary mental health workers work in a range of settings and in a variety of ways. They have been successful in reducing inappropriate referrals to specialist CAMHS and in developing the mental health skills of professionals whose core business is not child and adolescent mental health (Gale 1999; Gale & Vostanis 2003; Whitworth & Ball 2004). As well as signposting children and young people with complex, severe or persistent mental disorders to Tier 4 CAMHS, PMHWs also engage the voluntary sector and support young people to access services such as Connexions. This is the government's support service for all young people aged 13 to 19 in England. It aims to provide integrated advice, guidance and access to personal development opportunities for teenagers to make a smooth transition to adulthood and working life. Connexions embraces the work of the six government departments, along with their respective agencies and organisations, with voluntary sector, and with youth and careers services. Connexions services are delivered through local strategic partnerships working to national planning guidance.

Specialist CAMHS nurses

Nurses who work in primary services may sometimes need to refer a child or young person for specialist CAMHS assessment, treatment or management. Specialist CAMHS nurses come from a variety of backgrounds and work in a range of community and residential practice and agency settings at Tiers 2, 3 and 4. Although nurses are the largest single professional group and make up a quarter of the specialist CAMHS workforce (Audit Commission 1999), there is no single definition of a CAMHS nurse. Perhaps this is not surprising: CAMHS nurses have no single identity and there is huge variation in the background, qualifications and roles of nurses working in such specialist settings (Jones 2004; Jones & Baldwin 2004). There is a plethora of titles which include nurse in their title. These include staff nurse; nurse specialist; nurse practitioner; community nurse; nurse therapist; paediatric liaison nurse and consultant nurse. In addition, many professionals are practising as nurses but have completed additional training and are working in roles that are not defined in terms of nursing. These include roles such as cognitive behaviour therapist, family therapist and primary mental health worker. Despite the heterogeneity of the role, various authors have attempted to define CAMHS nursing. However, consensus has not yet been reached about the roles, responsibilities and primary functions of CAMHS nurses. As CAMHS have expanded and new ways of working have emerged, several authors have been concerned about the trend towards genericism and the demise of the specialist CAMHS nurse's professional identity and role (McMorrow 1990; 1995; Limerick & Baldwin 2000; Baldwin 2002). However, as Baldwin (2002) points out, it is possible to argue that there should not be a need to defend individual professional contributions to CAMHS if the aim is to create a team which together meets the needs of its users.

Table 1.1 Nurses in specialist CAMHS (England).

Grade	Number
A	228
B	280
C	37
D	128
E	491
F	260
G	627
H	332
I	70
Modern matron	19
Nurse consultant	23
Other	22
Total	**2517**

Source: CAMHS Mapping (Department of Health 2004).

It is difficult to estimate the size of the nursing workforce in CAMHS. Current figures suggest that there are about 6000 full-time equivalent specialist CAMHS professionals in England of which 2500 are nurses (Department of Health 2005a in press) (see Table 1.1). In a recent UK survey of nurses working in specialist CAMHS, half were registered mental health nurses (Jones 2004), but an increasing number are registered children's nurses. Most nurses in specialist CAMHS work autonomously. This means they practice and function independently, with the ability and recognised right to perform their total professional function on the basis of their own knowledge, skills and judgement (Baldwin 2002). Like all nurses, they are always accountable for their practice decisions and interventions. The grades at which nurses are currently working in specialist CAMHS are shown in Table 1.1. In addition to nurses in specialist CAMHS, there are an estimated 15 000 children's nurses (Royal College of Nursing 2002), 13 000 health visitors (DoH 2004b) and between 2000 and 2500 school nurses (DoH 2005b) who work in primary CAMHS and also have a role in meeting the mental health needs of children and adolescents.

However, as investment in CAMHS grows, there has been a significant shortage of appropriately trained nurses in specialist CAMHS, particularly in in-patient child and adolescent units (Griffiths & Lindsey 2003). This may be due to the lack of promotion opportunities within in-patient settings and the increasing loss of in-patient nurses to out-patient teams where they can work in new ways and enjoy family friendly hours (Scottish Executive 2004a). The lack of appropriately trained nurses in CAMHS has been consistently reported elsewhere (Lamb et al. 2004). Reasons for this include a long history of inadequate pre- and post-registration education and training programmes (Royal College of Nursing 1998; Hooten 1999; McDougall 2000; Townley 2002; Jones & Baldwin 2004; McDougall 2004); the lack of a defined career pathway from point of registration to senior nurse status (Royal College of Nursing 2002); a lack of appropriately prepared nurse teachers or lecturers (Davies et al. 2002); the lack of a national CAMHS nurse strategy in England (Griffiths & Lindsey 2003); and difficulties with the recruitment, retention and leadership of CAMHS nurses (Jones & Baldwin 2004; Royal College of Nursing 2004). Recruitment and retention of specialist CAMHS nurses depends on a number of factors including pay and conditions, job satisfaction, opportunities to practice therapeutically, and a respectful understanding of the many roles they fulfil within the multidisciplinary team.

Developments in Nursing

The twenty-first century has brought changing times for nurses in the UK. A number of significant Chief Nursing Officer (CNO) reviews have taken place during the preparation of this book. Some of these apply to nurses across the UK, whilst others are region-specific. Some apply to all nurses, midwives and health visitors, others to just one type of nurse. However, most of the key issues and recommendations have common currency for all nurses who work in CAMHS in the UK. First, the CNO review of the nursing contribution to vulnerable children issued a number of challenges to nurses, midwives and health visitors (DoH 2004c). These included the need to get better at safeguarding and protecting children, not only from abuse and neglect but also from educational failure, antisocial behaviour and mental ill-health. For too long, nurses in general and mental health nurses in particular have absolved themselves from child protection responsibilities. They have dutifully passed on their concerns to their social worker colleagues or the police, and then blamed them when things go wrong. This blinkered way of thinking must change and a review of the nursing contribution to the care of vulnerable children has helped set the scene in which the modernisation of children's services is evolving (McDougall 2003). The CNO review of the nursing contribution to the care of vulnerable children urged nurses to shed aspects of their traditional practice and replace them with modern, innovative and creative ways of working. The need for nurses and other professionals to improve services to safeguard children has also been highlighted in a number of other key reports. These include *Too Serious a Thing* (National Assembly for Wales 2002a) and *Every Child Matters* (Department for Education and Skills 2003). Published in the wake of the Victoria Climbie Inquiry (Laming 2003), *Every Child Matters* makes clear that nurses must strengthen links with their multi-agency colleagues to ensure that all children have every opportunity to reach their fullest potential.

Second are the government-led reviews of school nursing (Scottish Executive 2001; DoH 2005b). School nurses are uniquely placed to help children and young people reach their fullest potential because they are able to bridge health, education and social care boundaries. It is for this reason that the government wishes to widen and develop the role of school nurses to deliver their health and educational priorities. Of particular significance for nurses are the objectives and targets contained in the public health White Paper, *Choosing Health* (DoH 2004b). This strategy sets out the government's plans to enable all people, including children, to make informed and healthy lifestyle choices. *Choosing Health* recognises that children need more protection than others, and has championed school nurses as a key workforce to deliver these plans and objectives. This is to ensure that children make positive lifestyle choices by eating healthily, taking exercise and avoiding drugs and alcohol. *Choosing Health* recognises that good emotional health is of fundamental importance and aims to ensure that children have access to opportunities to nurture their mental health and emotional wellbeing. The Scottish Executive Government has also set the target that all schools will be *Health Promoting Schools* by 2007. School nurses are in key positions to help achieve this aspiration as well as implement the recommendations from *Nursing for Health* (Scottish Executive 2002). This was the report of the review of the nursing, midwife and health visiting contribution to improving public health. Both strategies contain standards on mental health and psychological wellbeing and explore ways in which nurses can meet the mental health needs of children in school.

Last, but by no means least are the two CNO reviews of mental health nursing currently underway in England and Scotland (DoH 2005c; Scottish Executive 2005). These are the largest of the CNO reviews and include children in their scopes. The purpose of both reviews is to create a new modern role for mental health nursing. The English review is evolving in tandem with new ways of working for other professionals such as psychiatrists (National Institute for Mental Health in England 2004) and allied health professionals (AHP), and is in keeping with a wider programme for the changing mental health workforce. As well as examining the impact of advanced and extended roles for mental health nurses such as nurse prescribing, the review will consider how mental health nurses can deliver NHS priorities and improve the service user experience. The CNO review of mental health nursing in England will also focus specifically on how mental health nurses working with all age groups can improve services to safeguard children. Since many of the 47 000 mental health nurses in NHS and independent sector services work with children and young people, the review will be an important opportunity to influence the future role of nursing care and practice in CAMHS (DoH 2005c).

It is not only the CNO reviews that have helped pave the way for the development of nursing in the UK. A number of other important publications have highlighted the role of nurses in improving the mental health of children and young people in all four UK regions. Whilst some have been led by government agencies, some have been initiated and undertaken by CAMHS nurses themselves. In 1999, the National Assembly for Wales published *Realising the Potential*, the strategic framework for nursing, midwifery and health visiting in Wales for the twenty-first century (National Assembly for Wales 1999). This was followed by a briefing paper and framework to help CAMHS nurses translate *Realising the Potential* into practice (National Assembly for Wales 2002b). The briefing paper, which set out a ten-year vision for CAMHS nurses, was produced by the All Wales Forum for Senior Nurses in CAMHS with the support of the CNO (National Assembly for Wales) and the Nurse Executive Wales Group. CAMHS nurses set themselves some key objectives to improve care and treatment including: to ensure high quality services for children and young people; to encourage independent practice; to develop new and existing career pathways; and to demonstrate the value of CAMHS nursing. As part of the modernisation of children's services across Wales, the CNO later made a number of key recommendations for all nurses who work with children, such as CAMHS nurses, including the need for nurses to help improve child protection, transition services and care pathways for all children and young people (Kennedy 2003).

In Northern Ireland, *Promoting Mental Health*, published by the Health Promotion Agency (HPA), whilst not focusing specifically on children and young people, produced a strategy that addressed mental health promotion and intervention with groups at higher risk of mental disorder (Health Protection Agency 2003). The differing needs of children and young people were recognised in the action plan, and a number of important recommendations were made that applied to all mental health professionals including nurses who work with children and adolescents. *Nursing for Health* (Scottish Executive 2002) identified mental health as a priority for improvement and highlighted the need for all nurses to get better equipped to promote good mental health, prevent mental health problems and support people with mental illness (Scottish Executive 2002). The particular roles that specialist CAMHS nurses can play were also described as recommendations for action. These included nursing children and young people with the most challenging mental health problems, and providing support and consultation to mainstream children's services and schools (Scottish Executive 2001).

Conclusion

A range of nursing strategies in England, Northern Ireland, Scotland and Wales have highlighted the important clinical and strategic roles that nurses have to play in helping to plan, deliver and evaluate modern and effective mental health services for children and young people. Nurses are in key positions to help meet the Public Service Agreement objectives, standards and performance targets that have been set for CAMHS. They have a lead role in helping to deliver the government's *Change for Children Programme: Every Child Matters* and in implementing strategies such as Sure Start, the Healthy Schools programmes and the Children's Fund initiatives. It is essential that nurses, midwives and health visitors take every opportunity to champion the needs of children with mental health problems (McDougall 2003; Masterson et al. 2004) through influencing local and national developments and ensuring that they become actively involved in local discussions and decision-making forums (Smith 2004).

CAMHS in all four regions of the UK are facing workforce pressures. These include significant challenges in the recruitment and retention of mental health nurses across England, Wales, Scotland and Northern Ireland (UKCC 1999; Shields & Ward 2001; Department of Health, Social Services & Public Safety 2002), and the fact that a substantial proportion of the exiting nursing workforce is approaching retirement is of concern (O'Donnell 2003). Government policy and strategy, CNO reviews and clear messages from service users, their families and carers have issued a number of challenges for nurses. It is nurses who have the most contact with children and young people with mental health problems. They are in key clinical, strategic and leadership positions to ensure that children and young people can be helped to reach their fullest potential.

References

Audit Commission (1999). *Children in Mind: a report on child and adolescent mental health services*. London: Audit Commission.

Baldwin, L. (2002). The nursing role in out-patient child and adolescent mental health services. *Journal of Clinical Nursing*, (11), 520–25.

Davies, J., Creswell, A. & Hannigan, B. (2000). Child and adolescent mental health services: rhetoric and reality. *Paediatric Nursing*, **14** (3), 26–28.

Department for Education and Skills (2003). *Every Child Matters*. London: HMSO.

Department of Health (2004a). *National Service Framework for Children, Young People and Maternity Services*. London: HMSO.

Department of Health (2004b). *Choosing Health: making healthier choices easier*. London: HMSO.

Department of Health (2004c). *The Chief Nursing Officer's review of the nursing, midwifery and health visiting contribution to vulnerable children and young people*. London: HMSO.

Department of Health (2005a). *National Child and Adolescent Mental Health Service Mapping Exercise*. London: HMSO.

Department of Health (2005b). *Chief Nursing Officer Review of School Nursing*. London: The Stationary Office.

Department of Health (2005c). *Chief Nursing Officer Review of Mental Health Nursing*. London: The Stationary Office.

Department of Health, Social Services and Public Safety (2002). *The Health and Wellbeing Survey*. Belfast: DHSSPS.

Gale, F. (2003). When tiers are not enough: developing the role of the child primary mental health worker. *Child and Adolescent Mental Health in Primary Care*, **1** (1), 5–8.

Gale, F., Hassett, A. & Sebuliba, D. (2005). *The competency and capability framework for primary mental health workers in child and adolescent mental health services (CAMHS)*. London: National CAMHS Support Service.

Gale, F. & Vostanis, P. (2005). Case study: the primary mental health team: Leicester, Leicestershire and Rutland CAMHS. In: Williams, R. & Kerfoot, M. (Eds) *Child and Adolescent Mental Health Services: strategy, planning, delivery and evaluation*. Oxford: Oxford University Press.

Green, H., McGinnity, A., Meltzer, H., Ford, T. & Goodman, R. (2005). *Mental health of children and young people in Great Britain*. London: Office of National Statistics.

Griffiths, P. & Lindsey, C. (2003). *A Comprehensive CAMHS: what are the training implications for those working with child and adolescent mental health issues? Report for the Mental Health and Psychological Wellbeing of Children and Young People External Working Group.* London.

Health Promotion Agency (2003). *Promoting Mental Health: strategy and action plan 2003–2008.* Belfast: HPA.

Hooten, S. (1999). *Results of a survey undertaken to establish the degree to which pre-registration programmes address child and adolescent mental health.* London: English National Board.

Jones, J. (2004). *The post-registration education and training needs of nurses working with children and young people with mental health problems in the UK: a research study conducted by the Mental Health Programme, Royal College of Nursing Institute, in collaboration with the RCN Children and Young People's Mental Health Forum.* London: RCN Institute.

Jones, J. & Baldwin, L. (2004). Tiers before bedtime: a survey shows post-registration CAMHS education is missing the mark. *Mental Health Practice,* **7** (6), 14–17.

Kennedy, R. (2003). *Report of the CNO focus visits to children's services in Wales: July–October 2003.* Cardiff: National Assembly for Wales.

Lamb, C., Riley, S. & Davies, G. (2004). Strategic thinking. *Young Minds Magazine,* (71), 15–16.

Laming, H. (2003). *The Victoria Climbie Inquiry: report of an inquiry.* London: The Stationary Office.

Limerick, M. & Baldwin, L. (2000). Nursing in out-patient child and adolescent mental health. *Nursing Standard,* **15** (13), 43–45.

McDougall, T. (2000). The role of the nurse specialist in raising the profile of children's mental health. *Nursing Times,* **96** (28), 37–38.

McDougall, T. (2003). Going Green: helping children reach their potential. *Mental Health Practice,* **7** (4), 37.

McDougall, T. (2004). Listen and learn: mental health. *Nursing Standard,* **19** (6), 58–59.

McDougall, T. & Crocker, A. (2001). Referral pathways through a specialist child and adolescent mental health service: the role of the specialist practitioner. *Mental Health Practice,* **5** (1), 16–20.

McMorrow, R. (1990). The new clinicians. *Senior Nurse,* **10** (3), 22–23.

McMorrow, R. (1995). An eclectic model of care; the role of the community psychiatric nurse in child psychiatry. *Child Health,* **3** (3), 95–98.

Masterson, A., Antrobus, S. & Smith, F. (2004). National service frameworks: from policy to practice. *Paediatric Nursing,* **16** (9), 32–34.

Meltzer, H., Gatward, R., Goodman, R. & Ford, T. (2000). *The Mental Health of Children and Adolescents in Great Britain.* London: The Stationary Office.

Mental Health Foundation (1999). *Bright Futures.* London: Mental Health Foundation.

National Assembly for Wales (1999). *Realising the Potential – A Strategic Framework for Nursing Midwifery and Health Visiting in Wales into the 21st Century.* Cardiff: National Assembly for Wales.

National Assembly for Wales (2002a). *The Review of Safeguards for Children and Young People Treated and Cared for by the NHS in Wales. Too Serious a Thing: the Carlisle Review.* Cardiff: National Assembly for Wales.

National Assembly for Wales (2002b). *Principles to practice – a framework for realising the potential of child and adolescent mental health nursing in Wales: improving the mental health of children and young people in Wales. Briefing Paper 5.* Cardiff: National Assembly for Wales.

National Assembly for Wales (2005). *National Service Framework for Children, Young People and Maternity Services in Wales.* Cardiff: National Assembly for Wales.

NHS Health Advisory Service (1995). *Together We Stand: the commissioning, role and management of child and adolescent mental health services.* London: HMSO.

National Institute for Mental Health in England (2004). *Guidance on New Ways of Working for Psychiatrists in a Multi-disciplinary and Multi-agency context: interim report.* London: HMSO.

O'Donnell, H. (2003). The future of mental health nursing in Northern Ireland: does anyone really care? *Mental Health Practice,* **7** (3), 30–33.

Royal College of Nursing (2002). *Children's Nursing Workforce (July 2002): a report to the Royal College of Nursing and the Royal College of Paediatrics and Child Health.* London: RCN.

Royal College of Nursing (2004). *Children and Young People's Mental Health: every nurse's business.* London: RCN.

Royal College of Nursing Child and Adolescent Mental Health Forum (1998). *Report of sub-committee on education and training: a review of post-registration education and training for CAMHS nurses* (unpublished). London: RCN.

Royal College of Psychiatrists (2005). *Building and sustaining specialist CAMHS: workforce, capacity and functions of Tiers 2, 3 and 4 specialist child and adolescent mental health services across England, Ireland, Northern Ireland, Scotland and Wales.* London: Royal College of Psychiatrists.

Rutter, M. & Smith, D. (1995). *Psychosocial disorders in young people: time trends and their causes.* Chichester: John Wiley.

Rutter, M., Giller, H. & Hagell, A. (1998). *Antisocial behaviour by young people.* London: Cambridge University Press.

Scottish Executive (2001). *Caring for Scotland: the strategy for nursing and midwifery in Scotland.* Edinburgh: Scottish Executive.

Scottish Executive (2002). *Nursing for Health: a review of the contribution of nurses, midwives and health visitors to public health.* Edinburgh: Scottish Executive.

Scottish Executive (2004a). *Child Health and Support Group: in-patient working group – psychiatric in-patient services.* Edinburgh: Scottish Executive.

Scottish Executive (2005). *National Review of Mental Health Nursing in Scotland: interim report.* Edinburgh: Scottish Executive.

Shields, M. & Ward, M. (2001). Improving nurse retention in the NHS in England: the impact of job satisfaction on intentions to quit. *Journal of Health Economics,* **20** (5), 677–701.

Smith, F. (2004). The NSF for children, young people and maternity services: an overview. *Paediatric Nursing,* **16** (8), 30–32.

Townley, M. (2002). Mental health needs of children and young people. *Nursing Standard,* **16** (30), 38–45.

United Kingdom Central Council (1998). *Fitness for Practice: The UKCC Commission for Nursing and Midwifery Education.* London: UKCC.

Whitworth, D. & Ball, C. (2004). The impact of primary mental health workers on referrals to CAMHS. *Child and Adolescent Mental Health,* **9** (4), 177–79.

Wolpert, M. & Wilson, P. (2003). Million dollar question. *YoungMinds Magazine,* (65), 28–29.

YoungMinds (1999). *Mental Health in Children and Young People: spotlight (No. 1 in a series of briefing papers).* London: YoungMinds.

Chapter 2

The Bigger Picture: CAMHS, nursing and the strategic context

Tim McDougall and Moira Davren

Key points

- Although children make up a quarter of the UK population, services to meet their mental health needs have historically been neglected, small, poorly coordinated and under-funded. However, there is evidence that this picture is changing. Child and adolescent mental health services (CAMHS) are receiving an increasing profile across England, Northern Ireland, Scotland and Wales.

- The *Change for Children Programme: Every Child Matters* and the National Service Framework (NSF) for Children, Young People and Maternity Services are ten-year developmental strategies which have set the scene in which CAMHS in England are developing.

- The *Mental Health and Learning Disability Review* in Northern Ireland has given CAMHS a high priority. The Expert Committee on Child and Adolescent Mental Health sets out a strategic vision for the development of comprehensive CAMHS and highlights key challenges in relation to their organisation, planning and delivery.

- The Scottish Needs Assessment Programme (SNAP) has made several key strategic recommendations in relation to child and adolescent mental health services. These included the need to mainstream CAMHS by focusing on mental health promotion and emotional wellbeing, preventing mental health problems and disorders, and strengthening local, regional and national services.

- The Welsh child and adolescent mental health strategy document *Everybody's Business* described the 'CAMHS Concept' as an overarching definition of child and adolescent mental health services. This is intended to promote the multiagency nature of CAMHS, to emphasise the roles and responsibilities of non-specialist CAMHS, and to encourage partnership working and a strategic approach to service commissioning and delivery.

- All four regions of the UK are facing significant CAMHS workforce challenges. Difficulties with recruitment and retention mean that mental health nurses with specialist CAMHS skills and competencies, in particular, are in short supply and high demand.

Introduction

Publications about children's services that aim to describe 'where we are now?' often start with 'where have we been?' and end with 'where are we going?' However, it is all but impossible to follow tradition and produce a comprehensive past, present and future account of CAMHS policy and strategy in the UK. This is because CAMHS in England, Northern Ireland, Scotland and Wales are at different stages in a constantly transforming process of evolution. It is therefore only possible to provide a snapshot, frozen in time and subject to inevitable change. Neither is it meaningful or indeed helpful to make regional comparisons. This is not only because there is a lack of comparable UK-wide data, particularly in relation to child and adolescent mental health, but also because major inequalities between England, Northern Ireland, Scotland and Wales mean that we would not be comparing like with like.

Furthermore, this chapter will not attempt to take stock of the history and development of CAMHS, as the rich tapestry of CAMHS' history has been summarised elsewhere (Black 1993; Cottrell & Abdullah 2005; Williams & Kerfoot 2005). Since the children's services modernisation agenda in England and Wales is a ten-year strategy, and since Northern Ireland and Scotland are developing similar programmes with long-term visions, it may be possible to make some general statements about where CAMHS might be heading in the future. However, whilst the general direction of travel may remain constant, we should expect that the slip-roads and exits might be renumbered. It is essential therefore that nurses, along with all children's professionals, scan the horizon for emerging developments and remain resilient during these times of change.

Background

Central devolution commenced in 1999 and has brought not only a raft of structural policy changes but also a strategic shift in the balance of power across the children's sector. As children's services have moved into the twenty-first century, children's policy has become fully devolved and the control of resources and delivery of CAMHS has moved away from central administrations into local organisations. This has been intended to empower local services and frontline staff by reducing bureaucracy and creating opportunities for innovation, growth and excellence. The three devolved UK governments and the Northern Ireland government, are developing their CAMHS along broadly similar lines. However, significant differences exist in terms of pace and scope of progress. The priority that CAMHS is given in England, Northern Ireland, Scotland and Wales, and the funding and resources that are allocated, is hugely variable. It should be no surprise that there are notable regional differences in children's policies (Jeffery 2004) and that each of the four regions of the UK is at a different stage in the strategic development, commissioning and delivery of their respective CAMHS.

England

Although there are nearly 12 million children living in England (Office for National Statistics 2002), services to meet their mental health needs have historically been neglected and services have been small, fragmented and under-funded (Health Select Committee 1997; McDougall 2000). This is despite one million children in the UK having a mental health problem serious enough to require professional help, and many more with significant mental health needs, including 400 000 children in need, nearly 60 000 children in care, and 320 000 disabled children (Nixon 2004), all of whom are at heightened risk of develop-ing mental health problems and disorders. It is only in the last ten years, and following publication of the HAS (Health Advisory Service) report, *To-gether We Stand* (Health Advisory Service 1995), that a strategic approach has been taken to the commissioning and delivery of CAMHS in England. Publica-tion of the HAS report followed an audit of child and adolescent mental health services in England, which highlighted the mismatch between resources and need (Kurtz et al. 1994). However, it was some time before a programme of proper investment began: for the first time in 1999, funds were allocated specifically for CAMHS through the Mental Health Specific Grant and the NHS (National Health Service) Modernisation Fund (DoH 1999), and this money has increased through year-on-year allocations until the present time at which the government has invested over £300 million in CAMHS allocated to local authorities and the NHS (see Table 2.1). In 2001 the Department of Health (DoH) issued further guidance to health and local authorities requiring them to develop a joint CAMHS development strategy to ensure local and national priorities were met. This meant that services could no longer be developed in isolation and local partnerships were required to produce joint commissioning and development strategies. In particular, health and local authorities were to provide assessment and a range of treatments without children and their families experiencing prolonged waiting periods, including in-patient care and treatment in age-appropriate specialist settings and local arrangements for 24-hour access and emergency intervention.

As part of the NHS Plan (DoH 2000) and *National Priorities and Planning Guidance 2003–2006* (DoH 2002) specific objectives have been identified for CAMHS. *Improvement, Expansion and Reform* (DoH 2002) sets out what organ-isations need to do over the next three years. It identifies national priorities and targets that local CAMHS need to factor into their local delivery plans

Table 2.1   CAMHS grant funding in England (1999–2008).

	Local Authority Revenue[1]	NHS Revenue	NHS Capital
1999/2000	–	£10m	–
2000/2001	£10m (£6m)	£10m	–
2001/2002	£15m (£11m)	£20m[2]	–
2002/2003	£20m (£16m)	–	–
2003/2004	£51m (£44m)	–	–
2004/2005	£67m (£63m)	£20m	£20m
2005/2006	£90m (£85m)	£50m[3]	£20m
2006/2007	£89m (£86m)		
2007/2008	£89m (£88m)		

1 Amounts in this column represent the total gross amount of CAMHS Grant payable. From 2003/2004 these monies have been separate from the CAMHS Grant. The net amounts payable to local authorities were lower than shown due to top-slicing for regional development workers and treatment foster care made prior to distribution to local authorities. The amounts actually allocated to local authorities are shown in brackets.
2 From 2002/2003 this amount for specific NHS CAMHS developments was included in baseline NHS funding to PCTs.
3 From 2006/2007 this amount for specific NHS CAMHS developments will be included in baseline NHS funding to PCTs.

(LDPs). Social services are identified as the lead services for improving life chances for children, and both health and social services together have a leading responsibility for mental health, in order to improve, expand and reform CAMHS. The priorities and planning framework includes a public service agreement (PSA) target, requiring commissioners to achieve comprehensive CAMHS in all areas by 2006 (DoH 2004). This means that there must be services available for mental health promotion, early intervention and timely crisis resolution for when children or young people do become unwell. Access to services must be improved, waiting times must be reduced and children and their families must have more choice about the CAMHS they receive. Mental health service outcomes are to be improved and life chances for children must be maximised.

Resources allocated in the last two spending reviews have been made according to the CAMHS PSA target. It is generally agreed that delivery of comprehensive CAMHS by the end of 2006 will not be easy to achieve. In some areas of England, specialist CAMHS remain patchy due to challenges in providing 24-hour services; services for 16 and 17 year-olds; and services for children and young people with learning disabilities. There are problems in recruiting appropriately trained CAMHS professionals from all disciplines, including nursing. A team of CAMHS regional development workers (RDWs), who together comprise the National CAMHS Support Service, has been charged with responsibility for helping local CAMHS partnerships achieve delivery of the comprehensive CAMHS target. The RDWs will also assist local CAMHS partnerships to review their progress against the delivery of National Service Framework (NSF) priority areas, and to facilitate networking, multiagency cooperation and the sharing of local good practice in CAMHS.

The National Service Framework for Children, Young People and Maternity Services

The NSF for Children, Young People and Maternity Services (DoH 2004) set new standards and defined service models for children across all NHS and social care settings. There are five core standards in the NSF which focus on various issues, including involving children and families, interagency working, competent commissioning and care pathways. In addition there are six specific standards which focus on children and young people with particular needs. These should be cross referenced and read in conjunction with the core standards. Nurses are encouraged not to read any of the chapters in isolation (see Box 2.1).

The publication of the NSF for Children, Young People and Maternity Services has transformed the context in which nurses practice. Services are no longer organised and delivered according to the needs of those who provide them: instead, the modernisation agenda places the needs of the children, and their family or carers, at the centre of all that nurses do in organising, planning and delivering mental health and other children's services (McDougall 2004; Smith 2004). The NSF is underpinned by an implementation strategy intended to provide support for parents and carers; early intervention and effective protection; accountability and integration; and workforce reform.

The NSF is part of a wider developmental strategy called the *Change for Children Programme: Every Child Matters* (Department for Education and Skills 2003). This cross-sector programme sets out a ten-year vision for the modernisation of children's services, which aims to support each and every child to be healthy, stay safe, enjoy and achieve, make a positive contribution and achieve economic wellbeing (DfES 2003). Several other important government strategies are part of the wider *Change for Children* programme. These include the *Quality Protects Programme,* focusing on disadvantaged and vulnerable children (DoH 1998); *Reform in Education to Promote Children's Mental Health in the Early Years* (DfES 2001) and the recently published Youth Green

Box 2.1   The NSF for Children, Young People and Maternity Services.

Standard 1: Promoting health and wellbeing, identifying needs and intervening early
Standard 2: Supporting parents
Standard 3: Child, young person and family centred services
Standard 4: Growing up into adulthood
Standard 5: Safeguarding and promoting the welfare of children and young people
Standard 6: Children and young people who are ill
Standard 7: Children in hospital
Standard 8: Disabled children and young people and those with complex needs
Standard 9: Mental health and psychological wellbeing of children and young people
Standard 10: Medicines for children and young people
Standard 11: Maternity services

Paper: *Youth Matters* (DfES 2005) which builds on the ambitions set out in *Every Child Matters*.

Northern Ireland

The *Health and Wellbeing Survey* (Department of Health, Social Services & Public Safety 2001) showed that people living in Northern Ireland are at greater risk of mental ill-health than people in England and Scotland (DHSSPS 2001). This is due to higher levels of socioeconomic deprivation and the ongoing 'troubles'. Over a quarter of Northern Ireland's population comprises children under the age of 18 (Northern Ireland Statistics and Research Agency 2002). However very little epidemiological information about the types and rates of mental health problems they experience is available. The widely cited research studies of 10 000 children published by the Office for National Statistics (Meltzer et al. 2000; Green et al. 2005) did not include those in Northern Ireland. Although rates of mental disorder across England, Wales and Scotland are thought to be broadly similar, Northern Ireland is distinguished by higher levels of socioeconomic deprivation, ongoing civil troubles, and higher rates of psychiatric morbidity in the adult population (Campbell 1999; Northern Ireland Association for Mental Health & Sainsbury Centre 2004). However, even at the lowest estimated prevalence rate of 10% (Meltzer et al. 2000; Green et al. 2005), approximately 45 000 children between 5 and 15 years of age living in Northern Ireland will have a moderate to severe mental health problem, or disorder that requires specialist CAMHS intervention.

At the time of writing this chapter CAMHS in Northern Ireland are having their profile raised. This is largely through the work of the Child and Adolescent Mental Health Expert Working Committee, which forms part of the mental health and learning disability review in Northern Ireland, commissioned by the Department of Health, Social Services and Public Safety (DHSSPS). In addition the report of the Child and Adolescent Mental Health Expert Working Committee sets out a strategic vision for the development of comprehensive CAMHS in Northern Ireland. Mental health services for children and young people in Northern Ireland have not always been highlighted as a priority area. CAMHS have previously been neglected, and the quality, consistency and accessibility of services have been inadequate and unsatisfactory. This is a result of chronic underinvestment and a previous lack of regionally coherent planning and investment. As funding for CAMHS in Northern Ireland is not dedicated, it is difficult to establish current expenditure on mental health services for children and young people. Although children under 18 years make up over a quarter of the population, the proportion of investment in CAMHS represents less than 5% of the total mental health budget for Northern Ireland (O'Rawe 2003).

Health and social services in Northern Ireland are managerially integrated, and responsibility for planning CAMHS lies with the DHSSPS. Responsibility for the governance of CAMHS is divided between four health and social services (HPSS) boards. A number of important political and strategic developments in relation to CAMHS in Northern Ireland came about in 2002, when the DHSSPS set planning priorities and actions for health and personal social services. The subsequent three-year service delivery plan set public service agreement targets for children's services. These included a target to improve CAMHS by providing a range of therapeutic interventions in the most appropriate settings. Also in 2002, the Northern Ireland Executive published a consultation report, *Investing for Health*. This highlighted mental health as a priority for action and noted an increasing concern about the high rates of mental health problems in children and young people (Northern Ireland Executive 2002a). Later in 2002 the Northern Ireland Executive published their strategy document, *Building on Progress*. This set out the priorities and planning framework for 2003–2006 (Northern Ireland Executive 2002b). Giving children the best start in life, safeguarding and protecting their needs and developing child and adolescent mental health services were all identified as key objectives. However, whilst recognising that the mental health of children and young people was crucial, the subsequent action plan for 2003–2008, *Promoting Mental Health* (DHSSPS 2003) did not give CAMHS such a high profile. The publication of *Building on Progress* coincided with commencement of the Regional Review of Mental Health and Learning Disability in 2002, which was later to include the Child and Adolescent Mental Health Expert Working Committee.

The tiered model of service delivery (HAS 1995) which is in use across England, Wales and parts of Scotland is broadly supported in Northern Ireland. However, resource constraints in terms of funding and workforce development have made implementation of the tiered model problematic. Consequently the planning, commissioning, delivery and management of CAMHS in Northern Ireland has not evolved in a strategic way. The last ten years have seen significant recruitment and retention problems within mental health nursing in Northern Ireland, both in adult mental health services and child and adolescent mental health services (O'Donnell 2003). Although those who are involved in the strategic CAMHS support the notion that CAMHS is everyone's business, many professionals and services in primary settings and projects established by social service departments, youth services and the voluntary sector do not see themselves as part of mainstream CAMHS. This is despite delivering what most would call prevention and early intervention CAMHS services. This has meant that developments at Tier 1 and Tier 2 have been limited and links with Tier 3 and Tier 4 services are stronger in some areas of the country than in others. Despite these constraints, there are many examples of good practice. A Tier 1, Sure Start early intervention programmes have been established across the four HPSS boards; statutory and voluntary family centres continue to be developed; and a range of voluntary and community organisations provide befriending schemes, advocacy services and educational input to schools. At Tier 2, a range of school-based CAMHS exist. Education departments are providing pastoral care and school-based counselling services. School nurses, educational psychologists, education welfare officers and emotional and behavioural support teams contribute to meeting the mental health needs of children in school. In addition, youth justice services are developing to support vulnerable young people with mental health needs.

Specialist CAMHS exist in each of the HPSS board areas but are managed by different directorates in children's services, in mental health and learning disability services, and in acute paediatric services in Northern Ireland. There are significant differences in the capacity, structure and operational policies of specialist CAMHS teams. Due to differences in legislation and responsibility for health, education and social services in Northern Ireland, the age limit for acceptance by Tier 3 or 4 CAMHS varies from 14 to 18 years old. This has inevitably led to gaps in services and at present, no services are adequately resourced to provide CAMHS for 16 and 17 year-olds. In some areas older adolescents have been treated in adult mental health services, whereas in other parts of the country this has not been possible due to increasing demands on adult services. Referral pathways also vary considerably. Although the core interventions provided by Tier 3 and Tier 4 services across the province are similar, differences exist in terms of which children and young people are accepted for treatment. Waiting list times vary, ranging from three months to 'closed except for emergencies'. This has led to a focus on waiting list initiatives such as the referral coordinator system and the development of a link workers system. Professionals with special interests and training opportunities have contributed to the development of emerging areas of speciality and interest in relation to working with young people with eating disorders, those with autistic spectrum disorders and children in care. A very small number of in-patient child and adolescent services in Northern Ireland are commissioned on a regional basis and delivered by separate provider services in health, education and social care settings.

A number of gaps in Tier 4 service provision that exist in other areas of the UK also exist in Northern Ireland. These include mental health services for young people with learning disabilities; alcohol and substance misuse services; and mental health services for young people in contact with the youth justice system. Increasingly, the lack of these specialist services is adding to the burden on specialist CAMHS, which are already stretched to capacity. Due to excessive demands placed on existing specialist CAMHS in Northern Ireland, out-of-hours and emergency CAMHS are lacking. Due to the problems of low capacity, it is not possible for Tier 3 services to provide 24-hour support to accident and emergency departments. In some areas, social services provide emergency services for children under 16, and adult mental health services for young people over 16.

The 20-year vision for health and wellbeing in Northern Ireland, published by the DHSSPS (2005), recognises that one of the most effective ways to im-prove the health and wellbeing of the nation is to invest early with children and their parents. Successful delivery of all the key outcomes set out in the vision, strategy and action plan depends crucially on the nursing workforce.

Targets that impact directly on both mainstream and specialist CAMHS include:

- Between 2001 and 2025 there is to be improvement in the mental health and wellbeing of young people aged 16 by one-fifth as measured by the General Health Questionnaire (GHQ).
- By 2015 no more than a quarter of those on specialist CAMHS waiting lists are to wait longer than three months for an appointment.
- By 2025 all children who need specialist CAMHS will be able to access them in three months or less.

Scotland

One in ten of the million children living in Scotland have mental health problems that interfere with their everyday lives (Public Health Institute for Scotland 2003). Just as the Health Advisory Report found in 1995 that CAMHS in England and Wales were patchy (HAS 1995), so too are CAMHS currently lacking in Scotland. However, rapid development of CAMHS in Scotland over the last three years has occurred in the context of a range of other policies and initiatives. *For Scotland's Children* (Scottish Executive 2002) sets out to ensure that every child matters and promotes the need for more effective and seamless services; and *Improving Health in Scotland* (Scottish Executive 2003a) is an overarching programme and focuses on intervention during the early years and adolescence. As funding for CAMHS in Scotland is not targeted, it is difficult to derive robust and comparable data on what local NHS Boards and their partner agencies are spending on CAMHS in Scotland (Public Health Institute for Scotland 2001). In 2003, an initial budget of £24 million was allocated by the Scottish Executive's *National Programme for Improving Mental Health and Wellbeing*. This was to be used by local services to achieve four key aims: to raise public awareness and promote positive mental health; to eliminate stigma and discrimination; to reduce suicide rates, particularly amongst young men; and to support recovery from mental illness. The national programme has also made improving the mental health and wellbeing of children and young people one of the main priority areas for action (Meier 2004). In 2004 a further £1 million was allocated over two years for CAMHS workforce development. This funding is to support nursing staff in Scotland's four in-patient services; to improve training and development; and to increase continuing professional development (CPD) opportunities for the increasing multiagency CAMHS workforce.

A small number of fundamental documents have paved the way for addressing the present deficiencies and inequalities in Scottish CAMHS. The most significant of these is the Scottish Needs Assessment Programme's (SNAP) *Report on Child and Adolescent Mental Health*. Commissioned by the Scottish Executive in 2000 and published by the Public Health Institute of Scotland (now NHS Scotland) in May 2003, the SNAP report made several key strategic recommendations. As well as a strong focus on involving children and their families or carers in the planning and delivery of CAMHS, a number of target areas for development were identified. These related to the need to mainstream CAMHS by focusing on mental health promotion and emotional wellbeing; on the early identification and prevention of mental health problems and disorders; on research; and on strengthening local, regional and national specialist CAMHS (Public Health Institute for Scotland 2003). The Scottish Executive's Child Health Support Group (CHSG) is responsible for the development of CAMHS as one of the five key themes in their work programme. The CHSG draws on the expertise of colleagues from NHS Scotland, education, social work and the voluntary sector.

Following publication of the SNAP report, an expert advisory group, the Child and Adolescent Mental Health Development Group was convened by the CHSG and charged with translating the outcomes of the SNAP report into action. The resulting template was called *Children and Young People's Mental Health* which set out a strategy and framework for mental health promotion, illness prevention and effective care delivery (Scottish Executive 2004a). The CHSG also established a separate in-patient working group, to consider the development of in-patient child and adolescent services and make recommendations about configuration, care models and commissioning arrangements. Their report was published by the Scottish Executive in December 2004 and recommended a phased increase in psychiatric in-patient beds for children and adolescents (Scottish Executive 2004b). Published alongside the SNAP report was the Scottish Executive's consultation document, *An Integrated Strategy for the Early Years* (Scottish Executive 2003b). This aimed to influence policy at a structural level and drew together existing policies in relation to childcare, health visitor services, preschool education and parenting skills, all of which embrace the evolving CAMHS agenda in Scotland.

A national project for child and adolescent mental health called *Heads Up Scotland*, was established by the Scottish Executive in 2004. This was to support the SNAP report recommendations by: ensuring active involvement of children, their families and carers; giving guidance to support local organisations who were delivering CAMHS; and strengthening partnerships and developing the CAMHS workforce. The Scottish Executive *National Programme for Improving Mental Health and Wellbeing* has provided leadership for the development of policy and implementation of CAMHS in Scotland. At government level, a National Director for Children and Young People's Mental Health is responsible for achieving improved integration across health, social work and education policy areas as it impacts on CAMHS. The National Director also oversees implementation of the SNAP recommendations. The Child and Adolescent Mental Health Development Group has made tackling workforce pressures one of its key priorities in helping deliver the SNAP report recommendations and building capacity in specialist CAMHS across Scotland. This will be assisted by a development framework published by NHS Education for Scotland to improve the capability and competence of the CAMHS workforce in order to deliver the SNAP recommendations (NHS Education for Scotland 2004). The framework document identified a range of core education and training standards that all professionals working with children in Scotland will be required to reach. As in the rest of the UK, workforce shortages are a key pressure on CAMHS in Scotland, where they arise from resource constraints and difficulties with recruitment and retention of nurses and other key workers.

Wales

There are over half a million children living in Wales and they make up almost one fifth of the total population (Welsh Office 1997; Hortron 2004). It is estimated that as many as a quarter have mental health problems but the majority do not receive specialist help due to low recognition rates and an overburden on specialist services, many of which are already overwhelmed and under-resourced (Welsh Office 1997; Davies et al. 2001). The strategic development of specialist CAMHS in Wales has been patchy and, until recently, CAMHS has not been recognised as a priority area (Cresswell et al. 2003). This is despite the 1995 HAS review recommendations made in relation to CAMHS which applied to Wales as well as England (HAS 1995). The most important landmark in the modernisation of CAMHS in Wales came with the publication of the All Wales CAMHS Strategy, *Everybody's Business* (National Assembly for Wales 2001). This ten-year comprehensive policy framework embraced the four-tier strategic concept based on the HAS framework and promoted inclusion, multidisciplinary working, interagency collaboration and user involvement. *Everybody's Business* described the CAMHS Concept, an overarching definition of child and adolescent mental health services. This was intended to promote the multiagency nature of CAMHS and encourage partnership working and a strategic approach to service commissioning and delivery. It can be argued that publication of *Everybody's Business* attempted to enable a cultural shift to occur in CAMHS. Whilst responsibility for the mental health of children and young people has been historically associated with specialist CAMHS, it is now acknowledged that all professionals who work with children share responsibility for their mental health and psychological wellbeing. However, whether recognition of this responsibility is realised at the level of practice remains to be seen.

Responsibility for commissioning specialist CAMHS in Wales is through Local Health Boards (LHBs) and Health Commission Wales (HCW). This is an executive agency of the National Assembly for Wales which is responsible for commissioning all highly specialist CAMHS at Tier 4 and some specialist CAMHS at Tier 3. All CAMHS at Tier 1 and some at Tiers 2 and 3 are commissioned and planned by LHBs and Children and Young People Framework Partnerships. These can be compared to the Local Strategic Partnerships that have been established in England in order to commission comprehensive CAMHS. Some limited funding for CAMHS in Wales has only recently been ring-fenced. Starting in 2004, £700 000 per year was allocated by the National Assembly for Wales to create emergency access to in-patient child and adolescent mental health services and community forensic CAMHS. However, these services have not yet been established. Money has also been allocated to develop primary mental health worker posts, establish specialist CAMHS training programmes and fund a small number of nurse consultant posts (Lamb et al. 2004). However, it is estimated that implementation of the recommendations in *Everybody's Business* will require around £10 million recurrent additional funding for the first three years to cover extra training, development of services and extra personnel (Royal College of Psychiatrists 2005).

The National Assembly for Wales has developed CAMHS along similar lines to government departments in England. Work on the National Service Framework for Children, Young People and Maternity Services, closely modelled on the English NSF, started in 2001 and was published in October 2005 (National Assembly for Wales 2005). This includes a module on mental health and psychological wellbeing of children and young people and key 'flagged actions' to be achieved by the Framework for Partnerships by March 2006. Progress against implementation of the NSF is to be reported to the National Assembly for Wales by all statutory agencies using the Self Assessment Audit Tool (SAAT) on an annual basis. The National Assembly for Wales has also set LHBs and NHS Trusts specific targets to reduce waiting times for specialist CAMHS to be achieved by March 2007. The NSF aims to help deliver the Welsh NHS Plan (National Assembly for Wales 2002), deliver the recommendations made in the Review of Health and Social Care in Wales (National Assembly for Wales 2003), and take forward the objectives set out in *Everybody's Business*.

Conclusion

This account of CAMHS policy and strategy in the UK represents a stocktake of what is currently being planned and provided in the UK. The picture is likely to change as all four UK regions implement their CAMHS strategies over the next few years. Historically, the four main regions of the UK have developed their CAMHS in isolation, and while this is to some extent inevitable, there are many opportunities that could be maximised by better cross-border collaboration. Through their cross-jurisdictional review group, the Royal College of Psychiatrists have led the way in taking a cross-border approach to the development of CAMHS in the UK as well as Ireland. This is a developmental group that aims to bring together common policies and themes, regardless of structural or policy differences (Maher 2004). Their aim is to work towards high quality, comprehensive, sustainable and equitable CAMHS in the UK. Increasingly, the Royal College of Nursing children and young people's forums, CAMHS nurse consultants and others in leadership positions are also collaborating across all four main regions of the UK. Although this development is very much in its infancy it is hoped that this will help reduce inequalities in CAMHS development and continue to raise the profile of nursing in CAMHS.

References

Black, D. (1993). A brief history of child and adolescent psychiatry. In: Black, D. & Cottrell, D. (Eds). *Seminars in child and adolescent psychiatry.* London: Gaskell.

Campbell, H. (1999). *The Health of the Public in Northern Ireland: Report of the Chief Medical Officer 1999: taking care of the next generation.* Belfast: DHSS.

Cottrell, D. & Abdullah, K. (2005). Growing up? A history of CAMHS (1987–2005). *Child and Adolescent Mental Health,* **10** (3), 111–17.

Cresswell, A., Davies, J., & Hannigan, B. (2003). Fit for mental health practice? *Paediatric Nursing,* **15** (1), 26–29.

Davies, A., Earles, C., Eaton, N., Luke, C. & Mills, A. (2001). Educating children's nurses in Wales. *Paediatric Nursing,* **13** (6), 21–24.

Department for Education and Skills (2001). *Promoting children's mental health within early years and schools settings.* London: HMSO.

Department for Education and Skills (2003). *Every Child Matters.* London: HMSO.

Department of Health (1998). *Quality Protects: transforming children's services.* London: HMSO.

Department of Health (1999). *NHS Modernisation Fund and Mental Health Grant for Child and Adolescent Mental Health Services 1999–2002.* London: HMSO.

Department of Health (2000). *The NHS Plan: a plan for investment, a plan for reform.* London: HMSO.

Department of Health (2002). *Improvement, Expansion and Reform: the next three years' priorities and planning framework 2003–2006.* London: HMSO.

Department of Health (2002). *Priorities and Planning Framework (2003–2006).* London: HMSO.

Department of Health (2003). *Improvement, Expansion and Reform: the next three years. Priorities and Planning Framework 2003–2006.* London: HMSO.

Department of Health (2004). *National Service Framework for Children, Young People and Maternity Services.* London: HMSO.

Department of Health, Social Services and Public Safety (2001). *Review of Nursing, Midwifery and Health Visiting Workforce: report of KPMG Consulting and DHSSPS Nursing and Midwifery Workforce Planning Initiative Steering Group.* Belfast: DHSSPS.

Department of Health, Social Services and Public Safety (2003). *Promoting Mental Health: strategy and action plan 2003–2008.* Belfast: Health Promotion Agency.

Department of Health, Social Services and Public Safety (2005). *A Healthier Future: a twenty-year vision for health and wellbeing in Northern Ireland: 2005–2025.* Belfast: DHSSPS.

Green, H., McGinnity, A., Meltzer, H., Ford, T. & Goodman, R. (2005). *Mental health of children and young people in Great Britain.* London: Office of National Statistics.

Health Select Committee (1997). *Fourth Report: Child and Adolescent Mental Health Services: report and proceedings.* London: HMSO.

Hortron, C. (2004). *Working with children: facts, figures and information.* London: Society Guardian and NCH.

Jeffery, C. (2004). *Devolution: what difference has it made?* London: Economic and Social Research Council.

Kerfoot, M. & Williams, R. (2005). Setting the Scene: perspectives on the history of and policy for child and adolescent mental health services in the UK. In: Williams, R. & Kerfoot, M. (Eds). *Child and Adolescent Mental Health Services: strategy, planning, delivery and evaluation.* Oxford: Oxford University Press.

Kurtz, Z., Thornes, R. & Wolkind, S. (1994). *Services for the Mental Health of Children and Young People in England: A National Review.* London: Department of Public Health, South West Thames Regional Health Authority.

Lamb, C., Riley, S. & Davies, G. Strategic thinking. *YoungMinds Magazine,* (71), 15–16.

McDougall, T. (2000). The role of the nurse specialist in raising the profile of children's mental health. *Nursing Times,* **96** (28), 37–38.

McDougall, T. (2004). Children First: The National Service Framework for Children, Young People and Maternity Services. *Mental Health Practice,* **8** (3), 35.

Maher, T. (2004). Border line. *YoungMinds Magazine,* (79), 10–11.

Meier, R. (2004). Snapping into place. *YoungMinds Magazine,* (70), 18–19.

Meltzer, H., Gatward, R., Goodman, R. & Ford, T. (2000). *The Mental Health of Children and Adolescents in Great Britain.* London: The Stationary Office.

National Assembly for Wales (1999). *Realising the Potential: a strategy for nursing, midwifery and health visiting in Wales into the 21st Century.* Cardiff: National Assembly for Wales.

National Assembly for Wales (2001). *Everybody's Business: improving mental health in Wales – a CAMHS strategy.* Cardiff: National Assembly for Wales.

National Assembly for Wales (2002). *The Welsh NHS Plan: improving health in Wales.* Cardiff: National Assembly for Wales.

National Assembly for Wales (2003). *The Review of Health and Social Care in Wales (advised by Derek Wanless).* Cardiff: National Assembly for Wales.

National Assembly for Wales (2005). *National Service Framework for Children, Young People and Maternity Services in Wales.* Cardiff: National Assembly for Wales.

NHS Health Advisory Service (1995). *Together We Stand: the commissioning, role and management of child and adolescent mental health services.* London: HMSO.

Northern Ireland Association for Mental Health & Sainsbury Centre for Mental Health (2004). *Counting the Cost.* Belfast: SCMH & NIAMH.

Northern Ireland Executive (2002a). *Investing for Health.* Belfast: Northern Ireland Executive.

Northern Ireland Executive (2002b). *Building on Progress: budget 03–06.* Belfast: Northern Ireland Executive.

Northern Ireland Statistics and Research Agency (2002). *Northern Ireland Census 2001.* Belfast: NISRA.

O'Donnell, H. (2003). The future of mental health nursing in Northern Ireland: does anyone really care? *Mental Health Practice,* **7** (3), 30–33.

Office for National Statistics (2002). *2001 Population Census.* London: Office for National Statistics.

O'Rawe, A. (2003). *Child and adolescent mental health: providing a service Northern Ireland style.* Paper presented at Include Youth Annual Conference: The Balancing Act. 16–17 October 2003.

Public Health Institute of Scotland 2003. *Scottish Needs Assessment Report on Child and Adolescent Mental Health.* Glasgow: PHIS.

Scottish Executive (2001). *Nursing for Health: a review of the contribution of nurses, midwives and health visitors to improving the public's health.* Edinburgh: The Stationary Office.

Scottish Executive (2002). *For Scotland's Children: towards better integrated children's services.* Edinburgh: HMSO.

Scottish Executive (2003). *An Integrated Strategy for the Early Years.* Edinburgh: Scottish Executive.

Scottish Executive (2004a). *Children and Young People's Mental Health: a framework for promotion, prevention and care.* Edinburgh: Scottish Executive.

Scottish Executive (2004b). *Child Health and Support Group: in-patient working group – psychiatric in-patient services.* Edinburgh: Scottish Executive.

Smith, F. (2004). The NSF for children, young people and maternity services: an overview. *Paediatric Nursing*, **16** (8), 30–32.

Welsh Office (1997). *The Health of Children in Wales.* Cardiff: Welsh Office.

Chapter 3

Nursing Children and Young People with Attention Deficit Hyperactivity Disorder

Noreen Ryan

Key points

- ADHD (attention deficit hyperactivity disorder) is a persistent and severe impairment of psychological development characterised by high levels of inattentive, restless and impulsive behaviour.

- ADHD rarely exists as a single disorder. In particular, comorbidity with conduct disorder is very common for those with ADHD, and attention should be paid to this when nurses are assessing children and young people.

- The causes of ADHD are complex and can be understood within biological, psychological and social constructs. There is evidence to support genetic, neurological and cognitive mechanisms involved in ADHD. However, it remains unclear how these factors interact to cause ADHD and what impact environmental factors may have.

- Nurses in mental health, paediatric and school settings are well placed to identify and recognise the symptoms of ADHD, with their knowledge and experience of child development.

- Interventions for the treatment of ADHD are varied and nurses usually provide these in the context of a multimodal treatment strategy, typically comprised of psycho-education, parent training and behaviour management, school-based interventions and psychopharmacology.

- Nurse prescribing is currently evolving and this will have a significant effect on the future role of nurses in the care of children and young people with ADHD.

Introduction

The symptoms of hyperkinetic disorder (HKD) have been well documented from the turn of the nineteenth century, highlighting a group of children presenting with a combination of attentional, motivational, motor control and learning deficits (Gillberg 2003). HKD is a topical and controversial subject. A wide variety of terms have been used to describe this syndrome, including hyperactivity, attention deficit disorder (ADD), attention deficit hyperactivity disorder (ADHD), and hyperkinetic disorder. ADHD will be used here as the generic term to describe the cardinal symptoms of inattention, overactivity and impulsivity associated with this disorder. This chapter will seek to address these issues and consider recent evidence regarding the aetiology, symptomatology, classification and prevalence of ADHD.

The development of mental health and paediatric nursing has offered opportunities for nurses to extend their role in the field of CAMHS (child and adolescent metal health services). With the development of CAMHS, from primary care to specialist services, the role of the nurse is varied. There have been numerous examples of the knowledge, skills and innovative practice developed by nurses to support child and adolescent mental health (Brown 2003; Brown & Bruce 2004; Kelly & Rounsley 2004). Nurse-led assessment and follow-up clinics are commonplace in the NHS (National Health Service) – nurses need to be able to evaluate the care they offer and ensure that it is evidenced-based. The use of protocols and integrated care pathways are a way of standardising care and will help ensure that nurses can deliver high-quality, comprehensive assessment and treatment interventions, as advised by the National Institute for Clinical Excellence (NICE) (NICE 2000).

What is ADHD?

There has been great debate about the recognition of this syndrome and much conjecture regarding the increase in the diagnosis of the disorder and the use of medication over the last half-century. This may be due to the broadening of diagnostic criteria and/or the use of biological influences on clinical assessment, rather than just the use of a sociological and psychological model of care. Views have tended to be polarised in relation to the belief that ADHD is either a medical and developmental disorder, or that it is associated with poor parenting and poor child-rearing practices (Schacher & Tannock 2002), and over the last half-century parallel concepts of ADHD have evolved. One such concept is that hyperactive children were judged to have a behavioural problem resulting from family and social discord, so such children were diagnosed with behaviour problems and conduct disorder and not ADHD.

ADHD is a persistent and severe impairment of psychological development characterised by high levels of inattentiveness, restlessness and impulsive behaviour (Taylor et al. 2004). These symptoms of inattention, restlessness and impulsiveness are common behavioural problems during preschool and school age, often persisting into adulthood (Schacher & Tannock 2002). Therefore, childhood sufferers of ADHD are at risk of learning, social and conduct problems, which may develop into serious impairments in adolescence and adulthood. It is important to reflect upon the complexity of the syndrome and on the different ways in which it presents. ADHD is one of the most common psychiatric disorders of childhood (Willoughby 2003) and is characterised by elevated levels of activity, poor concentration, increased impulsivity and distractibility. The prevalence of HKD, the more severe form of attentional/hyperactive and impulsive disorder, is 1%; and the prevalence of ADHD is 5% of school-age children (NICE 2000). ADHD rarely exists in isolation and children often have associated difficulties. Common associated difficulties include antisocial behaviour, learning difficulties, emotional disorders, autism, tics, coordination difficulties and poor self-esteem (Taylor et al. 2004).

There is a belief that ADHD is a childhood disorder. However, with increasing awareness and understanding of the developmental pathway of ADHD, it is now understood in terms of an enduring disorder with symptoms creating dysfunction in adult life (Willoughby 2003). A large quantity of literature has been written about ADHD and the definition, assessment, treatment and outcomes for young people with this disorder. It is clear that the consequences of ADHD in childhood into adulthood are widespread and severe. Willoughby (2003) writes that children with ADHD are at increased risk for high rates of psychiatric comorbidity, non-psychiatric medical difficulties, disrupted familial and peer relationships, academic failure, lower educational attainment and poor work histories.

ADHD has been conceptualised as a disorder of early and middle childhood, mainly affecting males (Willoughby 2003). However, as interest and research into ADHD has grown researchers have felt it necessary to reconceptualise ADHD as a chronic disorder in both sexes (Willoughby 2003). In terms of outcomes, Dalsgaard et al. (2002) followed up a cohort of young people diagnosed with ADHD over a twenty-year period. They found that of this cohort, nearly a quarter had experienced an acute adult psychiatric admission, and that the main diagnostic category for this group was personality disorder, followed by mood disorder. They also found that gender had a significant impact, but that it was girls diagnosed with ADHD that had a poorer psychiatric outcome than boys (Dalsgaard et al. 2002).

Diagnosing ADHD

In the UK most CAMHS clinicians use the ICD-10 diagnostic criteria (World Health Organization 1992) as a framework for the diagnosis of ADHD. The DSM-IV diagnostic category (American Association 1994) is also used, but this involves a broader set of characteristics and leads to a commoner diagnosis of ADHD. However, the behaviours are recognised by both diagnostic frameworks as being similar. The main difference between the two frameworks is that ICD-10 requires pervasive evidence of all the core symptoms of ADHD, i.e. hyperactivity, attentional difficulties and impulsivity, before a diagnosis of hyperkinetic disorder can be made. However, both sets of diagnostic criteria require that the symptoms of ADHD be:

- Pervasive with symptoms occurring in two or more settings (e.g. home and school).
- Present before the age of seven years, nearly always before the age of five years and frequently before the age of two years.
- Persistent for more than six months.
- Out-of-keeping with the child's developmental level.
- Maladaptive and produce impairment in the child's social, academic or occupational functioning.

In making an assessment of a child or young person for ADHD it is useful to consider both diagnostic criteria (Taylor et al. 2004).

ICD-10 criteria for diagnosing ADHD

In order to make a diagnosis of ADHD there must be evidence of at least six of the following nine symptoms of inattention over the past six months, which are maladaptive and inconsistent with the developmental level of the child (see Box 3.1).

Box 3.1   Inattention difficulties.

- Poor attention to detail/careless errors.
- Often fails to concentrate on tasks or play.
- Often appears not to listen.
- Often fails to finish things.
- Poor task organisation.
- Often avoids tasks which require sustained mental effort.
- Often loses things.
- Often distracted by external stimuli.
- Often forgetful.

There must also be evidence of at least three of the following five symptoms of disturbances of motor activity for at least six months, which are maladaptive and inconsistent with the developmental level of the child (see Box 3.2).

Box 3.2   Hyperactivity difficulties.

- Often fidgets with hands or squirms in seat.
- Often leaves seat when expected to sit still.
- Excessive inappropriate climbing or running.
- Is often unduly noisy in playing or has difficulty in engaging in leisure activities quietly.
- Persistent overactivity not modulated by request or context.

Evidence must also be available of at least one of the following four symptoms of impulsivity for at least six months, which are maladaptive and inconsistent with the developmental level of the child (see Box 3.3).

Box 3.3   Impulsivity difficulties.

- Often blurts out answers before the question is complete.
- Often fails to wait turn in groups, games or queues.
- Often intrudes into games or conversations.
- Often talks excessively without response to social appropriateness.

DSM-IV criteria for diagnosing ADHD

Box 3.4   Inattention.

- Often fails to give close attention to details or makes careless mistakes in schoolwork, work or other activities.
- Often has difficulty in sustaining attention in tasks or play activities.
- Often does not seem to listen when spoken to directly.
- Often does not follow through on instructions and fails to finish schoolwork, chores, or duties in the workplace (not due to oppositional behaviour or failure to understand instructions).
- Often has difficulty organising tasks and activities.
- Often avoids, dislikes, or is reluctant to engage in tasks that require sustained mental effort (such as schoolwork or homework).
- Often loses things necessary for tasks or activities (e.g. toys, school assignments, pencils, books or tools).
- Is often easily distracted by extraneous stimuli.
- Is often forgetful in daily activities.

Box 3.5   Hyperactivity.

- Often fidgets with hands or feet.
- Often leaves seat in classroom or other situations in which remaining seated is expected.
- Often runs about excessively in situations in which it is inappropriate (in adolescents or adults, may be limited to subjective feelings of restlessness).
- Often has difficulty playing or engaging in leisure activities quietly.
- Is often 'on the go', or acts as if 'driven by a motor'.
- Often talks excessively.

Box 3.6   Impulsivity.

- Often blurts out answers before questions have been completed.
- Often has difficulty awaiting turn.
- Often interrupts or intrudes on others (e.g. interrupts others' conversations or games).

DSM-IV is a more broadly defined set of symptoms and requires evidence of inattention and/or hyperactivity/impulsivity, thus leading to the possible diagnosis of:

(1)   ADHD combined type (symptoms of inattention and hyperactivity/ impulsivity criteria met).
(2)   ADHD predominantly inattentive type (six symptoms of inattention present, but criteria for hyperactivity/impulsivity not met).
(3)   ADHD predominantly hyperactivity-impulsive type (six of the symptoms of hyperactivity/impulsivity are present, but no evidence of inattention).

Comorbidity

We have heard that ADHD rarely exists as a single disorder. Comorbidity is very common for children with ADHD and attention should be paid to this when nurses are assessing children. Oppositional defiant disorder (ODD) (Jensen et al. 1997; Angold & Costello 2001) and conduct disorder (Dalsgaard et al. 2002) are both common additional disorders. It is estimated that half of all children with ADHD have difficulties with friendships and with relationships with parents, siblings and teachers (Nixon 2001). Behavioural disturbance may be attributed to the events of social rejection. One large study in the US – *The Multimodal Treatment Study of Child with Attention-Deficit/Hyperactivity Disorder* (MTA 1999) – found that children presenting with ADHD were also diagnosed with the following comorbidities: anxiety (33.5%); conduct disorder (14.3%); ODD (39.9%); affective (mood) disorder (3.8%); and tic disorder (10.0%).

Some children and young people who present with pervasive difficulties such as inattention, hyperactivity and impulsivity are more challenging for their parents to care for. Such children may also sometimes be challenging for teachers to manage, and they may come into conflict with the world around them. Day-to-day activities and functions may be more problematic. It may not be surprising therefore, that the consequences of their ADHD leads some children and young people to have family relationship difficulties, peer relationship difficulties, conflicts at school and self-esteem problems. Children who present with ADHD and comorbid difficulties are more likely to have severe problems and social dysfunction (Khune 1997).

Difficulties with diagnostic criteria and the interpretation of hyperactive behaviour are complex, and inattention, hyperactivity and impulsivity can be due to many factors. Behavioural symptoms, although suggestive of hyperactivity, could, for example, be due to anxiety and/or mood disorders, where children and young people become preoccupied and agitated and may appear hyperactive (Taylor et al. 2004). Attachment disorders, where children have had adverse early-life experiences, can lead to disrupted attachment relationships, which are characterised by indiscriminate clinging to adults, overly outgoing and undifferentiated relationships with adults and the inability to form long-standing trusting relationships (Taylor et al. 2004). Developmental disorders and learning difficulties can coexist with ADHD, but the nurse or other professional must try to evaluate whether the levels of inattention, hyperactivity and impulsivity are so severe that they cannot be accounted for by the child's development and history.

How common is ADHD?

ADHD is one of the most common disorders of childhood (Guevara 2001). Prevalence rates of ADHD depend on which diagnostic criteria are used. There has been much debate about this issue. Taylor et al. (2004) suggest that there is a prevalence of 1.5% for HKD in the primary school-age population and in European studies, a prevalence of between 0 to 2.5% recognised in practice. Attention deficit without hyperactivity is less well-researched, but is thought to be troublesome for another 1% of the school-age population (Taylor et al. 2004). NICE has stated in its technology appraisal that the prevalence of HKD is 1% of the school-age population and for a lesser diagnosis of ADHD, 5% of the school-age population (NICE 2000).

What causes ADHD?

As stated the aetiology of ADHD is complex and it can be understood within biological, psychological and social constructs. When these constructs exist individually or interact together, there is an increased risk of ADHD being present (Schacher & Tannock 2002). There is evidence to support genetic, neurochemical, neuropathological and cognitive mechanisms involved in ADHD (Green & Chee 1997; Schacher & Tannock 2002). However, it remains unclear how these factors interact to cause ADHD and what impact environmental factors may have. There is evidence from family, twin and adoption studies that there is a genetic susceptibility to ADHD (Schacher & Tannock 2002). Taylor et al. (2004) note that ADHD tends to aggregate within families and suggest a three- to five-fold increased risk for ADHD in first-degree relatives, but stress that high heritability should not be confused with genetic determinism.

The role of environmental factors in the aetiology of ADHD is also important. The effects of maternal stress during pregnancy, disrupted early care-giving, early fetal brain development, exposure to alcohol, drugs and environmental toxins, obstetric complications and prematurity all increase risks for neuro-biological hazards (Schacher & Tannock 2002). The role of the family has to be considered and the quality of family relationships and the environment of the child's school can be a protective or maintaining factor in the development of ADHD (Taylor et al. 2004).

Do children and young people grow out of ADHD?

Toddlers present with inattentive, hyperactive and impulsive behaviour as part of normal child development. Over time, these behaviours improve as the child learns and develops. It is therefore important for nurses to consider the developmental level of the child throughout all assessments. Those children who appear to have excessive levels of hyperactivity, impulsivity and poor concentration will require further assessment. Symptoms of ADHD are usually, but not always, noticed in the early years. What is now understood is that the symptoms of ADHD are not necessarily transient and that the symptoms can continue to cause impairment into adolescence and adulthood (Willoughby 2003). Young people with ADHD are at greater risk of developing substance abuse, antisocial behaviour, depression and anxiety, and of having completed significantly less education than their non-affected peers (Schacher & Tannock 2002).

What is the nurse's role?

The role of nurses in the assessment of ADHD is wide and varied. The symptoms of ADHD are often initially detected at the primary care level by school nurses, teachers or general practitioners, when the child is unable to meet the demands of the classroom (Schacher & Tannock 2002). Mental health, paediatric and school nurses are well-placed to identify and recognise the symptoms of ADHD with their knowledge and experience of child development. Teachers often seek the advice of school nurses in relation to disruptive behaviour in the classroom. Questionnaires may be used by nurses to assist the formulation of problems. An observation of the child in the structured classroom setting and the unstructured playground setting is very important. Discussions with the teacher regarding their observations of behaviour, taking particular note of inattention, hyperactivity and impulsivity, are also invaluable. Any concerns about physical health, such as problems with sight, hearing or growth and development should also be fully investigated. The impact of epilepsy, tic disorders and any concerns about disability should first be explored before making a referral to specialist services for a more detailed assessment. Only when the symptoms of inattention, hyperactivity and impulsivity cause family relationship difficulties and/or social and academic impairment, should referral to specialist services be made. The responsibility of specialist services is to respond to any queries for advice in consultation about cases, and to offer a comprehensive diagnostic assessment. The cornerstone of any nursing assessment is a carefully gathered, detailed history that includes the presenting concerns of the family/carer, the child's motor and cognitive development, family history, and the child's social development, physical health and school performance. The purpose of the assessment is to explore the child's difficulties within the context of their normal developmental milestones. A thorough nursing assessment should comprise a family interview, a parent or carer interview and a child interview.

The family interview

The assessment processes for ADHD are complex, requiring the nurse to use particular communication and observational skills. The aim of the assessment interview is to build up a picture of the child and his or her family or carers through the question-and-answer process. The interview not only acts as a medium for gathering information but also allows for a relationship to develop and forms the basis for a collaborative alliance to develop between the nurse and the child and family. This trusting relationship enables the nurse to consider which problems are amenable to change and is a medium through which to work with the child and their family to achieve this (Barker 1997).

During the assessment, the interview room should be well-equipped with toys that are appropriate to the developmental age of the child, and should be quiet, private and free from distractions. Observations made during the interview about the child's ability or inability to use the toys appropriately are useful. During the interview the nurse should also take note of the following:

- The child's activity levels and interactions in the small group and one to one.
- The child's ability to concentrate, levels of hyperactivity and impulsivity.
- The interactions between family members.
- Strategies used by the family members to manage behaviour in the interview.

The verbal component of the interview will also yield information to exclude concerns about mood, anxiety, learning, speech and language. There should be opportunity for the nurse to conduct a child-centred interview, as well as an opportunity for parents to discuss their concerns with the nurse on a one-to-one basis. During the parental interview, questionnaires that are helpful for the assessment of ADHD can be completed, including the Connors parent rating scale (CPRS) (Connors 1989) and the strengths and difficulties questionnaire (SDQ) (Goodman 1997).

The purpose of taking a detailed family history is to create an understanding of the family's methods of operating and to establish any other family difficulties. The family history may generate important information about parental conflicts, financial problems or difficulties with other family members. It is important to have an understanding of the ways in which the family copes with pressures and of their style of communication. It is also useful for the nurse to understand the language, emotions and behaviour exhibited by the family and to explore the social support systems that are in place. Using a genogram (family tree) is a useful way of enquiring about the extended family. This can help to facilitate a detailed understanding of the family history, the family belief systems and the development of family relationships over a period of time. The family history should be able to identify the following information:

- Who is in the family and who lives at home.
- Whether there is contact with absent parents.
- Family relationships and communication style.
- The coping style of the family.
- Family support systems.

- Distressing life events e.g. family separation, domestic violence, death of relatives, house and school moves.

The parent/carer interview

Parents or carers should always be given the opportunity to describe in their own words what their concerns are for their child. They should consider the duration of the difficulties and what they have tried to do to alleviate some of the problems, and whether anything has helped improve the situation. The parental interview should be conducted in order to ascertain the following:

- Their main concerns.
- Attempts by them to improve the problem.
- Impact of the problems on the family system.
- Parental communication.
- Parental questionnaires.

The child interview

Particular note should be taken of inattention, hyperactivity and impulsivity presented by the child on interview. The child interview should be used to assess the following:

- Ability to separate from caregivers.
- Physical appearance.
- Motor functioning.
- Speech and language comprehension and general use of language.
- Social interactions with family and interviewer dependant on the developmental level of the child.
- Mood.
- Child self-report if appropriate e.g. Conners Adolescent self-report (CASR) for children aged 12–18 (Conners 1987) and child SDQ for children aged 8–16 (Goodman 1997).

The developmental history

The need for a comprehensive account of the child's development is of fundamental importance when nurses are making an assessment for ADHD. It may be necessary to seek further information from other professionals, such as the health visitor, the school nurse, the GP (general practitioner) or paediatrician. An account of the following should be obtained:

- Maternal health during pregnancy (including information about conception; antenatal history; fetal growth; toxaemia; threatened miscarriage).
- Postnatal history (including birth complications; birth weight; neonatal complications).

- Use of medication during pregnancy (including drugs, alcohol and nicotine).
- Developmental milestones (including motor development; attachment; sleep; language development; growth and temperament).
- Medical history (including other developmental disorders; epilepsy and tics).
- School performance (including learning difficulties, ability to separate from parents at school age and comparison to developmental peer group at school).

Information from other sources

With the consent of the child and family, it is very helpful to obtain reports from the child's school. A telephone interview will provide the nurse with the necessary information about the child's academic, behavioural, developmental and social functioning in school. It will also provide some understanding of the coping style of the teacher and a sense of the teacher–child relationship. Use of standardised rating scales such as the Conners teacher rating scale (CTRS) and SDQ teacher report may provide useful information about the child's functioning. If necessary, more detailed information should be sought from speech and language therapists, educational psychologists, paediatricians and voluntary agencies to add important information in relation to the child's overall presentation.

Formulation and diagnosis

The care and attention to detail in the assessment of a child's difficulties suggestive of ADHD is crucial, focusing specifically on the symptoms and behaviours listed previously in the ICD-10 and DSM-IV diagnostic categories. The nurse should consider if there is a differential diagnosis and whether the presenting symptoms could be explained in terms other than ADHD. In order to make a diagnosis of ADHD there needs to be clear evidence of clinically-significant impairment in social, academic or occupational functioning. The use of the term 'impairment' suggests that the symptoms occur on a greater frequency and at a greater severity than would be expected of the child's developmental peer group and interfere with the child's day-to-day activities with their family, school and friends.

How can nurses help children and young people manage their ADHD?

Interventions for the treatment of ADHD are varied and a multimodal approach is often required. The consequences of the disorder can be far-reaching and the impact upon the child's life may be widespread. Each child and family will require different levels of input and this should be carefully negotiated. The following are the mainstay interventions currently used in the management of ADHD.

Psycho-educational measures

An important part of the nursing role is to provide education to parents, children, caregivers and teachers about ADHD. This will help the child and family to develop an understanding of the nature of the disorder and have more realistic expectations of their child. Teachers may benefit from information about a particular child's needs and difficulties. It is important to acknowledge the symptoms, aetiology, prognosis and treatment options.

Parent-training and behavioural interventions

Parent training programmes have been widely used to help parents and carers of children with ADHD (Taylor et al. 2004). The programmes utilise various approaches but are usually based on a combination of direct instruction, modelling and role-play. The programmes are designed to teach parents the need to reinforce positive behaviour, reduce the number of punitive strategies and suggest techniques to manage inappropriate and defiant behaviour. Parent training programmes have been shown to improve parental management of the child's behaviour, enhance parental self-confidence, reduce family stress and alleviate difficult behaviour (Schacher & Tannock 2002). During the treatment phase, nurses can help the family identify the areas of most concern and support them to employ appropriate management strategies that will be specific to their child's problems. The most commonly used techniques are those of paying positive attention to appropriate behaviour and compliance, giving clear commands effectively and using negative consequences for difficult behaviours (Taylor et al. 2004).

School-based behavioural and psychoeducational interventions

It is important that a child with ADHD is integrated into their peer group as much as possible. Schools may wish to seek advice from their specialist educational colleagues as to how best to help a child with ADHD access their education successfully. Factors such as classroom structure, providing manageable learning tasks that are frequently reviewed by the teacher, having the child placed near the teacher and implementing a range of behavioural strategies to address specific problem behaviours are all helpful. O'Regan (2002) has produced a book outlining classroom management techniques.

Psychopharmacological interventions

Psychopharmacology is used to relieve the core symptoms of inattention, hyperactivity and impulsivity and there have been many trials of effectiveness (Heyman & Santosh 2002).

Stimulants

Stimulants are used to increase attention and reduce hyperactivity. They are licensed for use in the UK for children aged six years and over. The most commonly used medication for ADHD is the stimulant medication methylphenidate (also known as Ritalin, Equasym, Equasym XL and Concerta XL). Almost half of all children with hyperkinetic disorder take methylphenidate (Green et al. 2005). According to NICE guidelines, methylphenidate should be used as part of a comprehensive treatment package after an intensive assessment by expert practitioners (NICE 2000). Other stimulants include dexamfetamine and pimoline, but these are not used widely in the UK. Taylor et al. (2004) recommend that the first-line treatment for ADHD should be methylphenidate and that this should be conducted as a trial.

However, stimulants have limitations since they are not an acceptable treatment choice for some families, and compliance with treatment plans affects effectiveness. Although considered to be generally safe, stimulants sometimes have unwanted side-effects which can lead to the discontinuation of treatment. Common side-effects of stimulant treatment include difficulty in falling asleep, decreased appetite, nervousness and dysphoria. Less common side-effects include nausea, headaches, weight loss, changes in blood pressure and skin rash; stimulants can also trigger tics or make tics worse if they already exist. It is a matter of clinical judgement and the wishes of the child and their family about whether stimulant treatment is discontinued in such cases.

It is important to explain the medication trial process to the child, parents or carers and teachers. This is because feedback regarding any changes in the child's presentation will assist the nurse in understanding whether there have been any positive or negative treatment effects. Treatment usually commences at a low dose and is gradually increased over a period of weeks until there is a positive treatment response, or until unwanted side-effects appear. Careful titration of doses needs to be considered in order to improve positive response to treatment. Nurses should be available to discuss parental or teacher concerns over the telephone throughout the trial. Some side-effects are short-lived but parents may often require support through the process of the trial. This support will help enhance the therapeutic relationship and ensure safe practice. Before a child with ADHD starts a medication trial it is important for the nurse to make a baseline assessment of:

- Height and weight: this should be plotted on a growth chart and used to assess growth and weight during the course of treatment.
- Blood pressure and pulse.
- Whether the child has any other physical or mental health disorders (for example methylphenidate is contraindicated in schizophrenia, hyperthyroidism, cardiac arrhythmias and glaucoma and should be used with caution in the presence of hypertension, depression, tics or family history of Tourette's syndrome, pervasive developmental disorders, severe mental retardation).
- Current medication, allergies and over-the-counter medications.

Monitoring treatment with stimulant medication

The use of rating scales for ADHD is helpful in trying to capture changes in inattention, hyperactivity, impulsivity and behaviour. However, questionnaires are not always sensitive enough to note changes. A meeting with parents and teachers to review the trial is a helpful way of gathering important information and to review the completed questionnaires about how the child's behaviour has changed during the trial. Following the review of the trial, a decision on whether to continue with methylphenidate is made. Nurses are well-placed to offer routine monitoring of medication and to provide other psychosocial interventions. Routine monitoring should focus on a general mental health assessment at each appointment, particularly noting possible tics, depression, irritability, social withdrawal or lack of spontaneity. The following factors should also be monitored:

- Blood pressure and pulse.
- Height and weight.
- Side-effects.
- Positive and negative responses to treatment.
- Progress at school.

The drug manufacturers of methylphenidate recommend periodic blood tests to review haematological status, but there is little evidence to support this practice, and it can be argued that the benefits of regular blood tests are outweighed by the distress caused to the child (Taylor et al. 2004). There is little guidance as to length of treatment: discontinuation of treatment is recommended periodically to assess the child's progress and the need to continue with treatment; treatment may continue into adult life and further research is required in this area.

Non-stimulants

There are other licensed non-stimulant treatments available. Atomoxetine is a norephinephrine re-uptake inhibitor. It is licensed for use in children over the age of six years. The advantages of this drug are that it provides all-day relief from symptoms and does not wear off like stimulant medication. However, data about the effectiveness of the drug is limited as atomoxetine has only recently been introduced into the UK and trials have been short in duration (Bailey 2003). The nurse plays an important role in the baseline and continued monitoring assessment of height, weight, blood pressure and pulse, effectiveness of treatment and any adverse side-effects. Other unlicensed treatments include tricyclic antidepressants (imipramine), antihypertensives (clonidine) and bupropion, but the evidence base for these treatments has been questioned due to the small scale of the studies and their methodological quality (Taylor et al. 2004).

How important is diet in the treatment of ADHD?

Currently there is not sufficient evidence-based information to support the restriction of diet as a treatment for ADHD. The Feingold diet in the mid-1970s supported the restriction of additives in the child's diet. However, this was not found to reduce symptoms of ADHD (Pliska et al. 1999). Some children may respond to caffeine in tea, coffee and carbonated drinks and become more active. The food dye tartrazine and food preservative benzoate can trigger worsening behaviour in children. Unfortunately there is no way of knowing which foods will create a reaction like this in certain children. It is helpful for parents to conduct their own trials restricting these substances to see if behaviour improves, and it would therefore be sensible for parents to continue to restrict a particular food if they consider their child's behaviour to be worse when taking it (Spender et al. 2001). As there is little evidence for restricting diet, healthier eating is advocated. This can be implemented by parents and may benefit the child's general wellbeing. However, more research into this area is required.

Nurse prescribing and ADHD

The introduction of nurse prescribing will have a dramatic effect on the role of the nurse with children and young people with ADHD. The concept of nurse prescribing in mental health nursing has been considered for many years, since the publication of the Cumberledge Report (DoH 1986) and the two Crown Reports (DoH 1989; 1999). However, its implementation has been slow. It has been suggested that nurses fear that the process of prescribing will alter their therapeutic relationship with the client (Nolan & Badger 2000). Currently, nurses engage mainly in supplementary prescribing for the management of mental health difficulties (Bradley & Nolan 2005). This can be defined as a voluntary prescribing partnership between an independent prescriber (IP) (doctor) and a supplementary prescriber (SP) (nurse or pharmacist), to implement an agreed patient-specific CMP with the patient's agreement (Department of Health 2002). For children and young people with a diagnosis of ADHD the implementation of supplementary nurse prescribing will provide more prompt care, reduce delays in initiating treatment, allow nurses to titrate doses and to stop one medication and commence another (DoH 2005b).

In order to gain the competence, skills and knowledge to be a supplementary nurse prescriber, nurses are required to undertake independent, extended and supplementary prescribing training. Supplementary prescribing is a collaborative process between the nurse, doctor, child and family (Shuttle 2004). With the extension of the nurse's roles in supplementary prescribing, and a move away from traditional nursing practice, clear frameworks to review the process of nurse prescribing need to be introduced within NHS Trust clinical governance structures (Jones & Harbone 2005). Nurses will need to engage in continued professional development to keep their knowledge up-to-date, to be aware of changes to the formulary and maintain their level of competency in nurse prescribing.

The challenges of nurse prescribing are evident in that it changes the therapeutic relationship between the nurse, doctor and patient. Not all specialist CAMHS nurses will want or need to become nurse prescribers, and not all child and adolescent psychiatrists will wish to take on the role of independent prescribers. It is important to ensure that nurses must continue to be bound by their professional code of conduct when implementing nurse prescribing, the core values of which are to 'do good and do no harm'; they should also involve children and young people in the process of obtaining consent to treatment and provide information accurately, truthfully and understandably (Nursing and Midwifery Council 2004). Though the pace of change in nurse prescribing has been slow, there has been further consultation with the Department of Health to consider extending the boundaries of nurse prescribing, and further developments are likely in the scope of nurse prescribing during the next few years.

Summary

ADHD is a complex disorder to assess and treat and this is not helped by the differing classification systems currently in use. It is not surprising, therefore, that there continues to be controversy around this disorder despite the recent advances in our understanding of the biological, genetic, psychological and social pathways. The long-term effects of ADHD diagnosis are widespread, particularly when the outcomes for this population extend into adulthood in terms of their mental health, work experience and long-term relationships. Further research is required into our understanding of the disorder and what interventions are helpful to children and families with ADHD.

Nurses have a vital role to play in the assessment, treatment and management of ADHD. They are well placed to gather clinical information from parents, children, teachers and other professionals, and communication and interviewing skills are an important part of the nursing assessment (Barker 1997). Knowledge of child development will assist the nurse in understanding atypical aspects of the child's development. These are the key areas to understand when conducting an assessment of the child's functioning. The type and severity of problems presented by the young person need to be evaluated in the context of the child's physical, emotional and cognitive development. School nurses are able to make observations of children in the school setting to assess the child's functioning in the school environment. They should consider the child's development in contrast with their peer group, thus giving an indication of the severity of the core symptoms of ADHD: hyperactivity, inattention and impulsivity; and the impact these have on the child's academic progress.

The nurse has a number of responsibilities in respect of the care of the child with a diagnosis of ADHD. They are required to gather clinical information to make a comprehensive assessment of the presenting problems. They also have a vital monitoring role when children are taking medication, including monitoring physical health (height, weight, blood pressure and pulse) and evaluating the effectiveness of medication and also any adverse side-effects of the medication treatment. Nurses are also in key positions to provide psychosocial interventions for the child and family to help ameliorate associated behavioural problems. It is important that nurses continue to update their skills and ensure that their knowledge and practice is evidenced-based. Full consideration should always be given to the professional code of conduct (United Kingdom Central Council 1998; Nursing & Midwifery Council 2004) and nurses should always work within their sphere of competence and acknowledge the limitations of their knowledge and skills. This also applies to the expanding role of the nurse and particularly supplementary nurse prescribing.

Edward

Edward's GP referred him to CAMHS. His teachers had expressed concern about his behaviour in the classroom, stating that he could not sit still and was distracting other pupils. Edward was reported to have difficulties with his behaviour at school generally. The referral information stated that he would not sit still, had poor concentration and was falling behind with his learning. His parents were said to find his behaviour a challenge, but felt that they had adapted their parenting style to manage his behaviour. The parents did not perceive him as being naughty; they described him instead as being a warm and loving child and a pleasure to be with. Edward had few friends at school or in his local area.

Family history

Edward is a seven year-old boy who lives at home with his mother Susan, and her partner Matthew, both aged 27. Edward does not have any contact with his natural father. His parents separated when Susan was three months' pregnant. Susan had returned to work soon after Edward's birth and he was cared for by his maternal grandmother, who was influential in his life. During the interview, Edward found it difficult to occupy himself with age-appropriate toys, seeking the assistance of the adults in the room to play with him. However, he was not disruptive or oppositional, but was active, restless and noisy. He was a planned pregnancy and was born full-term in a normal delivery, following a threatened miscarriage at 31 weeks' gestation. Edward and Susan lived with the maternal grandparents for the first 18 months of his life. Susan had untreated postnatal depression; however, his grandparents were alternative positive care providers. Susan was described by the grandmother as being like Edward when she was a child. She was described as being a live-wire, but more oppositional, and as failed at school.

Developmental history

There were no developmental concerns for Edward, as he walked at 14 months, talked fluently by two-and-a-half years, was sociable and separated well at nursery. He slept in the same bed as his mother until they moved into their own home where Susan was able to develop her own routine with Edward. The local nursery commented that at three-and-a-half years he appeared to be more hyperactive than his peer group and found it more difficult to settle on any activity. His family struggled to manage his demanding behaviour, but Susan felt it was normal as she had no other children with whom to compare. She reported that she felt that he was a little clumsy, but could ride a bike and fasten shoelaces. He fell over frequently, but this was due to rushing rather than a motor coordination problem. He is described as a healthy child, only having surgery for a hernia aged six weeks.

In reception class his teachers again described him as: hyperactive; excitable; running around the classroom; being frequently off-task; finding friendships troublesome; and standing out from the other boys in his class. By Year 1 his teachers commented as follows in his reports:

- 'Edward is unable to sit still, he makes loud noises and disrupts the class'.
- 'Lacks concentration, always racing ahead and can't remember what to do next'.
- 'Restless, inattentive and has a short attention span, compared to his peers'.
- 'Kind and sensitive to his peers, but has failed to form positive relationships with peers and adults'.

His parents reported that Edward did not have any habits or ritualistic behaviour and that his speech and language skills were good, even if he did speak rapidly. He was sleeping from 9:00 p.m., but rose early at 5:30 a.m. He is a fussy eater and has a restricted diet, which has improved since he started school. He does not have a friend and his parents report how he seems to irritate other children.

The family interview

The parents related in a warm, calm and consistent manner on interview. There were some differences in opinions between the parents and maternal grand-mother, but the family handled these in a sensitive way.

Interview with Edward

Edward separated readily from his family and did not appear shy or timid. He was active and restless in the room and he gave a verbal running commentary on what we did together. It was difficult to gain his eye contact and attention for any period of time; he found it hard to follow a train of conversation, choosing instead to tell the nurse interviewer lots of information about a recent school trip he had been on. He hurriedly drew a picture of himself, with little detail or showing any interest. He was warm and sociable if over-familiar. Edward was observed to have a slight facial motor tic on interview.

Information from other sources

No other professionals had seen the family prior to referral. Information from the school was already reported. The Conners Parent and Teacher Rating Scale questionnaires highlighted Edward's difficulties with inattention and hyperactivity. Also highlighted was the oppositional behaviour rated by teachers and parents. The SDQ highlighted more global difficulties that Edward was experiencing with his peer relationships, his difficult behaviour and hyperactivity at home and school, but did note that he presented as a warm and sociable child.

Conclusion

Edward is a seven year-old boy who presents with pervasive evidence of poor concentration, overactivity, impulsivity and distractibility in his development and on interview. He does not present with any evidence of social impairment, although he finds peer relationships difficult. He has a simple facial motor tic. These symptoms can be termed as attention deficit hyperactivity disorder (ADHD), as they cannot be accounted for in terms of his mother's postnatal depression as he had other positive caregivers (grandparents) during his early development. Clear and consistent behaviour management by his parents and school has not ameliorated his behaviour.

Management plan

(1) Psychological and information education to the parents and teachers about the symptoms of ADHD.
(2) Consultation with the educational psychologist and behaviour support service to assist the school in helping Edward to access his education fully.
(3) Trial of non-stimulant medication in view of the facial motor tic. This trial of non-stimulant treatment was unsuccessful in terms of reducing hyperactivity, impulsivity and inattention; however stimulants helped reduce hyperactivity, impulsivity and improve concentration without exacerbating facial motor tic. Regular review of medication management advised in nurse-led clinic.
(4) Continued behaviour management advice to the parents.

Outcome

Edward continues to take medication without any side-effects, and he is growing and gaining weight appropriately. His parents have been pleased with his progress and have made changes to their parenting style. At school Edward produces more work and at a better quality and appears more sociable and accepted by his peer group.

References

American Psychiatric Association (1994). *Diagnostic and Statistical Manual of Mental Disorders*. (4th edn). Washington DC: APA.

Angold, A. & Costello, E. (2001). The epidemiology of disorders of conduct: nosological issues and comorbidity. In: Hill, J. & Maughan, B. (Eds). *Conduct Disorders in Childhood and Adolescence*. Cambridge: Cambridge University Press.

Bailey, K. (2003). Pharmacological treatments for ADHD and the novel agent Atomoxetine. *Journal of Psychosocial Nursing*, **41** (8), 12–17.

Barker, P. (1997). *Assessment in Psychiatric and Mental Health Nursing: in search of the whole person*. Cheltenham: Stanley Thornes.

Bradley, E. & Nolan, P. (2005). Non-medical prescribing and mental health nursing: prominent issues. *Mental Health Practice*, **8** (5), 16–19.

Brown, G. (2003). Assessment of attention deficit hyperactivity disorder. *Nursing Times*, **99** (25), 34–36.

Brown, G. & Bruce, K. (2004) A nurse-led ADHD service for children and adolescents. *Nursing Times*, **100** (40), 36–38.

Conners, C. (1989). *Conners Adolescent Self Report Rating Scale Manual*. New York: Multi-Health System.

Conners, C. (1989a). *Conners Parent Rating Scale Manual*. New York: Multi-Health System.

Conners, C. (1989b). *Conners Teacher Rating Scale Manual*. New York: Multi-Health System.

Dalsgaard, S., BoMortensen, P., Frydenberg, M. & Thomsen, P. (2002). Conduct problems, gender and adult psychiatric outcome of children with attention-deficit hyperactivity disorder. *British Journal of Psychiatry*, (181), 416–21.

Department of Health (1989). *Report for the Advisory Group on Nurse Prescribing* (Crown Report). London: HMSO.

Department of Health (1999). Review of prescribing, supply and administration of medicines (Crown Report). London: HMSO.

Department of Health (2002) Supplementary Prescribing. London: HMSO.

Department of Health (2005b). *Improving Mental Health Services by Extending the Role of Nurses in Prescribing and Supplying Medication: a good practice guide*. London: HMSO.

Department of Health and Social Security (1986). *Neighbourhood Nursing: a focus for care (Cumberledge Report)*. London: HMSO.

Gillberg, C. (2003). ADHD and DAMP: a general health perspective. *Child and Adolescent Mental Health*, **8** (3), 106–113.

Goodman, R. (1997). The strengths and difficulties questionnaire: a research note. *Journal of Child Psychology and Psychiatry*, (38), 581–86.

Green, C. & Chee, K. (1997). *Understanding ADHD*. London: Ebury.

Green, H., McGinnity, A., Meltzer, H., Ford, T. & Goodman, R. (2005). *Mental health of children and young people in Great Britain*. London: ONS.

Guevara, J. (2001). Evidence-based management of attention deficit hyperactivity disorder. *British Medical Journal*, (323), 1232–35.

Heyman, I. & Santosh, P. (2002). Pharmacological and other physical treatments. In: Rutter, M. & Taylor, E. (Eds). *Child and Adolescent Psychiatry*. 4th edn. Oxford: Blackwell.

Jensen, P., Martin, D. & Cantwell, D. (1997). Comorbidity in ADHD: implications for research, practice and DSM-IV. *Journal of the American Academy of Child and Adolescent Psychiatry*, (36), 1065–79.

Jones, A. & Harbone, G. (2005). Supplementary prescribing in hospital settings. *Mental Health Practice*, **9** (1), 38–40.

Kelly, C. & Rounsley, C. (2004). Introducing a school-based monitoring system for children taking methylphenidate. *Royal College of Nursing: Nursing Minds*, (Autumn 2004), 6–7.

Khune, M., Schacher, R. & Tannock, R. (1997). Impact of comorbid oppositional or conduct problems on ADHD. *Journal of the American Academy of Child and Adolescent Psychiatry*, (36), 1715–25.

MTA Cooperative Group. (1999). A 14-month randomised clinical trial of treatment strategies for attention-deficit hyperactivity disorder. *Archives of General Psychiatry*, (56), 1073–86.

National Institute for Clinical Excellence (2000). *Technology Appraisal No 13 – guidance on the use of methylphenidate (Ritalin, Equasym) for attention deficit hyperactivity disorder (ADHD) in childhood*. London: NICE.

Nixon, E. (2001). The social competence of children with attention deficit hyperactivity disorder: a review of the literature. *Child Psychology and Psychiatry Review*, **6** (4), 172–80.

Nolan, P. & Badger, F. (2000). Mental health nurse prescribing: added chore or golden opportunity. *Mental Health Practice*, **4** (1), 12–15.

Nursing and Midwifery Council (2004). *The NMC code of professional conduct: standards for conduct, performance and ethics. Protecting the public through professional standards*. London. NMC.

O'Regan, F. (2002). *How to Teach and Manage Children with ADHD*. Cambridge: Learning Disabilities Association.

Pliska, S., Carlson, C. & Swanson, J. (1999). *ADHD with comorbid disorders: clinical assessment and management*. New York: Guildford Press.

Schacher, R. & Tannock, R. (2002). Syndromes of hyperactivity and attention deficit. In: Rutter, M. & Taylor, E. (Eds). *Child and Adolescent Psychiatry* (4th edn). Oxford: Blackwell.

Shuttle, B. (2004). Non-medical prescribing in a multidisciplinary team context. In: Courtenay, M. & Griffiths, M., (Eds). *Independent and Supplementary Prescribing: an essential guide*. Cambridge: Greenwich Medical Media.

Spender, Q., Salt, N., Dawkins, J., Kendrick, T. and Hill, P. (2001). *Child Mental Health in Primary Care*. Oxford: Radcliffe Medical Press.

Taylor, E., Doepfner, M., Sergeant, J., Asherson, P., Banaschewski, T., Buitelaar, J., Coghill, D., Danckaerts, M., Rothenberger, A., Sonuga-Barke, E., Steinhausen, H., & Zuddas, A. (2004). European clinical guidelines for hyperkinetic disorder – first upgrade. *Journal of European Child and Adolescent Psychiatry*, (13), Supplement 1, 1–30.

United Kingdom Central Council (1998). *Guidelines for Mental Health and Learning Disabilities Nursing*. London: UKCC.

Willoughby, M. (2003). Developmental course of ADHD symptomatology during the transition from childhood to adolescence: a review with recommendations. *Journal of Child Psychology and Psychiatry*, **44** (1), 88–106.

World Health Organization (1992). *The ICD-10 Classification of Mental and Behavioural Disorders: clinical descriptions and diagnostic guidelines*. Geneva: WHO.

Chapter 4

Self-Harm, Young People and Nursing

Marie Armstrong

Key points

- As many as 25 000 young people below the age of 20 present to general hospitals in England and Wales with problems involving self-harm. This represents an increase of almost 30% since the 1980s and repetition rates have doubled. Despite being alarmingly high, these figures are far from representative since most young people who self harm do not attend hospital for treatment.

- Nurses in CAMHS (child and adolescent mental health services) play a holistic role. This means they see the young person as a whole person and recognise that the child's and family's needs may be broad and varied. This insight is enabled by the nurse's well-developed communication skills and their ability to engage with the young person and their family.

- As well as understanding the significance of self-harm in the context of adolescent development, nurses should also be aware of the social context in which young people harm themselves. For some young people, self-harm may be symptomatic of a serious underlying problem; for others, it may be the result of experimentation as part of adolescent identity and self-image.

- Guidelines in England and Wales provide health professionals with evidence and standards for the assessment of young people who self harm. These can be applied by nurses across a range of paediatric, school, mental health and forensic settings.

- In order to help young people who self harm, the nurse must understand the problem and communicate this understanding and also create a therapeutic alliance which forms the bedrock for positive change.

- It is important that nurses who work with young people who self harm have regular clinical supervision. This is essential to ensure their practice is safe and effective, and also so that the nurse remains supported, up-to-date and professionally accountable for their work.

Introduction

Nurses in schools, hospitals, prisons and community settings may come into contact with children and young people who harm themselves. This chapter explores some of the myths and realities about self-harm and uses an evidence-based framework to guide nurses who are required to assess, treat and support such children in both frontline services and residential settings. Self-harm is heterogeneous, which means that it means different things to different people, therefore current evidence for the assessment of self-harm and clinical interventions are discussed. The development of mental health nursing in relation to self-harm is also described here and case vignettes are used to illustrate the different ways in which self-harm is understood and how a variety of nursing interventions can be used to meet young people's needs.

Terminology, distinctions and definitions

A range of terms are used to describe self-harm: self-injury, parasuicide and attempted suicide. In order to clarify what is meant by self-harm, Kerfoot (2000) uses the following distinctions:

- *Suicide:* those who intentionally kill themselves.
- *Attempted suicide:* those who self harm with the intention of suicide.
- *Parasuicide or self-harm:* those who self harm with little or no intention of killing themselves.

However, it is important to recognise that such definitions are far from straightforward. Categories often overlap, and the suicidal intent of young people may be changeable or unclear. The term self-harm is therefore often used to describe a young person's *behaviour* rather than their *intent*, and nurses and other professionals often use the term 'deliberate self-harm'. This may be misleading since the term 'deliberate' implies premeditation and wilfulness (Pembroke 1994). Indeed, self-harm is atypical, often spontaneous and obviously not preceded by awareness and conscious thought.

National Institute for Clinical Excellence (NICE) publication *Guidelines for the Short Term Physical and Psychological Management of Self-Harm in Primary and Secondary Care* (NICE 2004) has defined the following position which is adopted for use in this chapter:

> *Self harm:* Self-poisoning or injury, irrespective of the apparent purpose of the act.

How common is self-harm?

Rates of self-harm in the UK have increased over the last decade and are amongst the highest in Europe (NICE 2004). As many as 25 000 young people present to general hospitals in England and Wales with problems involving self-harm. Most have taken overdoses or cut themselves (Samaritans & Centre for Social Research 2002). This represents an increase of almost 30% since the 1980s and repetition rates (i.e. young people who harm themselves more than once) have doubled (Hawton et al. 2000). Despite being alarmingly high, these figures are far from representative: of a large survey of young people who self harmed, only 12% attended hospital (Hawton et al. 2002) and it is likely that most self-harm incidents will not reach the attention of services or professionals. Suicide trends over the last ten years have shown a 9% decrease in England and Wales, whilst rates in Scotland, Northern Ireland and the Republic of Ireland have increased by 13%, 27% and 26% respectively (Samaritans 2003). There are also significant differences in suicide rates according to race and cultural background. For example, the rate of suicide for Asian women in England and Wales is three times higher than for women of white British origin (Raleigh & Balarajan 1992). These trends clearly demonstrate the urgent need to find effective ways to help distressed young people.

Why is self-harm common in young people?

Adolescence

Adolescence marks the transition from childhood to adulthood. It is a period when young people experiment, question and try to make sense of physical, emotional and social changes in their lives. Adolescence is a developmental phase during which time a number of significant tasks are usually on the way to being achieved. These include the attainment of independence; the establishment of sexual orientation; the self-control of aggressive and oppositional impulses; and the formation of identity. Peer groups often become more intense and are important in terms of influencing interests and behaviour. The age-range which spans adolescence and the timing of specific developmental changes varies from one young person to the next.

Social context

As well as understanding the significance of self-harm in the context of adolescent development, it is also important to be aware of the social context in which young people harm themselves. For some young people, self-harm may be symptomatic of a serious mental health disorder such as major depression (Pfeffer et al. 1991). For others, it may be the result of experimentation as part of adolescent identity and self-image (Anderson et al. 2004). A significant proportion of young people who self harm experience difficulty in solving problems in non-destructive ways and may struggle with difficult and intolerable feelings (McLaughlin et al. 1996). Such feelings may be generated by current or previous abuse or trauma, or may be linked to problems with family, friends or school. Factors such as unwanted pregnancy, being bullied, parents who argue, abuse, rape and bereavement have all been associated with self-harm (NCH 2002). Self-harm by young people often occurs impulsively and with little thought about consequences. At other times, self-harm may be preceded by varying degrees of planning. It has been suggested that the media is responsible for perpetuating self-harm in young people. Various soap operas, artists and musicians have been criticised for increasing self-harm and suicide in young people.

Whilst these issues may help increase our understanding about why young people self harm, the thought that a child may want to die or harm themselves may be difficult for nurses to cope with. Until 1961 in the UK, and 1993 in the Republic of Ireland, suicide was a criminal offence (Hill 1995). Some of these communities may therefore regard suicide as shameful and treat relatives who have killed themselves accordingly. It is important for nurses to be aware that cultural issues may influence the young person's willingness to seek help.

National policy and guidelines

The Royal College of Psychiatrists (RCP) has produced council reports related to managing deliberate self-harm in young people (RCP 1982; RCP 1998). These reports recommend that young people who self-harm should be admitted to general hospital since the annual rate of repetition is higher for adolescents who are not admitted (Hawton & Fagg 1992). Despite the national guidelines described above, a review of protocols for the management of self-harm by young people revealed that many services fail to implement the recommendations (Dorer 1998). These findings are consistent with the research of Armstrong (1995) who explored the management of young people who self harm. In this study, nine hospital departments and six GP (general practitioner) practices were asked about their referral and treatment guidelines. The study found that only four services had formal guidelines. More recently, NICE guidelines for the management of self-harm have been produced (NICE 2004). Emphasis is placed on short-term intervention within 48 hours. Special consideration has been given to children and young people in terms of guidance in relation to paediatric triage assessment. It remains to be seen how these guidelines impact on the inconsistent and patchy practice that has been described previously.

The prevention of suicide has also been the subject of national guidelines (Health Advisory Service 1994). These guidelines were followed by a national suicide prevention strategy (Department of Health 2002) and an annual progress report (DoH 2003). These reports identify the year following an incident of self-harm as a high-risk time for young people, and include the need to reduce access to significant quantities of medicines and promote the responsible representation of suicidal behaviour by the media. Standard 9 of the National Service Framework (NSF) for Children, Young People and Maternity Services (DoH 2004) also identifies standards for good practice applicable to self-harm. These include mental health promotion, early intervention, partnership working and easy access to local services.

Assessing young people who self harm

National guidance provides nurses with evidence and standards for the assessment of all young people who self harm (Health Advisory Service 1994; RCP 1998; NICE 2004). This can be applied across a range of settings by different professionals who work with young people.

Nurses in primary settings

School nurses and youth workers as well as other primary care professionals come into contact with many young people who self harm (HAS 1995; Hawton et al. 2002). NICE guidelines recommend that primary care workers should assess the urgent physical and mental health needs of young people who have self harmed during the previous 48-hour period (NICE 2004). In the case of self-poisoning, primary care workers should refer the young person to the emergency department and also consider referral for other forms of self-harm such as cutting. Referral of a young person to the emergency department will depend on the severity, intention, and frequency of the cutting. The need to inform parents or carers may need to be discussed with the young person. Sometimes referral to the emergency department is not made as the assessment of risk by the primary worker is low, and their needs can be met more appropriately elsewhere. Where school nurses and other primary workers suspect that a young person is harming themselves, they should consider discussing this with a colleague in a specialist CAMHS team. This may result in a formal consultation and the referral of the young person for a specialist CAMHS assessment.

Nurses in emergency departments

The overarching principles of the NICE guidelines (2004) for emergency departments include the following:

- Professionals should be respectful and understanding.
- Paediatric staff should undertake physical and mental health triage in a specific area for children and young people.
- Young people should normally be admitted to a general paediatric or adolescent hospital ward.
- Once admitted, consideration should be given to making a referral to the specialist child and adolescent mental health service for a comprehensive psychosocial assessment.

Nurses in specialist CAMHS

Specialist CAMHS provides a comprehensive psychosocial risk assessment which involves talking with the young person individually, meeting with the parents or carers and then making a collaborative management plan. Specialist

CAMHS professionals will consult with the paediatric team and, as necessary, social services, education and other agencies. The primary aim of the assessment is to engage the young person and family in a therapeutic process, whilst considering knowledge of risk factors, child protection issues and the needs of the young person. Information about the following factors should be sought:

- Family tree.
- Peers, school and hobbies.
- Other agencies/professionals involved.
- Developmental history.
- Physical health, mental wellbeing and any history of abuse or neglect.
- Alcohol or substance misuse.
- Relationships and support systems.
- History of previous self-harm, including the child's knowledge of others who self-harm.
- Detailed account of presenting episode of self-harm including precipitating factors, intentions, how the child feels now and if they think they are likely to do it again.
- Hopefulness and hopelessness.
- What the young person thinks needs to change to improve their situation.

Standardised risk-assessment tools such as the Beck Depression Inventory and Suicidal Intent Scale are among others reviewed by Steer & Beck (1988), which can be used to aid the clinical assessment and inform risk status. However, risk assessment measures should not be used to justify not offering a service to a person considered to be low risk. Details of the assessment and management plan should be clearly documented in the young person's case notes. With appropriate consent, this plan should be communicated to all professionals and other workers involved in the young person's care, welfare and education. It is now considered good practice to copy such letters to young people and their parents unless there are good defensible reasons why this would not be in their best interests (DoH 2000).

What does the research tell us about young people who self harm?

A major systematic review of the efficacy of psychosocial and pharmacological treatments for the prevention of repetitive self-harm has been reported elsewhere (Hawton 1998). This meta-analysis evaluated a series of 20 randomised controlled trials. However, only one study specifically involved adolescents (Cotgrove et al. 1995). This study assessed the value of readmission to hospital on demand and found that the intervention failed to have a positive effect. Since this systematic review, further studies have been published. A randomised trial of home-based family intervention for young people who had self poisoned did not result in better outcomes than the 'routine care' provided to the control group (Harrington et al. 1998). However, a moderate decrease in suicidal ideation was identified in the subgroup without major depression. In this study the term routine care was used to describe a diverse range of interventions provided in the hospital setting. Harrington et al. (2000) set out to explore why a brief family intervention worked well with some young people and not with others. The follow-up results showed that improvements in the group of young people who were not depressed were not related to changes in family functioning. A nursing service in Glasgow has implemented an adapted version of the home-based intervention model described above (Fyfe & Dale 2002).

A randomised controlled nurse-led trial has reported on the impact of group therapy for adolescents who repeatedly harm themselves (Wood et al. 2001). The results showed no reductions in levels of depression or suicidal thinking but it did report reduced rates of self-harm. However because of the small sample size of this study, confidence intervals were wide, which means that up to 14 young people may need the group intervention before one is prevented from repeating self-harm. This study is currently being repeated with a larger sample through the Assist trial due to report in 2006. Depression and measures of depressive behaviour are often core elements of quantitative research. This is because major depression is a strong predictor of outcome in relation to young people who harm themselves (Pfeffer et al. 1991). Hopelessness has been found to be another significant factor reported by young people who self harm, even after the effects of depression have been taken into account (McLaughlin et al. 1996). This study also identified problem-solving difficulties in young people who harm themselves and suggested that this should be a focus for intervention.

Research on the use of cognitive behavioural therapy (CBT) with young adults has suggested that the intervention is no more effective than routine care in reducing depression, hopelessness and suicidal ideation (Linehan et al. 1991). Dialectic behaviour therapy (DBT) is used to help adults who engage in repetitive self-harm and is associated with helping people who have borderline personality characteristics (Linehan 1993). DBT is designed to help people learn skills to cope with life stresses and to understand and resist their urges to self harm. Some of these skills have now been incorporated into adolescent group work (Wood et al. 2001), which is currently being researched. Impulsiveness also seems to be a key factor. In a follow-up study of 48 young people who had attempted suicide, Keinhorst et al. (1995) suggested that suicidal behaviour in young people was commonly a 'phasic' desire for relief rather than a reasoned and long-standing decision. Hence the importance in follow-up of trying to reduce impulsive behaviour, as delaying self-harm by even half-an-hour may be sufficient to implement an alternative safer strategy and therefore prevent a potential suicide attempt. During this crucial (impulsive) period the reduction of access to tablets through the safe storage of medicines is also known to assist in the prevention of overdoses by young people (Hawton et al. 2004).

What do young people tell us about self-harm?

Various consultation exercises have been undertaken to elicit young people's views about the services they receive. A project for young people aged between 13 and 25 in Leeds sought to understand the factors that make protective services for self-harm effective (Neill 2003). Confidentiality, having choice and being respected were identified as important factors. A further study with young people aged between 15 and 25 looked at their views of self-harm protection (Spandler 1996). A key theme that young people reported was the need for control, both of the self-harm and of the meaning this had for them. Young people explained that when control was taken away from them, this often felt like abuse. This had the paradoxical effect of the young person harming themselves more. A qualitative research study by Le Surf & Lynch (1999) set out to understand the perceptions and attitudes of young people towards counselling. The need for confidentiality as highlighted by Neill (2003) was a consistent theme. This was often associated with stigma and the effects of having counselling, as well as a deeper experience of shamefulness. This implies that young people may often not want others to know they are having counselling for their self-harm.

A summary of the evidence of what works for young people who self harm suggests that a good service should involve:

- Removal of access to means to self-harm such as medication.
- Identifying and treating depression.
- Identifying and responding to hopelessness and impulsivity.
- Strategies to enhance problem-solving.
- Group work.
- Alternative coping strategies.
- Maintaining confidentiality.
- Enabling choice.
- Respect.
- Collaboration rather than control.
- Addressing stigma and shame.

Since problems surrounding self-harm are diverse, it is important that nurses adapt these markers of good practice according to the needs of each young person at any one time.

Child and adolescent mental health nursing

The role and function of mental health nurses has generated much debate. Mental health nursing has gone through a significant period of change in the last 20 years (Jackson & Stevenson 2000). During this period, Schon (1987) observed a move away from a practical, task-orientated role towards reflexive involvement with patients. Michael (1994) suggests that this shift has made it more difficult for nurses to recognise and define their role. This is because working alongside patients means their skills have become less visible. A focus-group study facilitated by Jackson and Stevenson (2000) asked nearly 100 people to explore what people need mental health nurses for. Their results suggested that service users valued nurses who were able to move across domains and dimensions in response to need. The focus groups reported that nurses were experienced by service users as both friend and professional, and wanted them to be intimate and also have professional knowledge. Mental health training requires nurses to spend significant periods of time with patients and fosters closeness and an approach to mental health care that is different from that of other professionals, such as psychiatrists (Baldwin 2002).

The role of nurses in child and adolescent mental health services (CAMHS) is no better defined in the literature. This is despite concern that such a lack of clarity may lead to the loss of the role (McMorrow 1995). The unique contribution that nurses make remains undefined but implicitly accepted. Indeed, they are considered to be core members of the CAMHS multidisciplinary team (HAS 1995). Nurses in CAMHS play a holistic role. This means they see the young person as a whole person and recognise that the child's and the family's needs may be broad and varied. This insight is enabled by the nurse's well-developed communication skills and their ability to engage with the young person and their family.

So how does this translate into nursing young people who self harm? The following case vignettes are used to illustrate how self-harm can be imbued with a range of meanings. Each vignette focuses on different nursing interventions that are used to help young people and their families or carers. It is intended that these descriptions of practice go some way to depict part of the essence of child and adolescent mental health nursing.

Ann

Ann, aged 15, is a dual heritage white/black Caribbean British girl who has taken an overdose of 28 paracetamol tablets. Ann was assessed by a CAMHS self-harm nurse on a general paediatric ward in accordance with national and local guidelines. The overdose had been precipitated by a recent disclosure of sexual abuse and a family bereavement. Ann reported that she had been feeling down for a couple of weeks and explained that she felt she did not have much to live for.

Nursing is in part about *being* with a person. A fundamental component of all interventions with young people is to establish a good therapeutic relationship. In order to understand Ann's self-harming behaviour the nurse sought first to understand what it was like to be Ann. The nurse aimed to make Ann feel at ease by listening to her thoughts and feelings and encouraged her to share her distress and fears. The better the knowledge about a young person, the better the risk assessment. Prior to asking detailed questions about self-harm, the nurse collected some background information about family and friends, school and other professionals who were involved. A brief assessment of mood and mental state were also undertaken. In order to understand Ann's self-harming behaviour, a series of questions were used to explore the overdose incident, assess risk and inform the intervention strategy:

- How much medication was accessible/available/taken?
- Were drugs or alcohol involved? If so, which drugs or alcohol and how much?
- Was the overdose planned or impulsive?
- Was the overdose taken whilst the young person was alone? If not, who was present?
- How much does the young person know about the lethality/harmful effects of the overdose?
- Was a suicide note written?
- Did the young person tell anyone before or after the overdose?
- Is the young person regretful or disappointed to be alive?
- Would the young person be likely to take another overdose?
- Is the young person actively planning to take another overdose?
- How hopeful/hopeless does the young person feel about the future?

Involving the parents or carers of young people who self harm

Parents often have a different understanding than their child about why the self-harm has occurred. Ann's mother strongly believed that her daughter's disclosure of sexual abuse explained the self-harm. Ann herself thought that recent changes in family relationships were more significant. The disclosure of sexual abuse can generate many strong emotions in parents such as anger, guilt and shame (Jones 2003). After meeting her, the nurse became aware that Ann's mother also needed support and arranged this with a local voluntary organisation. Ann was clear that she wanted her session work to remain confidential. Whilst she did not want anyone at school to know about her overdose, Ann gave permission for the nurse to inform the GP about the overdose and ongoing support she was receiving. Ann accepted that her mother had a duty to ensure she was safe. The nurse explained to Ann's mother that most overdoses by young people are impulsive, and therefore the importance of safe storage of medicines was discussed.

The importance of follow-up

By asking Ann a series of questions about her intentions and thoughts and feelings before, during and after the overdose it is possible to form an opinion about risk. After interviewing Ann, the nurse assessed the risk of further self-harm as medium and the risk of suicide low. One of the outcome aims of the assessment was to enable Ann to feel more hopeful about the future than she was at the time of the overdose. During the interview it became apparent that Ann had high expectations of herself and rarely allowed herself to feel sad, upset or angry. Giving a young person permission to cry and acknowledging their feelings in a safe, supportive environment can be both validating and liberating for them. All young people who self harm should be given at least one follow-up appointment. Ann has fortnightly sessions to discuss her thoughts, feelings and fears and has not harmed herself further.

Sally

Sally, aged 16, is a white British girl who took five Temazepam tablets in order 'to sleep a prolonged period'. She had no intention of killing herself. Sally has a two-year history of cutting her arms and legs, and described feeling unloved by her family who have multiple social problems. Her attendance at school was poor and Sally left school with no qualifications. After briefly attending college, Sally dropped out and was told to leave the family home. At this time she began to get regularly drunk and engage in petty crime. The police and Youth Offending Team became involved.

When Sally was assessed by the nurse specialist it became apparent that many of Sally's peer group were involved in self-harming behaviour. She had previously cut herself at the same time as her friends and believed them to be supportive and understanding of how she felt. This was in contrast to some of the adults and professionals who Sally had encountered, and who had disapproved of her cutting. One of the biggest challenges faced by young people who self harm is the stigma and negative attitudes they can encounter. This is addressed in the NICE guidelines on self-harm which state that people who self harm should be treated with the same care, respect and privacy as any patient, whilst taking into account the likelihood of their additional distress (NICE 2004).

Reducing self-harm through alternative coping strategies

After the nurse had completed an initial assessment of mental state and risk, Sally reported that she wanted help to stop cutting herself. Cutting can be compared to other behaviours such as smoking, eating or exercising in that a person has to want to change their behaviour or they will continue as before. Even if a young person wants to change their self-harming behaviour it is important to remember that this may be difficult for them. Cutting has developed as a coping strategy and as such young people will need to identify a different coping strategy to replace this. In the meantime, young people are likely to continue to self harm and the nurse should enable them to feel more accepted, less judged and better understood. Sally and the nurse met again on several sessions. This was to help Sally to understand the situations and triggers that precipitated the cutting. Sally used a diary to help her remember the circumstances that had led her to cut. This assisted the nurse in recognising the patterns and identifiable triggers for this self-harm.

Working as part of a specialist CAMHS team, nurses can bring and access a wealth of experience and knowledge about young people who self harm. Whilst maintaining confidentiality, this breadth of experience can often be shared to benefit young people who self harm. Sally appeared to gain hope and confidence from knowing that other young people had been able to reduce or stop cutting. This was a belief that was shared by Sally and the nurse throughout her sessions. As well as identifying risk situations that appeared to trigger cutting, a range of alternative coping strategies were discussed and explored by Sally. These included distraction techniques, ventilating emotions and the use of alternative or safer pain, which are methods described as helpful by people who self harm (Crisis Recovery Unit 1998). Sally decided to combine several components of these strategies which involved leaving the house, having a freezing shower and blasting her music when faced with a situation which made her want to cut. Some young people report that snapping an elastic band on the wrist, tightly holding ice cubes and snapping wood are ways of inflicting pain or discomfort on themselves. Some young people also draw on themselves with a red marker pen or use ketchup or red food colouring to replicate self-harm in a way that is less destructive and permanent than cutting.

Whilst Sally was being supported to use alternative coping strategies the cutting continued but became less frequent. As recommended by the NICE guidance on self-harm, the nurse provided advice about harm minimisation. Sally was encouraged to replace cutting with broken glass with a sterile blade to reduce the risk of infection and scarring. Education about first aid was provided and the need to have access to clean wound care supplies was recommended. During the course of treatment it became apparent that the social and family factors that made Sally feel sad were unlikely to change. The focus of therapeutic sessions was to enable Sally to identify a positive future and support her in achieving independence. The nurse supported Sally in making a housing application, made links with an organisation called Connexions in order for her to return to college and arranged transport for appointments. Noticing positive changes and rewarding these with praise and encouragement made notable differences to Sally's self-esteem.

Jackie

Jackie, aged 13, is a black British Caribbean girl. Although this is her first admission to hospital after an overdose of codeine, the assessment reveals that Jackie has taken several small overdoses and has cut herself on numerous occasions. Jackie is unclear about why she took the 6 tablets. She reports feeling unhappy, hates herself and does not want to live any more. Jackie feels that life is a struggle but cannot think of any particular reason why. Jackie describes a need to punish herself and reports that self-harm helps her release tension. She does not like being at home or school and has recently begun to truant. Jackie is offered individual sessions to explore the reasons why she is unhappy and self harming. It soon becomes apparent that there are family relationship problems and that Jackie often gets angry, refuses to talk or runs away for short periods.

In terms of adolescent development, it is important to remember that adolescents often do not have a breadth of life experience to draw on. Their personalities are developing and they are not able to put things into perspective in the way adults might be able to do. Jackie, like many young people her age, was struggling with the developmental task of controlling her emotions and constructing her self-identity (Hoare 1993; Anderson et al. 2004).

Family therapy

Although Jackie did not initially want her parents involved in her care, the nurse enabled her to recognise that their involvement was crucial to therapeutic change. Had Jackie, at age 13, continued to refuse to share her self-harm with her parents, the nurse would still have had a child-protection responsibility to inform her parents. However, Jackie had a choice about whether to engage in family therapy and her consent was required. Working with young people in a collaborative way is a key function of the nurse. This involves supporting them in decision-making and in planning and evaluating the care programme. Inevitably there are different views about the usefulness of family therapy between the young person, their parents and the nurse. This was addressed in this case by explaining the process in advance, visiting the room in which family therapy would take place and talking about the one-way screen and observation suite.

In the first session Jackie said nothing at all. However she heard other family members say things she had never heard before and managed to stay in the room. As the sessions progressed, family members developed a growing understanding of each other. Where rigid beliefs had become entrenched, these were replaced with new meanings and explanations. Jackie's 'bad' behaviour, previously met with hostility and criticism, became understood as a sign of distress and was met with care and compassion. One positive change led to another and as well as a general improvement in family relationships, Jackie's self-esteem and confidence increased. The issue of self-harm did not often feature during the family therapy. Instead, the focus was on improving relationships and enhancing communication.

Ben

Ben, aged 14, is a white British boy who took a serious overdose of 80 paracetamol tablets with the clear intention of dying. The overdose was discovered when Ben was heard vomiting by his younger brother. It was two weeks before he was medically fit to be assessed by the nurse specialist from the CAMHS self-harm team. This was because the possibility of a liver transplant was being discussed by the paediatric team. When Ben recovered sufficiently, his story was clear. He was intimidated by a local gang and feared for his life. Ben made a decision to kill himself before the bullies killed him. Ben's family were distraught, but shared Ben's fears as their house had been vandalised and a window had recently been smashed.

Therapeutic relationships

Fear often features in young people's accounts of their self-harming behaviour. This can be generated by a number of factors including bullying, exam stress or pregnancy. Of fundamental importance for Ben, the nurse needed to help create a plan where Ben felt safe, protected and supported. In order to help him feel safe, Ben was initially encouraged to bring one of his parents to the sessions. After just a few sessions he felt more relaxed and reassured that the nurse understood his fears and was there to help him.

Part of establishing a therapeutic relationship involves decisions about how much self-disclosure by the nurse is appropriate. Ben asked the nurse whether she had children and if they had been bullied. In keeping with the theory of practice where nurses move across domains of intimate friend and knowledgeable professional (Jackson & Stevenson 2000), the sharing of personal information can sometimes be appropriate and helpful. Initially Ben did not feel safe to leave his house. Sessions with the nurse took place in the family home. Flexibility about where to see young people can increase their control and responsibility and is an important part of the collaborative therapeutic process. After initially meeting at Ben's house, his confidence improved and he utilised and valued the support of his family and friends. Ben became more socially included and joined clubs outside of his immediate neighbourhood. In time, Ben was able to reflect on his overdose and felt confident that he could keep himself safe when faced with difficult situations.

The importance of clinical supervision

Clinical supervision is essential for the provision of safe and accountable nursing practice and the governance of CAMHS. It is important that nurses who work with young people who self harm have regular clinical supervision. This is to ensure their practice is safe and effective, and so that the nurse remains up-to-date and professionally accountable for their work. Supervision can take many forms and can take place across a range of settings. Nurses can receive supervision individually, in groups and from nurses or other colleagues with understanding of the key issues in relation to young people and self-harm. Ben's nurse discussed his case with the specialist multidisciplinary team. This provided evidence-based reflection on practice, helped to develop a case management plan and supported the nurse in the individual work he was doing with Ben.

Conclusion

This chapter has described and illustrated that self-harm by young people is increasing. The case studies have illustrated that self-harm is heterogeneous and means different things to different people. An overview of national strategy in relation to the assessment and management of self-harm was discussed, and a range of interventions by nurses to support young people, their families or carers were described. The chapter has aimed to capture some of the essence of nursing care which is notoriously difficult to articulate. Theoretical concepts such as caring and understanding were defined in terms of practical interventions and psychological approaches that nurses can undertake in order to engage, help and support young people who self-harm. Of fundamental importance has been the message that to help any young person who self-harms, the nurse must understand, communicate this understanding and create a therapeutic alliance which is the bedrock for change. A range of nursing skills such as the ability to listen, be accepting and appropriately use self-disclosure were identified as crucial in terms of helping young people who self harm.

References

Anderson, M., Woodward, L. & Armstrong, M. (2004). Self-harm in young people: a perspective for mental health nursing. *International Nursing Review*, (51), 222–28.

Armstrong, M. (1995). *The Management of Self-harm in Children and Adolescents* (Unpublished thesis). Lancaster: University of Lancaster.

Armstrong, M. (2002). *Self-harm Management Guidelines for Children and Adolescents*. Nottingham: Nottinghamshire Health Care Trust.

Baldwin, L. (2002). The nursing role in out-patient child and adolescent mental health services. *Journal of Clinical Nursing*, **11**, 520–25.

Brock, A. & Griffiths, C. (2003). Trends in the mortality of young adults aged 15–44 in England and Wales 1961 to 2001. *Health Statistics Quarterly*, (19), 22–31.

Cotgrove, A., Zirinsky, L., Black, D. & Weston, D. (1995). Secondary prevention of attempted suicide in adolescents. *Journal of Adolescence*, **18**, 569–77.

Crisis Recovery Unit (1998). *Working with the Work: our approach to working with individuals who self-harm, based on our experience*. London: (CRU – unpublished).

Department of Health (2000). *The NHS Plan: a plan for investment, a plan for reform*. London: HMSO.

Department of Health (2002). *National Suicide Prevention Strategy for England*. London: HMSO.

Department of Health (2003). *National Suicide Prevention Strategy for England: annual report on progress*. London: HMSO.

Fyfe, M. & Dale, M. (2002). Hope in the city. *Mental Health Practice*, **5** (6), 18–21.

Harrington, R., Kerfoot, M., Dyer, R., McNiven, F., Gill, J., Harrington, V., Woodham, A. & Byford, S. (1998). Randomised trial of home-based family intervention for children who have deliberately poisoned themselves. *Journal of American Academy of Child and Adolescent Psychiatry*, **37** (5), 512–18.

Hawton, K. (1998). Deliberate self-harm: systematic review of efficacy of psychosocial and pharmacological treatments in preventing repetition. *British Medical Journal*, Aug 15. Online http://www.findarticles.com (14/01/02).

Hawton, K. & Fagg, J. (1992). Deliberate self-poisoning and injury in adolescents: a study of characteristics and trends in Oxford 1976–1989. *British Journal of Psychiatry*, **161**, 816–23.

Hawton, K., Fagg, J., Simkin, S., Bale, E. & Bond, A. (2000). Deliberate self-harm in adolescents in Oxford: 1985–1995. *Journal of Adolescence*, **23**, 47–55.

Hawton, K., Rodham, K., Evans, E. & Weatherall, R. (2002). Deliberate self-harm in adolescents: self report survey in schools in England. *British Medical Journal*, **325**, 1207–11.

Hawton, K., Simkin, S., Deeks, J., Cooper, J., Johnston, A., Waters, K., Arundel, M., Bernal, W., Gunson, B., Hudson, M., Suri, D. & Simpson, K. (2004). UK Legislation on analgesic packs; before and after study of long-term effect on poisonings. *British Medical Journal*. Published 29th October, downloaded from bmj.com, 1–5.

Health Advisory Service (1994). *The Challenge Confronted: suicide prevention.* London: HMSO.

Hill, K. (1995). *The Long Sleep: young people and suicide.* London: Virago.

Hoare, P. (1993). *Essential Child Psychiatry.* New York: Churchill Livingstone.

Jackson, S. & Stevenson, C. (2000). What do people need psychiatric and mental health nurses for? *Journal of Advanced Nursing*, **31** (2), 378–88.

Jones, D. (2003). *Communicating with Vulnerable Children: a guide for practitioners.* London: Gaskell.

Kerfoot, M. (2000). Youth suicide and deliberate self-harm. In: Aggleton, P., Hurry, J. & Warwick, I. (Eds). *Young People and Mental Health.* Chichester. John Wiley.

Kienhorst, I.C.W.M., De Wilde, E.J., Diekstra, R.F.W. & Wolters, W.H.G. (1995). Adolescents' image of their suicide attempt. *Journal of the American Academy of Child and Adolescent Psychiatry*, **34**, 623–28.

Le Surf, A. & Lynch, G. (1999). Exploring young people's perceptions relevant to counselling: a qualitative study. *British Journal of Guidance and Counselling*, **27** (2), 231–43.

Linehan, M. (1993). *Cognitive-Behavioural Treatment of Borderline Personality Disorder.* New York: Guilford.

Linehan, M., Armstrong, H., Suarez, A., Allmon, D. & Heard, H. (1991). Cognitive behavioural treatment of chronically parasuicidal borderline patients. *Archives of General Psychiatry*, (48), 1060–64.

McLaughlin, J., Miller, P. & Warwick, H. (1996). Deliberate self-harm in adolescents: hopelessness, depression, problems and problem-solving. *Journal of Adolescence*, (19), 523–32.

McMorrow, R. (1995). An eclectic model of care: the role of the community psychiatric nurse in child psychiatry. *Child Health*, **3** (3), 95–98.

Michael, S. (1994). Invisible skills. *Journal of Psychiatry and Mental Health Nursing*, **1** (5), 56.

National Children's Home (2002). *Look Beyond the Scars: understanding and responding to self-harm.* London: NCH.

NHS Health Advisory Service (1995). *Child and Adolescent Mental Health Services: together we stand.* London: HMSO.

National Institute for Clinical Excellence (2004). *Guidelines for the Short-Term Physical and Psychological Management of Self-Harm in Primary and Secondary Care.* London: NICE.

Neill, L. (2003). Market forces: listening to what young people want. *YoungMinds Magazine*, (62), 20–22.

Pembroke, L.R. (1994). Self-harm: perspectives from personal experience. *Survivors Speak Out.* October.

Pfeffer, C., Klerman, G., Hunt, S., Lesser, M., Peskin, J. & Siefker, A. (1991). Suicidal children grown up: demographic and clinical risk factors for adolescent suicide attempts. *Journal of the American Academy of Child Psychiatry*, **30**, 609–16.

Raleigh, V. & Balajaran, R. (1992). Suicide and self-burning among Indians and West Indians in England and Wales. *British Journal of Psychiatry*, **129**, 365–68.

Royal College of Psychiatrists (1982). The management of parasuicide in young people under sixteen. *Psychiatric Bulletin*, **6**, 182–85.

Royal College of Psychiatrists (1998). *Managing deliberate self-harm in young people*. London. Council Report CR64.

Samaritans (2003). Suicide in the United Kingdom and the Republic of Ireland. http://www.samaritans.org/know/suicide_stats.shtm

Samaritans & The Centre for Social Research (2002). *Youth and Self Harm: perspectives*. Oxford University Press.

Schon, D. (1987). *Educating the Reflexive Practitioner*. San Fransisco: Jossey-Bass.

Spandler, H. (1996). *Who's Hurting Who?: young people, self harm and suicide*. Manchester: 42nd Street (unpublished).

Wood, A., Trainor, G., Rothwell, J., Moore, A. & Harrington, R. (2001). Randomised trial of group therapy for repeated deliberate self harm in adolescents. *Journal of American Academy of Child and Adolescent Psychiatry*, **40** (11), 1246–53.

Chapter 5

Nursing Children and Young People with Emotional Disorders

Sharon Leighton

Key points

- Depression has been identified as the leading cause of disability amongst 15–44 year-olds worldwide.

- Anxiety disorders are the most prevalent disorders reported for children in the general population.

- Coexisting problems within the family and with peers increase the risk of depression substantially as the child may view all relationships as unsupportive.

- Nurses should obtain a comprehensive history from several sources, using different methods and reliable diagnostic criteria.

- Formal studies of treatment for emotional disorders in children are in their infancy, with the majority occurring within the research community.

- Further research is required to explore the links between anxiety, depression and suicide and a greater understanding of adolescent suicide is needed.

Introduction

This chapter provides a brief overview of the enormous body of knowledge concerning emotional disorders in children and adolescents. This is an area in which intense scholarship continues in order to address what has become an immense social problem. The chapter focuses on defining the various emotional disorders, identifying risk and protective factors and exploring issues around assessment, treatment and prevention from the perspective of nurses working in a range of child and adolescent mental health services (CAMHS). Core knowledge and skills will be identified. Case studies and a reflective exercise are provided to link theory with practice. All will be placed within the current political and social context.

The word children is used to denote both children and adolescents unless it is deemed necessary to use both terms. Current diagnostic classification schemes include the DSM-IV (American Psychiatric Association 1994) and ICD-10 (World Health Organization 1996), but in order to avoid complicating the issue, reference is made to the former diagnostic classification system. Key texts for further reading and internet resources are listed at the end of the chapter.

The current context

The emotional disorders of childhood have generated much research in recent decades. This was preceded by a long period when cursory attention was paid to the subject and debates were held about whether such disorders actually existed. However, the study of historical evidence demonstrates that these disorders have been in existence for centuries. Recent studies have highlighted risk and protective factors, developmental differences, age-specific factors and uncertainty in relation to continuities throughout life (Parry-Jones 2001; Treffers & Silverman 2001).

Psychosocial problems amongst children in Western society have increased considerably in recent decades. Some of the main factors that have been found to have contributed to the problem include the breakdown of traditional communities, changes in family structure and expanding inequalities in income (Davidson & Manion 1996; Adelman et al. 1997; Mental Health Foundation 1999). In the UK there are approximately 12 million children of whom at least 20% are reported to be experiencing mental health problems at any given time. Despite the scale of the problem, epidemiological studies indicate that less than one-fifth of the children who need mental health services actually receive them. Of the one in five children and young people who will have a mental health problem, 4% will have an emotional disorder (Mental Health Foundation 1999; Meltzer et al. 2000; Green et al. 2005). Such problems have a negative impact on a child's physical, emotional, social and cognitive development (Mental Health Foundation 1999; Meltzer et al. 2000; Department of Health 2005). Suicide rates have also increased among young people, especially in young males, and a link has been suggested between the increase in emotional disorders amongst young people and the increased rate of suicide. (Flisher 1999; Hawton et al. 1999). Additionally, tremendous emotional, social and financial costs to families and society are incurred (Appleton & Hammond-Rowley 2000; de Wilde et al. 2001).

With some clinicians there exists an erroneous belief that children do not experience anxiety or depression. Symptoms such as irritability are sometimes misunderstood as difficult behaviour and the psychological basis of some somatic problems is not fully explored. This creates professional uncertainty about what to do with depressed children and young people (Department for Education and Skills 2001). There are clearly serious implications if the emotional disorders of children remain undetected and untreated. However, there are many obstacles that hinder service development that need acknowledging.

First, stigma still pervades issues associated with mental health, with negative and critical beliefs rife. Failure to address and challenge stigmatising views amongst children has serious implications for the mental health of society's youth (Richardson & Partridge 2003). Second, spending in the UK on mental health services in general is low in comparison with other medical services. Historically CAMHS have been under-funded and under-resourced, with a huge variation in service configuration and activity, service provision by different agencies is disjointed and input at Tier 1 limited (Health Advisory Service 1995; Mental Health Foundation 1999). Whether recent investment in CAMHS and plans outlined in the Children's National Service Framework (NSF) (DoH 2004) have a positive impact on funding, resources and structure remains to be seen.

All professionals working with children and their families require an understanding of the assessment, detection, treatment and management of mental health problems in children (DoH 2004). Nurses work across a range of settings and across the tiers in CAMHS (HAS 1995); they are involved in all of the above activities to varying degrees and are therefore in a position to influence the service children and young people receive. Guidance for reform of the children's workforce highlights staff training issues and the need for the development and acquisition of a common core of skills and knowledge (DfES 2003; DoH 2004), all of which are pertinent when addressing the issue of emotional disorders in children. Ideally, child and adolescent mental health training for nurses should include preregistration training programmes, post-registration programmes for those working at Tier 1 such as health visitors and school nurses, and specialist training opportunities for nurses working in paediatric settings and in specialist CAMHS (Royal College of Nursing 2004).

Emotional Disorders

Emotional disorders consist of both mood disorders and anxiety disorders. These encompass a variety of diagnoses and refer to conditions where disordered emotion is a central feature (American Psychiatric Association 1994; Kovacs & Devlin 1998). There is increasing evidence that emotional disorders often start in childhood, that they are recurrent and that they carry an increasing risk of lifelong disability or suicide (Kovacs & Devlin 1998; Flisher 1999; Hawton et al. 1999; Costello et al. 2002).

Mood disorders

The DSM-IV classifies mood disorders as consisting of three categories of depressive disorder (major, dysthymic and atypical); and bipolar disorder (involving episodes of both mania and depression). Diagnosis can be assigned regardless of age (American Psychiatric Association 1994).

Depression

Depression has been identified as the leading cause of disability amongst 15–44 year-olds worldwide (WHO 1996). Evidence suggests that though childhood depression is rare (about 1% of total population), it carries a high risk for recurrence during adolescence and adulthood (Angold & Costello 2001; Costello et al. 2002). The prevalence of depression in post-pubertal adolescents is about 3%, with females twice as likely as males to be affected (2% and 1% respectively). Prior to puberty there appears to be no age-by-gender difference (Angold & Costello, 2001; Costello et al. 2002).

Feelings of sadness of varying intensity and duration are a normal part of life for most children. However, clinical depression is characterised by unpleasant mood and feelings, thoughts and behavioural and physical changes. Depressed mood (dysphoria) is pervasive, persistent and severe enough to disrupt daily functioning, with pleasure derived from life significantly reduced. An irritable rather than depressed mood can sometimes dominate (American Psychiatric Association 1994). Thoughts may be negative and self-critical, and hopelessness and helplessness pervade. Concentration is often impaired, attention span reduced and decisions may be difficult to make. In addition, suicidal ideation may be present (Asarnow et al. 2001; Kolvin & Sadowski 2001). Behavioural and physical changes include physical slowing down (psychomotor retardation) or agitation; sleep disturbances; significant appetite and weight changes; and loss of energy and social withdrawal (Asarnow et al. 2001; Kolvin & Sadowski 2001). The clinical features of depression vary according to the age and developmental level of the child. Adolescent depression most closely resembles adult depression, and distress and negative emotions can manifest behaviourally. In younger children, somatic symptoms such as aches and pains are more common (Kolvin & Sadowski 2001).

Bipolar Disorder

Bipolar disorder is an intermittent, potentially lifelong and damaging disorder characterised by mood swings that cycle between depression and mania (or its more common and milder variant, hypomania). Hypomanic episodes include elation, pressure of speech, irritability and disinhibited behaviour. Delusions and, more rarely, hallucinations may occur (Graham 1991). Bipolar disorder is thought to result from the effects of abnormal neurological activity in the brain on mood, thinking and behaviour (von Hahn 2004). Estimates regarding prevalence remain unclear due to variations in definitions used and controversy over differences in clinical presentation between childhood and adult bipolar disorder (Costello et al. 2002; von Hahn 2004). It has been suggested that although bipolar disorder is uncommon in children and adolescents, its prevalence is actually as widespread as in the adult population (von Hahn 2004). Available data suggest that bipolar disorder in adolescents follows the remitting–relapsing course seen in adults. Childhood bipolar disorder appears to be a more chronic condition, presenting with major depression and without the relapse–remission seen in adults (Harrington & Dubicka 2001; von Hahn 2004). It is often difficult to diagnose bipolar disorder in very young children. Preschool children may present with prolonged states of emotional arousal that occur with minimal stimulation. Explosive and unmanageable temper tantrums, hypersexuality and grandiosity can also occur during childhood (von Hahn 2004). Other psychiatric conditions such ADHD (attention deficit hyperactivity disorder), conduct disorder and some medical and neurological disorders can mimic bipolar disorder and contribute to difficulties in diagnosis (von Hahn 2004).

Anxiety disorders

Although anxiety is the most common mental disorder of childhood (Coghill 2003), it is a normal human response to the perception of danger. Anxiety presents differently in childhood as compared to adulthood. Different types of anxiety will be experienced normally by children as they attempt to accomplish developmental tasks. For example, separation is an issue for infants, academic performance can cause anxiety during middle childhood and peer rejection is a source of fear for adolescents (Moore & Carr 2000; Stock et al. 2001).

The DSM-IV identifies several anxiety disorders. One of these is separation anxiety, which typically presents in childhood and affects approximately 0.9% of boys and 0.7% of girls (Meltzer et al. 2000). The other anxiety disorders can be assigned irrespective of age and include: phobias (subdivided into specific, social and agoraphobia); generalised anxiety disorder; post-traumatic stress disorder (PTSD); and obsessive compulsive disorder (OCD) (American Psychiatric Association 1994). Anxiety disorders, at 6–10%, are the most prevalent disorders reported for children in the general population. The figure for those adversely affected in daily life by their symptoms is about 2% (Verhulst 2001). Anxiety disorders are more prevalent in girls and in older children (Verhulst, 2001). The clinical features of anxiety disorders include feelings of uneasiness and apprehension. A range of physiological symptoms such as palpitations, breathlessness, dizziness, sweating and nausea are symptomatic. Associated difficulties include: concentration impairment; impulsive and aggressive behaviour; social withdrawal; and isolation (Moore & Carr 2000; Stock et al. 2001).

How do anxiety disorders differ?

The following distinctions illustrate some of the differences between anxiety disorders:

- *Separation anxiety*: is characterised by inappropriate and excessive anxiety when separated from caretakers.
- *Phobic anxiety*: is the experience of intense fear when confronted with an object, event or situation, which is out of proportion to the danger posed

by the stimulus leading to repeated avoidance. Specific phobias include those associated with animals, the natural environment and particular situations. Social phobia is the fear of being evaluated negatively by others. Agoraphobia is an intense fear of being in public spaces where one fears escape will not be possible.

- *Generalised anxiety disorder*: is characterised by an ongoing dread that the world is unsafe and disaster is imminent.
- *Panic disorder*: is more likely to start in late adolescence than in childhood (Biederman et al. 1997) and involves recurrent unexpected panic attacks, which are experienced as acute and distressing episodes of intense anxiety lasting a few minutes or longer.
- *Post traumatic stress disorder (PTSD)*: occurs in many children and adolescents following a catastrophic trauma, which the child perceived as life threatening. Symptoms of PTSD vary according to the nature of the trauma, but increased anxiety, intrusive or recurring thoughts, visual flashbacks and avoidant behaviour are common hallmarks.
- *Obsessive compulsive disorder (OCD)*: is typically characterised by distressing obsessive thoughts and compulsive rituals, which reduce the anxiety associated with the obsessions. Whilst adults often recognise that their obsessions or compulsions are irrational, children may not possess the cognitive abilities to reach this judgement. OCD has been reported to occur in abut 2% of adolescents and onset of symptoms is earlier in boys than in girls (Meltzer et al. 2000).

Comorbidity

Comorbidity with depression and other disorders, especially anxiety disorders, ADHD and conduct disorders is high (Angold & Costello 2001; Brooks-Gunn et al. 2001; Fonseca & Perrin 2001; Kolvin & Sadowski 2001; Verhulst 2001). Additionally, anxiety often precedes depression (Brooks-Gunn et al. 2001; Kolvin & Sadowski 2001). The high levels of comorbidity between anxiety and depression have led to the hypothesis that they may be considered part of a wider construct of emotional distress rather than two distinct disorders (Kolvin & Sadowski 2001; Verhulst 2001). Comorbid anxiety and depression increase the severity and duration of a depressive disorder, leading to an increase in suicidal behaviour and psychosocial problems (Kolvin & Sadowski 2001). Despite these high rates of cormorbidity, little is known about the relationship between anxiety and suicidal behaviour (de Wilde et al. 2001). While there is insufficient evidence to explain the pathways between depression and suicide, a range of psychosocial factors are thought to be influential. These include: life stresses; cognitive distortions; a sense of hopelessness; an inability to tolerate negative emotions; and impulsivity. All have been associated with suicide in depressed children (Kolvin & Sadowski 2001). Increased rates of suicide are also seen in children with untreated bipolar disorder (von Hahn 2004).

Risk and protective factors

Risk factors

Risk factors can be divided into environmental and individual risks. However, although their mode of interaction remains unclear, risk factors rarely act in isolation (Goodyer 2001; Manic Depression Fellowship 2003). A previous episode of depression or anxiety disorder is a risk factor for further episodes of the same general type of disorder (Kolvin & Sadowski 2001). There is increasing evidence that the pattern and degree of risk varies with development, severity and number of illness episodes. Reasons for this are thought to include neurobiological changes that occur in the brain (Goodyer 2001; Harrington & Dubicka 2001; Le Doux 2003).

Environmental risk

Social adversity, high life stress, family problems, abuse, physical illness and poor academic achievement are generally associated with childhood psychopathology (Angold & Costello 2001). Specific high risks for depression include: parental marital difficulties; emotional difficulties between the child and a parent; child abuse; severe acute events within the family such as sudden death; and friendship difficulties (Goodyer 2001). Parental mental illness, especially depression is also a high risk factor (Beardslee et al. 2003). Coexisting problems within the family and with peers increase the risk substantially as the child may view all relationships as unsupportive (Goodyer 2001). Insecure attachment relationships and high levels of parental anxiety are associated with increased risk of anxiety disorders in children (Manassis 2001; Prins 2001). Stressful life events and relationship difficulties have been identified as risk factors in bipolar disorder (Manic Depression Fellowship 2003).

Individual risks

Low self-esteem and depressive cognitions are viewed as general risk factors (Angold & Costello 2001). Specific temperamental traits represent a risk for the development of symptoms of anxiety and depression in children. High levels of factors that reflect negative affectivity (the degree of dissatisfaction with life and associated feelings of distress) appear to place children at risk for both anxiety and depression. Low levels of factors associated with positive affectivity (the level of pleasurable engagement in life and the extent to which the individual feels enthusiastic and involved) appear to represent a specific risk for the development of depressive symptoms (Lonigan et al. 2003). The temperamental trait of behavioural inhibition (reluctance in new situations) is linked to mood and anxiety disorder (Oosterlaan 2001; Lonigan et al. 2003). Cognitive distortions such as negative self-evaluation (self-criticism) and a ruminating thinking style (dwelling on situations) are risk factors for depression and anxiety in children (Alloy & Abraamson 1999; Manassis 2001; Prins 2001; Muris et al. 2003). Biological factors including genetic and brain-chemistry imbalances, and medical disorders, can increase the risk of bipolar disorder (Manic Depression Fellowship 2003). Emotional disorders in children and young people with learning disabilities are often overlooked (Royal College of Psychiatrists 2004). This is because they are often masked by behavioural problems or missed by clinicians who do not possess the specialist skills required to assess mood and anxiety disorders in this population of young people.

Protective factors

Protective factors against the development of psychopathology in children include higher intelligence, an easy temperament, secure family attachments, positive school experiences and strong interests and attachments to adults outside of the family (Rutter 1999). Protective factors against depression specifically include a secure attachment relationship with one or both parents, good non-deviant friendships, and a strong relationship with a sibling (Goodyer 2001). Social support and individual coping skills can provide protection for those at risk for anxiety disorders (Donovan & Spence 2000). Higher intelligence and good premorbid functioning are identified as protective factors for children with bipolar disorder (Fonagy et al. 2002).

Nursing assessment

The nurse's professional expertise will influence the quality of the assessment (Benner 1984). A nurse working in a specialist CAMHS would be expected to complete a more thorough, holistic assessment and planned treatment programme, than a school nurse with limited mental health experience working in a primary setting. Nevertheless, with appropriate training, non-specialist nurses can become skilled in early and accurate identification of emotional disorders and suicidal risk (Horowitz et al. 2001). Nurses who are assessing children and young people for emotional disorders should have a good knowledge of child and adolescent development, paediatric emotional disorders, and risk and protective factors for mental health problems in general. This is in addition to understanding cultural issues and legal and ethical issues (Graham 1991; Hoghughi 1992). A comprehensive nursing assessment should aim to obtain the following information about the young person and their presenting problems and needs:

- Identification of the problems including duration, intensity and frequency.
- The effects on everyday life and functioning.
- Identification of any intrinsic, family and environmental factors which trigger and maintain the problem.

- Analysis of the relationship between different variables.
- Identification of specific risk factors.
- Assessment of the child and family's capacity to participate in treatment.
- Establishment of a therapeutic relationship with the child and their family or carers.

Nurses should be aware of the different assessment methods that are available and how to use them (Scahill & Ort 1995). Core skills include good communication and negotiation skills, active listening skills and the ability to identify barriers to change, such as maternal depression or difficulties with motivation (Herbert 1991). Specific skills include an ability to undertake assessment for risk of suicide (de Wilde et al. 2001) and identifying comorbidity (Stock et al. 2001).

A comprehensive history should be obtained from several sources. Depending on issues of age and consent this should include the child, their parents and siblings and teachers. Children are often wary of answering questions about their thoughts and feelings in front of parents, and therefore it can be helpful to see them individually as well as with their families where possible (Jones 2003). A range of assessment methods should be utilised. These might include interviews, observations and use of rating scales. Specific rating scales which nurses can use to assess for mood and anxiety disorders include the Children's Depression Inventory (Kovacs 1992); the Revised Children's Manifest Anxiety Scale (Reynolds & Richmond 1978); and the Washington University Kiddie Schedule for Affective Disorders and Schizophrenia (KIDDIE-SADS) (Geller et al. 1996).

Since adolescents with bipolar disorder often present with a mix of psychotic and affective symptoms, it is important for the nurse to assess whether psychotic symptoms are mood congruent. Irritability (Geller et al. 2002), ADHD (Lewinsohn et al. 2003) and substance misuse (Geller & Luby 1997) are each specific symptoms and disorders that make diagnosis of bipolar disorder during adolescence difficult. Referral for physical examination and appropriate physical investigations will also be required for bipolar disorder and day or in-patient observation may also be necessary (Fonagy et al. 2002).

Risk assessment

Nurses should always perform a risk assessment. The assessment of suicide risk involves an exploration of behaviour across several domains including school, interpersonal relationships and social functioning. The presence of acute and chronic stress factors should be identified and recorded. Primary risk factors, including mood disorder, should be explored using direct questioning. This is to assess current ideation, intent and planning. Secondary risk factors, such as substance abuse, and situational factors, such as family functioning, social support, and major life events, all need to be explored using multiple methods and involving different people (Stanard 2000).

Treatment

Treatment approaches have been addressed elsewhere in this book. In this chapter different approaches to the specific treatment of emotional disorders are outlined. The core skills identified previously also apply here. Additional skills relate to training in different therapeutic techniques and specific treatment packages and to knowing what options are available in an individual situation. Nurses also need an understanding of the possible side-effects of any medication that may be prescribed.

It has been suggested that the effectiveness of therapeutic interventions is largely attributable to client variables and environmental factors, followed closely by the quality of the therapeutic relationship. A combination of specific therapeutic techniques and placebo effects reportedly count for less than a third of the improvement in client situations (Silverman & Berman 2001). Formal studies of treatment for emotional disorders in children are in their infancy, with the majority occurring within the research community (Silverman & Berman 2001; Costello et al. 2002; Fonagy et al. 2002). As yet, reliable evidence-based protocols for the management of emotional disorders in children have not been developed. Clinical guidelines published by the National Institute for Clinical Excellence (NICE) relating to emotional disorders in children were published in October 2005. These provide recommendations for good practice based on the best available evidence of clinical and cost effectiveness. These are the only NICE guidelines that have been written specifically for children (NICE 2005). The PTSD draft guideline has a chapter dedicated to children (NICE 2004a). The scope of the bipolar disorder guideline is the management of bipolar disorder in adults and adolescents (NICE 2003b). The scope of the NICE OCD guideline includes adults and children (NICE 2003c). The anxiety guideline is specifically for adults with generalised anxiety disorder and panic attacks and does not refer specifically to children (NICE 2004b).

The current treatment of emotional disorders usually involves a combination of treatment strategies, including medication, cognitive behaviour therapy (CBT), short-term psychotherapy, creative therapies, support and education for families, and possible in-patient treatment for mood disorders (Fonagy et al. 2002). Electroconvulsive therapy (ECT) may be considered for severe depression. However it is rarely used with this age-group and its use is controversial (Graham 1991). The treatment of acute mania in bipolar disorder is largely psychopharmacological (Fonagy et al. 2002). The issue of nurse prescribing and emotional disorders in children is an area of contention. Currently there are no antidepressant drugs licensed for use with children and off-label prescribing is therefore carried out. At present, nurses are not permitted to prescribe off-label drugs and it may be some time before the issue of nurse prescribing for emotional disorders is fully addressed.

Prevention

The NSF for Mental Health (DoH 1999) identified mental health promotion and suicide prevention as part of the mental health agenda, identifying that key local organisations need to work to a common agenda to reduce suicide rates. The NSF for Children, Young People and Maternity Services (DoH 2004) also identified the need for coordinated and integrated local partnership working across agencies to help meet the mental health needs of children. This ten-year strategy includes preventative interventions for mental health, early intervention and suicide reduction (DoH 2004). What is not clear is from where the necessary resources will be obtained in order to achieve this laudable aim. Society-wide, or at least local support is necessary in order for this to be achievable.

Nevertheless, should preventative intervention be a viable option within local resources, then children who are undiagnosed but deemed to be at high risk for emotional disorders may be targeted in one of two ways. First, identifying those where life events, demographic factors and other variables have been shown to increase risk (Gillham et al. 2001); and second, identifying children who display some of the symptoms of depression or anxiety (Klingman 2001). It can be argued that nurses working in primary settings are ideally placed to undertake preventative work, although health promotion has been identified as a task for professionals working in all settings (HAS 1995). Additionally, all childcare professionals are now being encouraged to work in multidisciplinary teams based in and around schools (DfES 2003), providing scope for all nurses who work with children to undertake more of a preventative role in relation to addressing the issue of emotional disorders of children.

There are few controlled preventative trials reported for depression in children. The Preventive Intervention Project is a large-scale efficacy trial in the USA of a manual-based intervention programme for use in public health settings by a variety of professional groups including health visitors, school nurses and CAMHS nurses. It targets children of depressed parents and intervention results to date have been promising (Beardslee et al. 2003). Although research into the prevention of anxiety disorders in children is also in its infancy, initial findings look hopeful. Donovan & Spence (2000) identified that knowledge about risk and protective factors, developmental considerations and intervention strategies are increasingly available. Psychoeducational interventions based on the stress vulnerability model have previously been described for use with children and families in primary care settings (Asarnow et al. 1991). This intervention is designed to enhance understanding of depression through a working model that links stress to effects on feelings, thoughts and behaviour which if left unchallenged can spiral into depression (Asarnow et al. 2001). Such a working model warrants further consideration by nurses who are in a position to undertake preventative work in relation to paediatric emotional disorders.

Case Studies

Case scenarios are used here to demonstrate clinical practice, with a reflective exercise for readers at the end of the section. The young people and their families willingly gave their consent and their identities have been changed for reasons of confidentiality.

Tom – Chronic PTSD in a 10 year-old boy

Tom was referred to CAMHS with symptoms of anxiety following his involvement in a car crash 18 months previously. The assessment involved Tom and his parents. Identified symptoms included frequent nightmares where the crash was reexperienced with flashbacks of the accident. These occurred if Tom was unoccupied and led him to rumination about 'what if . . .' He became increasingly reluctant to attend school and became worried about using public transport. He refused to travel by aeroplane or boat and thus holiday options were limited. Tom had stopped riding his bike, leading to some social isolation and he was reported to have become a nervous and irritable child. This was attributed to both the accident and his age, and had improved recently, although travel by car was still an ordeal. Tom would only go out with a parent, and had to sit in the nearside back seat. If another car was travelling too fast (over 35 mph) or was too close, he would become distressed, crying uncontrollably. He met the criteria for a diagnosis of chronic PTSD.

Risk factors identified during the initial assessment included a ruminating thinking style and high levels of parental anxiety. Being endowed with higher intelligence was identified as a protective factor. Treatment consisted of a short series of desensitisation sessions with Tom and his mother. These included completing a hierarchy of anxiety-provoking situations related to the trauma, teaching a relaxation technique, guided imagery, practice in between sessions, providing literature and an explanation of the physiological basis of anxiety, and identifying strategies that Tom could use to control his anxiety, especially when in the car. At the six-month review, Tom reported that he was no longer experiencing flashbacks or nightmares. He still felt anxious on occasions, but could control his anxiety in the car most of the time. He had started at grammar school and was enjoying it.

Mary – Panic attacks and secondary depression in a 15 year-old girl

Mary was referred by her GP with a 16-month history of panic attacks, which started after her father developed anxiety and depression. The first panic attack had left her feeling nauseous and dizzy and increasingly reluctant to socialise with others. She had been receiving help from her mother and her GP (general practitioner) over a two-month period, using a thought-stopping technique and a breathing exercise, with some success. At the time of assessment the situation was improving with the panic attacks abating.

Risk factors identified during the assessment included temperamental traits of behavioural inhibition and high negative affectivity; parental mental health problems (the father suffered from depression and the mother had experienced panic attacks during late adolescence); and relationship difficulties at home. Protective factors included a close and supportive relationship with her mother and Mary's membership of the county youth orchestra.

Initially it appeared that a couple of sessions focusing on anxiety and anxiety management were all that would be required. Unfortunately this was not so, and there were occasions over the next year when the situation deteriorated, the panic attacks increased and symptoms of depression led to a diagnosis of secondary depression. The treatment involved Mary individually, with her mother joining later on in the sessions. The model used was CBT, within a therapeutic relationship. Literature, information and explanation were provided about anxiety, anxiety management, panic attacks and parental mental illness. Strategies for coping with stress and anxiety in general and panic attacks in particular were identified and practised. Patterns of negative thinking were identified and challenged and pleasurable activities identified and promoted. Small, achievable goals were set with the mother providing support. A letter was sent to the school requesting consideration of Mary's mental health problems in her GCSEs. At discharge Mary had completed her exams, left school, started her first job and was leading an active social life. (See Appendix 1 for Mary's report.)

Kim – Agoraphobia and depression in a 13 year-old girl

Kim was referred to the nurse specialist by her GP with symptoms of agoraphobia and school refusal. She was seen with her mother during the assessment, and was reluctant to be seen individually (though this did occur as therapy progressed). Kim presented with a five-month history of gradual refusal to go out with her friends and increasing reluctance to attend school. Her symptoms included nausea, shakiness and inability to concentrate. She was preoccupied with negative thoughts about going out, had sleep and appetite disturbance and had lost enthusiasm and interest in life. Despite having severe symptoms of depression, Kim denied feeling suicidal.

Risk factors identified included a paternal history of depression (his current illness episode, which started 18 months previously, was Kim's first experience of this); temperamental traits of behavioural inhibition, high negative affectivity and low positive affectivity; a ruminative and self-critical cognitive style. Protective factors included higher intelligence and close, supportive relationships with her mother and older brother who shared her love of music.

Therapy with Kim lasted over three years, with the frequency of sessions gradually decreasing. Several professionals were involved, including the educational welfare officer, home tutor, GP, consultant psychiatrist (to prescribe and monitor antidepressant medication); and later, a Connexions worker. A mixture of psychosocial and pharmacological approaches was employed within the context of a therapeutic relationship with both Kim and her mother. These included monitoring mood and medication, providing education about stress, anxiety and depression; exploring and teaching anxiety management techniques with Kim e.g. relaxation, positive self-talk; encouraging social interaction; identifying and engaging in pleasurable activities; setting small, achievable goals; contingency management and anxiety management for the mother.

Tina – Generalised anxiety disorder in an 11 year-old girl, followed by conduct disorder and depression at 13 years

Tina was first referred by her GP at 11 years of age, with symptoms of generalised anxiety disorder. She was described as having always been a fiery child who responded negatively to new situations. Her mother had experienced similar problems as a child and had ended up as an out-of-control adolescent in care. The mother did not want Tina to experience similar difficulties.

Several risk factors were identified, including maternal depression, paternal alcoholism and ongoing parental acrimony, despite being divorced. Her relationships with her parents were identified as being insecure. She displayed temperamental traits of behavioural inhibition, high negative affectivity and low positive affectivity. Higher intelligence was identified as a protective factor by her mother. Tina and her mother were seen on three occasions, with the focus being on individual and family management of Tina's symptoms of anxiety. The mother and the daughter viewed the treatment as successful and Tina was discharged.

A social worker re-referred Tina two years later, with complaints of conduct disordered behaviour, including lying, stealing, mixing with deviant peers, drug-taking and running away from home. Tina and her parents attended the initial interview. Animosity between all three was high and Tina appeared angry and belligerent, insisting on her privacy, but disrespectful of her parents' right to the same. She presented with symptoms of depression, including sleep and appetite disturbance, persistent low mood, lack of energy, a pervading sense of hopelessness and helplessness. Additional risk factors included the separation of mother and stepfather, leading to less income and moving to a poorer neighbourhood, poor relationships within the family and mixing with a deviant peer group. She also demonstrated a ruminative and self-critical cognitive style.

Minimal interagency collaboration and difficulty in engaging the father in the process hindered the treatment. The mother tried to be supportive, and changed her attitude towards Tina, but her own mental health problems, social circumstances and lack of support made this difficult. Tina was ambivalent about help this time. She demanded support, pushed the boundaries of therapy and was resentful when pre-agreed consequences were carried out. Tina had been prescribed antidepressant medication, but had continued to smoke cannabis despite being provided with evidence of the risks associated with this. When the professions involved liaised and the decision was made to stop the antidepressant medication, Tina's response was one of 'so what'. Though Tina continued to attend for several sessions, attempts to explore thoughts and feelings and identify negative thinking patterns were unsuccessful. Tina preferred to talk in an emotionless manner about how everything was always somebody else's fault and what was the point in trying to change fate. At 10 years old she had hoped to become a lawyer, but by 13 years any job would do, provided that it funded clothes, cigarettes and drugs.

Poppy – Anxiety and depression in a vulnerable 15 year-old girl

Poppy was referred by her GP following the suicide of a friend. She had a past history of anxiety and self-harm. Poppy was described as having always been a sensitive child who had found life's stressors difficult to cope with, especially in social situations. She had frequent and powerful low moods, which adversely affected her thinking and behaviour. Negative thinking and the attitudes and behaviour of others also easily influenced her mood. She was often caught in a downward spiral of self-criticism, rumination, low mood, irritability and social withdrawal. After her friend's death, she had also experienced several symptoms of depression, but these had subsequently lessened. She had also made a decision to stop using self-harm as a coping strategy, but was unsure what to do instead.

Risk factors included temperamental traits of behavioural inhibition, high negative affectivity and low positive affectivity; a ruminative and self-critical cognitive style; parental marital conflict due to work-related stress; bereavement; and being a long-term victim of bullying in school. Protective factors included higher intelligence; a close relationship with her mother; a supportive extended family network. Therapy with Poppy lasted for ten months, involving both the mother and the daughter, at Poppy's request. Written information on bereavement was provided and discussed. A CBT model was used within the context of a therapeutic relationship. This included: exploring and practising strategies for learning to recognise and cope with various types of stress; identifying and challenging negative thinking patterns (her mother was immensely helpful with this task); an exploration of strategies to lift mood, including identifying and participating in pleasurable activities; and assertiveness training. A psychiatric assessment was undertaken due to the persistent prevalence of depressive symptoms. The possible use of an antidepressant medication was discussed, but neither Poppy nor her mother wanted to consider medication as a treatment option. A letter was sent to her school requesting consideration of Poppy's mental health problems in her GCSEs and she took extended study leave. At discharge Poppy appeared to be learning to recognise and cope with her vulnerabilities and build on her strengths, and was looking forward to studying art at the local college.

Case study exercises

- Consider each case in terms of diagnostic criteria and evidence-based guidelines

- Identify and reflect on similarities and differences in relation to:
  - presentation
  - risk and protective factors
  - treatment
  - outcome.

- What factors might account for some of the similarities and differences?

- If Ben, Mary, Kim, Tina or Poppy had been referred to their school nurses initially, what might their role and intervention(s) have been?

- Might there have been a preventative role for the health visitor or school nurse in the early years if temperamental vulnerabilities had been identified? If so, what might the role have entailed?

- What issues might have been considered had a referral to Tier 4 in-patient services been required for Kim?

- How might different professionals and agencies work together across the tiers to best help children and adolescents with emotional disorders?

Conclusion

Many unanswered questions remain to be explored in relation to emotional disorders in children and adolescents, and the context in which nurses work continues to evolve. It is a sobering indictment that not only have emotional disorders and suicide increased in this population, but also the majority of young people suffering from emotional disorders go undetected in the community. With appropriate training, the necessary knowledge and skills, and support and resources mental health and non-mental health nurses are able to engage in identification, assessment, treatment and preventative interventions for children with, or at risk of, emotional disorders. Further research is required to explore the links between anxiety, depression and suicide, and a greater understanding of adolescent suicide is needed. Training is required to develop nurses' ability to both participate in and use research in an informed and critical manner. They would then be in a stronger position to contribute to training and to the research agenda in order to impact, where possible, on the high rate of emotional distress experienced by society's young people.

References

Adelman, H., Taylor, L., Bradley, B. & Lewis, K. (1997). Mental health in schools: expanded opportunities for school nurses. *Journal of School Nursing,* **13** (3), 6–12.

Alloy, L. & Abraamson, L. (1999) Depressogenic cognitive styles: predictive validity, information processing and personality characteristics and developmental origins. *Behaviour Research and Therapy,* **37** (6), 503–31.

American Psychiatric Association (1994). *Diagnostic and Statistical Manual of Mental Disorders.* 4th edn. Washington DC: American Psychiatric Association.

Angold, A. & Costello, E. (2001). The epidemiology of depression in children and adolescents. In: Goodyer, I. (Ed.) *The Depressed Child and Adolescent* (2nd edn). London: Cambridge University Press.

Appleton, P. & Hammond-Rowley, S. (2000). Addressing the population burden of child and adolescent mental health problems: a primary care model. *Child Psychology and Psychiatry Review*, **5** (1), 9–16.

Asarnow, J., Jaycox, L. & Thompson, M. (2001). Depression in youth: psychosocial interventions. *Journal of Clinical Child Psychology*, **30** (1), 33–47.

Beardslee, W., Tracy, R., Gladstone, E., Wright, M. & Cooper, A. (2003). A family-based approach to the prevention of depressive symptoms in children at risk: evidence of parental and child change. *Pediatrics*, **112** (2), 119–31.

Beiderman, J., Faraone, S., Marrs, A., Moore, P., Garcia, J. & Abion, J. (1997). Panic disorder and agoraphobia in consecutively referred children and adolescents. *Journal of the American Academy of Child and Adolescent Psychiatry*, (36), 214–23

Benner, P. (1984). *From Novice to Expert: excellence and power in clinical nursing practice.* London: Addison Wesley.

Brooks-Gunn, J., Auth, J., Petersen, A. & Compass, B. (2001). Physiological processes and development of childhood and adolescent depression. In: Goodyer, I. (Ed.) *The Depressed Child and Adolescent* (2nd edn). London: Cambridge University Press.

Coghill, D. (2003). Current issues in child and adolescent psychopharmacology. Part 2: anxiety and obsessive-compulsive disorders, autism, Tourette's and schizophrenia. *Advances in Psychiatric Treatment*, (9), 289–99.

Costello, E., Pine, D., Hammen, C., March, J. & Plotsky, P. (2002). Development and natural history of mood disorders. *Society of Biological Psychiatry*, (52), 529–42.

Coyle, J., Pine, D., & Charney, D. (2003). Depression and bipolar support alliance consensus statement on the unmet needs in diagnosis and treatment of mood disorders in children and adolescents. *Journal of the American Academy of Child and Adolescent Psychiatry*, **42** (12), 1494–1503.

Davidson, S. & Manion, I. (1996). Facing the challenge: mental health and illness in Canadian youth. *Psychology, Health and Medicine.* **1** (1), 41–55.

de Wilde, E., Kienhorst, I. & Diekstra, R. (2001). Suicidal behaviour in adolescents. In: Goodyer, I. (Ed.) *The Depressed Child and Adolescent* (2nd edn). London: Cambridge University Press.

Department for Education and Skills (2001). *Promoting Children's Mental Health Within Early Years and School Settings.* London: HMSO.

Department for Education and Skills (2003). *Every Child Matters.* London: DfES.

Department of Health (1999). *The National Service Framework for Mental Health.* London: HMSO.

Department of Health (2004). *The National Service Framework for Children, Young People and Maternity Services.* London: HMSO.

Donovan, C. & Spence, S. (2000). Prevention of childhood anxiety disorders. *Clinical Psychology Review*, **20** (4), 509–31.

Farnfield, S. & Kaszap, M. (1998). What makes a helpful grown-up?: children's views of professionals in the mental health services. *Health Informatics Journal*, (4), 3–14.

Flisher, A. (1999). Annotation: Mood disorder in suicidal children and adolescents: recent developments. *Journal of Child Psychology and Psychiatry*, **40** (3), 315–24.

Fonagy, P., Target, M., Cottrell, D., Phillips, J. & Kurtz, Z. (2002). *What Works for Whom? a critical review of treatments for children and adolescents.* London: Guilford Press.

Fonseca, A.C. & Perrin, S. (2001). Clinical phenomenology, classification and assessment of anxiety disorders in children and adolescents. In: Silverman, W.K. & Treffers, P.D.A., (Eds) *Anxiety Disorders in Children and Adolescents: research, assessment and intervention.* Cambridge: Cambridge University Press.

Geller, B., Williams, M., Zimerman, B., & Frazier, J. (1996). *Washington University in St Louis Kiddie Schedule for Affective Disorders and Schizophrenia (WASH-U-KSADS).* St Louis: Washington University Press.

Gellèr, B. & Luby, J. (1997). Child and Adolescent Bipolar Disorder: a review of the past 10 years. *Journal of the American Academy of Child and Adolescent Psychiatry,* **36** (9), 1168–76.

Geller, B., Craney, J., Bolhofner, K., Nicklesburg, M., Williams, M., & Zimerman, B. (2002). Two-year prospective follow-up of children with a prepubertal and early onset bipolar disorder phenotype. *American Journal of Psychiatry,* **159**, 927–33.

Gillham, J. Shatte, A. & Freres, D. (2000). Preventing depression: a review of cognitive-behavioral and family interventions. *Applied & Preventative Psychology,* (9), 63–88.

Goodyer, I. (2001). Life events: their nature and effects. In: Goodyer, I. (Ed.). *The Depressed Child and Adolescent* (2nd edn). Cambridge: Cambridge University Press.

Graham, P. (1991). *Child Psychiatry: a developmental approach* (2nd edn). London: Oxford Medical Publications.

Green, H., McGinnity, A., Meltzer, H., Ford, T. & Goodman, R. (2005). *Mental health of children and young people in Great Britain.* London: Office of National Statistics.

Harrington, R. & Dubicka, B. (2001). Natural history of mood disorders in children and adolescents. In: Goodyer, I. (Ed.) *The Depressed Child and Adolescent* (2nd edn). Cambridge: Cambridge University Press.

Hawton, K., Houston, K. & Shepperd, R. (1999). Suicide in young people: study of 174 cases aged under 25 years based on coroners' and medical records. *British Journal of Psychiatry,* (175), 271–76.

Herbert, M. (1991). *Clinical Child Psychology.* London: John Wiley.

Hoghughi, M. (1992). *Assessing Child and Adolescent Disorders: a practice manual.* London: Sage.

Horowitz, L., Wang, P., Koocher, G. & Burr, B. (2001). Detecting suicide risk in a pediatric emergency department: development of a brief screening tool. *Pediatrics,* **107** (5), 1133–38.

Jones, D. (2003). *Communicating with Vulnerable Children.* London: Department of Health.

Klingman, A. (2001). Prevention of anxiety disorders: the case of post-traumatic stress disorder. In: Silverman, W. & Treffers, P. (Eds) *Anxiety Disorders in Children and Adolescents: Research, Assessment and Intervention.* Cambridge: Cambridge University Press.

Kolvin, I. & Sadowski, H. (2001). Childhood depression: clinical phenomenology and classification. In: Goodyer, I. (Ed.) *The Depressed Child and Adolescent* (2nd edn). Cambridge: Cambridge University Press.

Kovacs, M. (1992). *Children's Depression Inventory (CDI) Manual.* Pittsburg: Multi-Health Systems.

Kovacs, M. & Devlin, B. (1998). Internalizing disorders in childhood. *Journal of Child Psychology and Psychiatry,* **39** (1), 47–63.

Le Doux, J. (2003). *Synaptic Self: how our brains become who we are.* London: Penguin.

Lewinsohn, P., Seeley, J. & Klein, D. (2003). Bipolar disorders during adolescence. *Acta Psychiatrica Scandinavica*, (108), (suppl 418), 47–50.

Lonigan, C.J., Phillips, B.M. & Hooe, E.S. (2003). Relations of positive and negative affectivity to anxiety and depression in children: evidence from a latent variable longitudinal study. *Journal of Consulting and Clinical Psychology*, **71** (3), 465–81.

Manassis, K. (2001). Child-parent relations: attachment and anxiety disorder. In: Silverman, W. & Treffers, P. (Eds). *Anxiety Disorders in Children and Adolescents: research, assessment and intervention*. Cambridge: Cambridge University Press.

Manic Depression Fellowship (2003). *Bipolar Disorder in Children and Young People*: London: Manic Depression Fellowship.

Meltzer, H., Gatward, R., Goodman, R. & Ford, T. (2000). *The Mental Health of Children and Adolescents in Great Britain*. London: The Stationary Office.

Mental Health Foundation (1999). *Bright Futures: promoting children and young people's mental health*. London: Mental Health Foundation.

Moore, M. & Carr, A. (2000). Anxiety disorders. In: Carr, A. (Ed.) *What Works with Children and Adolescents?* London: Routledge.

Muris, P., Schouten, E., Meesters, C. & Gijsbers, H. (2003) Contingency-competence-control-related beliefs and symptoms of anxiety and depression in a young adolescent sample. *Child Psychiatry and Human Development*, **33** (4), 325–39.

National Institute for Clinical Excellence (2003b). *Bipolar Disorder: the management of bipolar disorder in adults and adolescents in primary and secondary care (Scope)*. London: NICE.

National Institute for Clinical Excellence (2003c). *Obsessive-Compulsive Disorder in Adults and Children in Primary and Secondary Care (Scope)*. London: NICE.

National Institute for Clinical Excellence (2004). *Core Interventions in the Treatment and Management of Anorexia Nervosa, Bulimia Nervosa and Related Eating Disorders*. London: NCCMH.

National Institute for Clinical Excellence (2004a). *PTSD (Post-traumatic stress disorder): the management of PTSD in primary and secondary care (1st draft)*. London: NICE.

National Institute for Clinical Excellence (2004b). *Anxiety: management of generalised anxiety disorder and panic disorder (with or without agoraphobia) in adults in primary, secondary and community care (draft for second consultation)*. London: NICE.

NHS Health Advisory Service (1995). *Together We Stand: the commissioning, role and management of child and adolescent mental health services*. London: HMSO.

Oosterlaan, J. (2001). Behavioural inhibition and the development of childhood anxiety disorders. In: Silverman, W. & Treffers, P. (Eds). *Anxiety Disorders in Children and Adolescents: research, assessment and intervention*. London: Cambridge University Press.

Parry-Jones, W. (2001). Historical aspects of mood and its disorders in young people. In: IM Goodyer (Ed.) *The Depressed Child and Adolescent* (2nd edn). Cambridge University.

Prins, P. (2001). Affective and cognitive processes and the development and maintenance of anxiety and its disorders. In: Silverman, W. & Treffers, P. (Eds). *Anxiety Disorders in Children and Adolescents: research, assessment and intervention*. Cambridge: Cambridge University Press.

Reynolds, C. & Richmond, B. (1978). What I think and feel: a revised measure of children's manifest anxiety. *Journal of Abnormal Psychology*, **6** (2), 271–80.

Richardson, G. & Partridge, I. (Eds) (2003). *Child and Adolescent Mental Health Services: an operational handbook*. London: Gaskell.

Royal College of Nursing (2004). *Children and Young People's Mental Health: every nurse's business*. London: RCN.

Royal College of Psychiatrists (2004). *Psychiatric services for children and adolescents with learning disabilities: council report CR123*. London: Royal College of Psychiatrists.

Rutter, M. (1999). Resilience concepts and findings: implications for family therapy. *Journal of Family Therapy*, **21** (2), 119–44.

Scahill, L. & Ort, S. (1995). Selection and use of clinical rating instruments in child psychiatric nursing. *Journal of Child & Adolescent Psychiatric Nursing*, **8** (3), 33–34.

Silverman, W. & Berman, S. (2001). Psychosocial interventions for anxiety disorders in children: status and future directions. In: Silverman, W. & Treffers, P. (Eds) *Anxiety Disorders in Children and Adolescents: research, assessment and intervention*. London: Cambridge University Press.

Stanard, R. (2000). Assessment and treatment of adolescent depression and suicidality. *Journal of Mental Health Counseling*, **22** (3). 204–17.

Stock, S., Werry, J. & McClellan, J. (2001). Pharmacological treatment of paediatric anxiety. In: Silverman, W. & Treffers. P. (Eds) *Anxiety Disorders in Children and Adolescents: research, assessment and intervention*. Cambridge: Cambridge University Press.

Treffers, P. & Silverman, W. (2001). Anxiety and its disorders in children and adolescents before the twentieth century. In: Silverman, W. & Treffers, P. (Eds). *Anxiety Disorders in Children and Adolescents: research, assessment and intervention*. London: Cambridge University Press.

Verhulst, F. (2001). Community and epidemiological aspects of anxiety disorders in children. In: Silverman, W. & Treffers, P. (Eds). *Anxiety Disorders in Children and Adolescents: research, assessment and intervention*. London: Cambridge University Press.

Von Hahn, L. (2004). Bipolar disorder: an overview. *The Exceptional Parent*, **34** (5), 56–61.

Westenberg, P., Siebelink, B. & Treffers, P. (2001). Psychosocial developmental theory in relation to anxiety and its disorders. In: Silverman, W. & Treffers, P. (Eds) *Anxiety Disorders in Children and Adolescents: research, assessment and intervention*. Cambridge: Cambridge University Press.

World Health Organization (1996). *The Global Burden of Disease*. Geneva: WHO.

World Health Organization (1992). *The ICD-10 Classification of Mental and Behavioural Disorders: clinical descriptions and diagnostic guidelines*. Geneva: WHO.

Recommended Reading

Dogra, N., Parkin, A., Gale, F. & Flake, C. (2002). *A Multidisciplinary Handbook of Child and Adolescent Mental Health for Front-line Professionals*. London: Jessica Kingsley.

Fonagy, P., Target, M., Cottrell, D., Phillips, J. & Kurtz, Z. (2002). *What Works for Whom? a critical review of treatments for children and adolescents*. London: Guilford Press.

Goodyer, I. (2001). *The Depressed Child and Adolescent* (2nd edn). Cambridge: Cambridge University Press.

Royal College of Nursing (2004). *Children and Young People's Mental Health: every nurse's business*. London: RCN.

Richardson, G. & Partridge, I. (2003). *Child and Adolescent Mental Health Services: an operational handbook*. London: Gaskell.

Silverman, W. & Treffers, P. (2001). *Anxiety Disorders in Children and Adolescents: research, assessment and intervention*. Cambridge: Cambridge University Press.

Stallard, P. (2003). *Think Good – Feel Good: a cognitive behaviour therapy workbook for children and young people*. London: John Wiley.

Appendix 5.1

Written report by a fifteen year-old girl suffering from panic attacks and secondary depression

When I have bad days I feel very low, depressed, tearful, on edge. It sometimes happens when I'm under pressure, amount of schoolwork. I sometimes feel I can't eat, can't get anything down. I feel like I just want to be on my own. I do panic, palms of hands go sweaty, feel dizzy, dry mouth, feeling tired, hot and feel sick. When I feel like this I have to do something to get rid of these feelings and not to think about these feelings. I must put my relaxation techniques into practice. It does help and calm you down. You must keep going that also does help. Don't think about it. Do things you enjoy – walking relieves stress; pampering yourself; doing what you want to do to cheer yourself up. If you feel you are going to have a panic attack walk away for a minute or so; don't think about it; putting a brown paper bag over your nose and mouth, breath into it, it's meant to help the carbon dioxide levels. Do the relaxation exercises regularly because when an attack happens you then use them automatically.

Chapter 6

Nursing Children and Young People with Eating Disorders

Lisa Lewer

Key points

- Eating disorders are involuntary, complex and sometimes life-threatening illnesses involving an unhealthy and unconventional view of and relationship with food, weight and shape.

- Anorexia nervosa is primarily a psychological disorder characterised by a number of physical, behavioural and psychological factors. It is a serious, life-threatening illness with one of the highest mortality rates of any psychiatric disorder.

- The most obvious sign of anorexia nervosa is severe weight loss. Most of the physical complications associated with this disorder are a direct result of starvation, malnutrition and dehydration.

- Bulimia nervosa is characterised by chaotic patterns of eating and food avoidance, and episodes of overeating or bingeing, during which young people experience a sense of loss of control.

- The National Institute for Clinical Excellence (NICE) has published guidelines for the treatment and management of anorexia nervosa, bulimia nervosa and related eating disorders. The guidelines set out overarching principles that nurses should consider when providing services for children and young people with eating disorders.

- Physical assessment and continuous monitoring are integral to the treatment of eating disorders. However, physical symptoms cannot be managed effectively without an understanding of the young person's underlying psychological difficulties.

Introduction

The task of nursing a child or young person with an eating disorder is a challenging experience that demands incredible curiosity, patience, persistence, resilience and humour. Young people with eating disorders often possess extraordinary strengths, talents and capacities and have futures well worth living for. However, in their relentless pursuit of thinness, the eating disorder hijacks all of these. The initial role of the nurse is to engage with the young person, listen to them and understand their symptoms. Having established this, the task is then to help the young person find meaning and words so that what needs to be expressed can be done so safely to those who need to hear it. This chapter explores this fascinating task, and describes a psychodynamic approach to assessment and treatment that the author has found useful in nursing young people with eating disorders.

Background

The spectrum of eating disorders in young people is wide and varied (Lask & Bryant-Waugh 2000). The term 'eating disorder' is used to refer to a range of conditions, many of which are on a continuum. These include: anorexia nervosa; bulimia nervosa; binge eating disorder; compulsive eating; obesity; selective eating; pervasive refusal; food refusal; and food avoidance emotional disorder. The term 'eating disorder not otherwise specified' (EDNOS) is also used to refer to a clinically heterogeneous group, but for the purpose of this chapter, only anorexia nervosa and bulimia nervosa will be discussed in detail. The chapter is structured in two sections. The first part provides a brief over-view of eating disorders, including how they are understood, who suffers from them and why. The second part examines aspects of assessment and treatment that are to be considered and addressed by the nurse on the young person's journey through care and treatment. This is alongside guidance for nurses on how to engage young people and assist them towards recovery.

The reader is taken on the young person's journey from first contact to discharge. Although the views offered are mostly those involving the in-patient experiences, nurses may be able to adapt much of the information to suit a range of practice settings. Whilst the focus is on nursing work, the import-ance of working alongside a multidisciplinary team and the young person's family or carers cannot be overestimated. Young people with eating disorders often have complex needs, and they therefore require interventions as part of a comprehensive multidisciplinary treatment package.

What are eating disorders and who suffers them?

Eating is influenced by a combination of individual, social and cultural factors. Appetite, culture and religious beliefs all affect what one chooses to eat. The media, fashion, friends and family all shape attitudes to food and eating. The seemingly simple act of providing food and eating, apart from being necessary for sustaining life, is also an enormously symbolic and powerful one (Williams et al. 2003). From the facilitation of attachment to our mothers, to the conveyance of religious and cultural beliefs and identity, the significance of food and eating is individual, meaningful and complex, and is often performed at an unconscious level. Most problems with food are not serious; indeed, food fads are common during childhood and it is not unusual for children to temporarily go off food or simply refuse to eat. Nurses who work with children in hospital will notice that children often struggle with eating. This is perhaps not unusual. Feeling ill causes a loss of appetite and being away from home brings a change of routine. Food may be unfamiliar and eaten at different times to those the child is accustomed to. By comparison, some children eat more if they are worried, anxious or depressed. Such temporary changes in eating are rarely a cause for concern. Rather, they usually occur as part of a change of routine or trauma and will usually resolve without professional intervention.

By comparison, an eating disorder is an involuntary, complex and sometimes life-threatening illness involving an unhealthy and unconventional view of and relationship with food, weight and shape. Young people with such eating disorders are often highly sensitive, competitive, perfectionist, self-hating and low in self-esteem, and frequently have significant difficulty in putting feelings into words (Wood & Lewer 2004). The manifestation of an eating disorder can be viewed as external physical symptoms that signal an internal psychological difficulty. Having an eating disorder can be described as being trapped in a fierce dispute between two opposing sides: growth and life on one, death on the other. Young people with eating disorders have described feeling compelled and addicted to their physical symptoms as they experience a sense of safety and achievement through self-denial and punishing control of the body (Krautter & Lock 2004). The symptoms also exert power and control over others (Bryant-Waugh & Lask 2004), meaning the young person can feel 'in charge'. This results in a sense of oneself, which overcomes existing feelings of helplessness and despair. A vicious cycle can therefore be established whereby the illness seems to take on a life of its own, relentlessly taking control of the young person by splitting off their rational thinking mind from their body.

Despite the increasing number of reports and the emphasis on thinness in the popular press, it is hard to know whether rates of eating disorders are increasing in young people (Fombonne 1995). However, what is known is that the increase of media interest has led to the myth that eating disorders are due to the general increase in dieting behaviours and weight sensitivity in our culture. It is not true that this necessarily leads to the development of eating disorders. An eating disorder is a way of showing that the self hurts, demonstrated by both the closing of the mouth to food, and the shutting out of others. Magagna (2000) argues that young people, driven by an acute dread of taking something in, have closed their minds to emotional experiences and relationships and have withdrawn from the social world in a bid to form a protective shell. The possibilities for being nurtured by food and emotional experiences are shut out and the young person effectively forms a 'no entry' system of protection (Williams 1997). Eating disorders tend to get worse if they are not treated. Without help, young people may place both their physical and mental health at risk. Depression, low self-esteem and self-hatred are all long-term psychological effects from untreated eating disorders.

Anorexia nervosa

Anorexia and anorexia nervosa are not the same thing. Whilst anorexia literally means loss of appetite, anorexia nervosa is a serious, life-threatening illness with one of the highest mortality rates of any psychiatric disorder. After asthma and obesity, anorexia nervosa ranks as the third most serious health problem in adolescent girls (Gowers 2002). One in ten cases of anorexia nervosa lead to premature death, either by cardiac arrest, starvation, other medical complications or suicide (National Eating Disorders Screening Programme 1999). Anorexia nervosa is primarily a psychological disorder with physical manifestations. In most cases, starvation results in life being threatened, and in extreme cases can result in death. It is a disorder characterised by determined attempts to lose weight or avoid weight gain at times when such weight gain is necessary for growth and development. This occurs through avoiding food or hydration, exercising excessively, abusing laxatives or inducing vomiting. Young people with anorexia nervosa may claim to be fat even when they are significantly underweight. Typically, a preoccupation and dissatisfaction with body shape and size occurs. Young people often feel grossly fat which leads to a focus on food intake, and a variety of reasons for refusing food are given. Though the most common of these include fear of fatness and concerns about weight and shape, difficulties in swallowing, nausea, feeling full, loss of appetite and abdominal pain have also been reported (Fosson et al. 1987).

In addition to physical symptoms, associated psychological problems can also occur. These include depression (North & Gowers 1999) and obsessive compulsive disorder (OCD) (Herpertz-Dahlmann & Remschmidt 1993). Young people and their families experience considerable distress and disruption to their lives in response to these addictive behaviours, and also as a result of some of the feelings that the disorder elicits. These feelings may include blame, guilt, shame, hopelessness or anger. Despite being relatively well understood, anorexia nervosa remains the subject of a number of misconceptions and myths (see Box 6.1).

Who suffers from anorexia nervosa?

Anorexia nervosa affects people of all ages including pre-pubertal children and young people. The disorder most commonly affects girls in early adolescence, with the average age of onset being fourteen (Lask & Bryant-Waugh 2000). However, there is an increasing recognition that boys are also affected. In a survey of over 1000 calls to Childline about eating disorders, half were from boys (Childline 2003). Boys appear to be less concerned about weight and are

Box 6.1   Anorexia nervosa: fact or fiction?

Anorexia nervosa only affects white, middle class girls
Fiction: Anorexia nervosa is an international disorder affecting all social classes. Whilst the majority of those who suffer from eating disorders are female, anorexia nervosa also affects boys and men.

Anorexia nervosa is a diet that has gotten out of control
Fiction: Though there are similarities between dieting and anorexia nervosa, there are also significant differences. For example, young people on diets usually set themselves a target for weight loss. By comparison, those with eating disorders continue to lose weight despite being told they are underweight.

Young people can die as a result of anorexia nervosa
Fact: Anorexia nervosa is responsible for the highest number of deaths from psychiatric disorder.

Young people with anorexia nervosa lose their appetite and do not get hungry
Fiction: Hunger, appetite and satiety are controlled by the hypothalamus. Young people with anorexia nervosa retain their appetite and feel hunger.

Nearly all the physical complications caused by anorexia nervosa are reversible
Fact: Though many of these are reversible, there are a number of permanent effects caused by this disorder during childhood. Pre-pubertal anorexia nervosa may permanently impair the child's physical development and sexual maturation. Children with anorexia nervosa are also at higher risk of developing osteoporosis than adolescents or adults.

Young people with anorexia nervosa can literally stop growing
Fact: Growth slows down and can even stop altogether during starvation. It is generally agreed that 'catch-up growth' can occur but to what extent is unclear. There have been reports of young people going through puberty in their mid to late twenties.

instead preoccupied with shape and attempts to avoid 'flabbiness'. Rather than set out to lose weight, boys are likely to over-exercise and avoid particular foods such as those regarded as unhealthy or fattening. However, as with anorexia in girls, there is subsequent weight loss.

Susan

Susan, 13, has two younger sisters aged 12 and 9, and lives with both parents. She describes feeling close to her mother but says she has a difficult relationship with her father. At assessment, parents described Susan as 'perfect' – bright, cheerful, popular and successful both academically and at sport. Her father had noticed 18 months ago, on holiday in Spain, that she looked thin but he was told off by Susan and her mother for being critical. After her holiday Susan began to limit certain foods, saying that she wanted to be healthy for her netball team. She continued to restrict her diet until a school nurse became concerned about Susan's low weight and advised her parents to take Susan to the GP (general practitioner). Her GP, alarmed at an 8kg weight deficit referred her to the local CAMHS who diagnosed anorexia nervosa. Susan denied there was a problem and continued to lose weight, despite weekly out-patient sessions. She was referred to an in-patient adolescent unit where she deteriorated further, isolating herself and refusing to eat. Susan's mood was low and she spent a lot of her time crying and writing in her diary. Eventually, Susan required nasogastric feeding.

In relation to the social and cultural aspects of eating disorders, there have been some relatively small-scale studies of early onset anorexia nervosa, but analysis of these two areas show that further investigation is required before conclusions can be reached. On one hand, it has been suggested that there may be some over-representation of eating disorders in socially advantaged and affluent families. On the other, it has been suggested that rather than affluence *per se*, it might be the pressure to achieve that is associated with eating problems. Eating disorders are no longer considered to be culture-bound syndromes affecting only western Caucasians. They are universal disorders that have been identified in many countries and in a variety of cultures (Bryant-Waugh & Lask 1995). It has been suggested that young people from minority ethnic backgrounds who develop anorexia are more likely to socialise primarily with others of the same racial origin, meaning that young people have to assimilate their experiences of home life with their experiences at school and elsewhere (Lask & Bryant-Waugh 2000). Interestingly, eating disorders have not been identified in cultures where food is scarce.

Signs and symptoms of anorexia nervosa

Physical signs

The most obvious sign of anorexia nervosa is severe weight loss. Most of the physical complications associated with this disorder are a direct result of starvation, malnutrition and dehydration. Other physical changes associated with anorexia nervosa may be less immediately obvious. Prolonged calorie restriction leads to widespread physiological disturbance. Hormonal and endocrine changes are associated with a range of gastro-intestinal, cardio-vascular and gynaecological problems. Onset of anorexia nervosa before puberty can result in delayed growth. In older children, the risk of infertility and damage to internal organs increases into adult life. Children with anorexia nervosa are particularly at risk of osteoporosis (brittle bones). This is because children develop peak bone density and strength during their adolescence. Disruption to nutritional and mineral metabolism before puberty and during adolescence can also lead to osteoporosis and other problems in adulthood. Nurses may notice that the skin and hair of young people with anorexia nervosa is in poor condition. There may also be chilblains and calluses on the hands. This arises from the malnutrition caused by starvation. When a young person suffers severe weight loss, their body introduces a range of survival mechanisms. Young people with anorexia nervosa may complain of feeling cold and experience numbness in their hands and feet. This is caused by low body temperature, poor circulation and a lack of body fat. In extreme cases this may lead to hypothermia.

Behavioural signs

Since the majority of interpersonal communication is nonverbal, nurses should be aware of a number of behavioural clues that young people may be suffering from anorexia nervosa. Wearing big, baggy clothes may be an attempt to hide a body that has become emaciated and young people may engage in excessive exercise in an attempt to burn off calories and lose weight. Behaviour before, during and after meals is often indicative of a problem with eating. Prior to meals, young people may become anxious or preoccupied. During meals, nurses may notice that eating is methodical, ritualistic and often very time-consuming. Young people may be visibly distressed and may make themselves sick before and/or after their meal.

Psychological signs

Psychological signs and symptoms of anorexia nervosa are more difficult to detect as young people can often mask their feelings in an attempt to hide their eating disorder. However, talking about eating may reveal a preoccupation with body shape, size and weight as well as an intense fear of weight gain and fatness. Young people with anorexia nervosa may also be obsessive, have poor concentration and experience mood swings (see Table 6.1).

NICE has published guidelines for the treatment and management of anorexia nervosa, bulimia nervosa and related eating disorders (NICE 2004). These set out overarching principles that professionals and services should consider when providing services for children and young people with eating disorders. Whilst each child or adolescent has their own individual needs, the NICE guidelines make clear recommendations on the types of treatment that should be available and sets out structured pathways of care. As far as possible, young people with anorexia nervosa should be managed as out-patients. This is to avoid disruption to school and family life. In-patient treatment should

Table 6.1 Signs and symptoms of anorexia nervosa.

Physical	Behavioural	Psychological
Extreme weight loss	Wearing big, baggy clothes	Mood swings
Malnutrition	Over-exercising	Preoccupation with body shape, size and weight
Dry or rough skin	Self-induced vomiting	Intense fear of weight gain
Hormonal changes	Use of laxatives or diuretics	Intense fear of fatness
Delay in onset of puberty	Secrecy	Obsessive thinking
Amenorrhoea (irregular periods)	Methodical eating	Fear of eating
Stomach ache or constipation		Poor concentration
Tiredness		
Feeling cold		
Osteoporosis (brittle bones)		
Myopathy (muscle wastage)		
Dental erosion		

only be sought if more rigorous physical management and psychological therapy in the form of the in-patient therapeutic milieu is required (Crouch 1998). Wherever possible, children and young people admitted to hospital for treatment of their eating disorder should receive this is an age appropriate setting (NICE 2004).

Signs and symptoms of bulimia nervosa

Bulimia nervosa is an illness that is rare in young people under the age of 12 (Lask & Bryant-Waugh 2000). Though it affects boys too, bulimia nervosa is most likely to affect adolescent girls and young women. It is characterised by chaotic patterns of eating; food avoidance; and episodes of over-eating or 'bingeing', during which young people experience a sense of loss of control. Bulimia nervosa is not always easy for nurses and other professionals to recognise. Although young people are usually of normal weight, attempts to avoid weight gain are made through self-induced vomiting, laxative or diuretic abuse and appetite suppressants. Whilst there are many overlapping features with anorexia nervosa, the destructiveness of bulimia nervosa is more easily concealed from others. But similarly, young people may deny they have a problem and be evasive about eating.

One of the more obvious signs of bulimia nervosa is bingeing, i.e. eating large quantities of food in a short period of time. The young person may only stop eating when they cannot physically eat any more food. After bingeing, the young person may feel anxious, guilty about weight gain and out of control. To regain control they usually make themselves sick or over-exercise. Intense shame may follow bingeing and young people often feel distressed by their symptoms. An intense preoccupation with food develops which progressively interferes with educational and social activities. Whilst young people with bulimia nervosa present different images from those of young people with anorexia nervosa, many of the psychological features are the same, that is, the provision of safety through control. In bulimia nervosa this is shown by the distinctive patterns of gorging or bingeing followed by evacuation (see Table 6.2).

The NICE guidelines for the treatment and management of eating disorders (NICE 2004) make several recommendations for assessment that are common to both anorexia nervosa and bulimia nervosa. The majority of patients suffering from bulimia nervosa can be successfully treated in out-patient settings, needing only in-patient mental health treatment if they are at risk of severe self-harm or suicide (Schmidt & Treasure 1997). Indications for admission to hospital due to medical complications caused by bulimia nervosa include oesophageal tears, intractable vomiting and hypothermia. The treatment of choice is cognitive behavioural treatment (CBT) for bulimia nervosa (NICE 2004) and some nurses in specialist CAMHS have been trained to use this approach. Nurses using CBT for children and young people with bulimia nervosa will need to adapt their approach to suit the age, circumstances and developmental needs of the child.

Table 6.2 Signs and symptoms of bulimia nervosa.

Physical	Behavioural	Psychological
Frequent weight changes	Bingeing (eating large quantities of food in a short space of time)	Negative attitudes to weight, shape and size
Stomach pains	Being sick after eating	Obsession or preoccupation with food
Swollen salivary glands	Misuse of medication to 'control' weight	Low self-esteem
Dental erosion/tooth decay	Over-exercising	Guilt and shame
Mouth infections/ulcers	Dieting	Mood swings
Oesophagitis	Secretive eating	Anxiety and depression
Amenorrhoea (irregular periods)		Impulsivity
Dry or poor skin		
Sore throat		

Why do eating disorders develop?

An eating disorder stems from a complex integrated model that is made up of predisposing, precipitating and perpetuating factors, which interact and maintain the disorder (Lask & Bryant-Waugh 2000). These factors are unique to each individual, and attention will need to be paid to them in treatment. Long-term healthy outcomes demand a reconnection of the body to the mind, where the eating disorder has severed this link. Both physical and psychological issues must be addressed in the context of a relationship with an adult who can remain thoughtful, robust and containing in the face of the young person's rejection and withdrawal. This is at the heart of what really helps these young people and their families, and is the focus of the rest of the chapter.

Esme

Esme, 16, was the youngest child of four and her parents had recently separated. Emse lived with her mother. Her oldest brother was musically talented and lived away at university. Esme's father lived in the next village with his new wife and baby and saw Esme fortnightly. Esme described herself as 'a disappointment' to her family, feeling that she was not bright. Esme reported that her difficulties began when she was called a pig by a friend at school. This was around the same time as her brother left home. Esme stopped eating at school, and instead ate large amounts of food in the evenings. She began to put on weight, which made her feel bad, and so she began vomiting and her weight stabilised. Having secretly lived like this for 18 months, Esme began to get scared as she was vomiting blood. She confided in an aunt, who informed her mother some six months later when Esme's attempts to stop were unsuccessful. Esme embarked on an out-patient programme, met a specialist nurse every week and managed to reduce her bingeing and vomiting to twice a week. She talked at length about her feelings of failure and 'not being good enough' in comparison to her brother and her schoolfriends.

The assessment process

With the publication of the NICE guidelines on the assessment and management of eating disorders, nurses and other health professionals as well as young people and their families or carers, now have access to evidence-based interventions (NICE 2004). These include specific interventions for children and young people and provide a helpful framework for how services should be organised and what service users should expect. Evidence-based interventions in this area and age-group are weak, and the guidelines do not provide specific guidance in how to nurse these young people. Individualised goals aside, there are some goals that are vital to address for all eating-disordered young people and their families, which will be addressed in the context of a relationship with the nurse and team. Assessment of children and young people with eating disorders should be comprehensive and include physical, psychological and family needs. The following careplan gives an illustration of the objectives for treatment of anorexia nervosa:

Individual treatment goals

- Weight and normal eating patterns will be restored to enable development and growth. For most young people with anorexia nervosa this means an average weekly weight gain of 1kg if they are in hospital and 0.5kg if they are being treated in the community.
- Personal strengths and capacities will be affirmed to enhance identity and self-esteem.
- Motivation for change will be identified and utilised.
- An emotional language will be developed and the voice will be used to express feelings and resolve conflicts.
- Ability to use support and helping relationships will be developed.
- Confidence in relating to peers will be developed.

Family treatment goals

- Affirming existing capacities and strengths.
- Developing coping skills and persistence.
- Developing a network of support.
- Supporting hopefulness.

Assessment and treatment are about providing a holistic experience – addressing the whole of the young person and not simply bits of them. An initial assessment in a comfortable setting is therefore vital. This sets the stage for the rest of treatment. There are a number of components to a thorough assessment, focusing on the young person, their family or carers, physical health and school. Thorough assessment in all of these domains will require the skills of additional professionals. The overall aim of an assessment is to gather information so that a complete picture of the young person can begin to be established; to enable the young person to give meaning to their story; to give the young person an opportunity to share their sense of identity; and to make an immediate assessment of physical status and risk to self.

Assessment should be understood as a two-way process. Not only is the nurse making their assessment, but the family and patient will be assessing the nurse for trustworthiness, knowledge and understanding. It is therefore vital to facilitate a climate of support where the family will feel heard and understood. It is also important for the nurse to demonstrate that they understand the family across the breadth of their development and in the immediate context of their relationships, expectations and environments (Farrell 2000). Hopes and fears must also be discussed and understood, and expertise should be shared. To facilitate this, it should be made clear that there is more than one way of viewing the young person's problems. Instead of attributing blame, the nurse should be interested in how the difficulties have developed and discuss what needs to happen in order to address them. Through openness, honesty, collaboration and support, relationships between parents and professionals will develop and the young person's eating disorder can be positively addressed (Geller et al. 2001). Equally important during engagement is to make clear that taking a collaborative approach does not mean that the nurse and young person will never disagree nor have times when things feel unbearably tense and uncomfortable. The nurse, young person and their families or carers should agree to be as honest and open as possible.

The nurse's primary task in the assessment process is to act like a magnet does to iron filings. This is to draw together all the fragmented pieces that have previously been uncoordinated and separated off. This usually involves contacting other professionals for further information. The whole story should be listened to with close attention and sincere interest. In doing this, the young person is given an experience of adults working together in the interest of understanding their eating disorder. It is useful to meet the young person alone after seeing the family together. This is so that things can be shared in privacy if the young person so wishes.

Involving families and carers

NICE guidelines for the assessment and treatment of eating disorders state that families and carers should be involved at every stage during the assessment and treatment process (NICE 2004). This is to negotiate care and treatment objectives, share information about progress and to provide advice on behavioural management. Often, parents blame themselves for their child developing an eating disorder (Honig 2000). If they are to support their child back to health, they need to understand why their child is refusing to eat, and that this is not because their child is bad, naughty or troublesome, but rather because the control of eating is a way of coping with difficulties and a means of self-protection. Parents often need support to give up blaming themselves. They will often feel very angry and frustrated with trying to support their child to eat. Parental attitudes and beliefs should be explored, as these provide insight into issues that may have become inextricably linked to eating and weight loss (Dare et al. 1994). The nurse needs to gather enough information to enable a sense of what it might feel like to be the parents or carers of the young person, and a sense of what they may find helpful.

While the issues of eating and weight are clearly very important, it can be helpful to address these directly towards the end of the assessment meeting. Suggested areas for assessment include:

- What is currently pertinent for the young person? Have these issues changed and how have they impacted on the young person and family life?
- How does the young person feel about themselves?
- Who is important to them, who most understands them, and whom do they trust?
- Who are they most like in their family?
- What do they want to change if anything, what motivates them?
- What are their strengths and what do they like doing/how do they spend their time?
- What gives them pleasure and what are their hopes for the future?
- How has school been?
- Who are their friends, and how often do they see them?
- What are the young person's feelings about growing up?
- What are the expectations they feel are placed upon them, and by whom?

The importance of a physical assessment

The most obvious symptom of anorexia nervosa is severe weight loss. This can lead to a range of physical complications that are a direct result of starvation and malnutrition. Physical assessment and continuous monitoring are integral to the treatment of eating disorders (Nicholls et al. 2000). However, physical symptoms cannot be managed effectively without an understanding of the underlying psychological difficulties (Robinson & McHugh 1995). It is usually preferable for the nurse to undertake the physical assessment after hearing the young person's story. This is so that a context is understood for the physical condition the young person may be in. At this stage, young people may feel vulnerable and they may want to be accompanied by a parent or carer. However, the nurse should remember that the young person may have concealed their body for many months. Parents or carers may therefore need to be prepared for how emaciated their child has become. Nurses should always respect the young person's safety, privacy and dignity when performing physical assessments. This means that due attention should be paid to the young

Box 6.2 How can I work out a young person's body mass index (BMI)?

Establishing the body mass index (BMI) is only one part of the assessment of anorexia nervosa. It is a measure of weight-to-height relationship. BMI measurement is not an exact science, due to developmental variations and differences in body shape, size and age. There are also minor sex differences in BMI calculations. To work out a young person's BMI you must carefully measure their height and weight. The BMI score is calculated by dividing weight in kilogram's by height in metres squared (BMI = kg/m^2). For example, if a young person weighs 35kg and is 1.5m in height, their BMI equals 15.6. Individual BMI scores should be plotted on BMI reference curves, i.e. population norms for boys and girls. Like height and weight charts, ranges are set in centiles, which allow the nurse to plot a young person's BMI according to their age and sex.

person's age, sex and gender and it is good practice for nurses not to perform physical assessments in isolation. Physical examination should include weighing the young person on digital scales and measuring their height. This is to work out their body mass index (BMI) which will indicate how underweight they are. However, nurses should remember that BMI is only one indicator of physical risk and it is an unreliable measure in young people, especially children (NICE 2004) (see Box 6.2).

Taking an accurate recording of weight is of paramount importance and must be non-negotiable. This is often an area of strong resistance. A balance has to be struck between maintaining firmness and showing respect for the young person. Reluctance to be weighed is common and often linked to feelings of shame that the young person has about lying, or being secretive and concealing difficulties from parents. Young people may find it comforting to hear explicit acceptance from the nurse such as:

'We understand that eating disorders make young people engage in destructive behaviours. We also know that you feel badly about these things, but we do not blame you for them.'

It is not unusual for nurses to feel cruel and bullying in being necessarily persistent in relation to physical examination. However, it is important to remember that something is being communicated in the young person's resistance. In persisting, the nurse challenges the eating disorder and fulfils their duty of care towards the young person. It is unhelpful to get into battles about this, as it is how the patient feels, and this must be validated by making such statements as:

'It must feel so uncomfortable to live in a body that you hate so much at the moment.'

Compromise can be a very useful skill in these situations. The nurse may want to suggest that the young person stands on the scales backwards, covering the numbers or that a parent weighs their child with the nurse in the room.

Guidelines for physical assessment

Nurses may find it helpful to consider the following guidelines as part of the physical assessment process:

- Observe the young person's general appearance. Are they wearing clothing to hide their body? Are they looking after themselves and attending to appearance? What is the condition of hair, skin and nails?

- Measure height and weight to work out the young person's BMI.

- Record blood pressure, pulse and temperature.

- Examine the body for muscle wastage, signs of dehydration or evidence of self-harm.

- Examine head, eyes, ears and throat (for swollen saliva glands, dental corrosion, or tiny haemorrhages in back of throat).

- What is the young person's complaint about weight? When did they first become concerned? Have they used vomiting, laxatives or diuretics to control weight?

- What have been the young person's highest and lowest weights? What were the circumstances?

- What does the young person typically eat in a day?

- What is the young person's experience of hunger? Do they have urges to eat? Do they binge? If so, what on? How does it start and end and what is felt afterwards?

- What is a young person's typical day like in terms of eating? Is it ritualised? Does the young person eat alone or in company?

- Does the young person use excessive exercise to control weight? If so, what kind, how often and for how long?

Treatment stage 1: engagement

Once the assessment process is completed, goals for treatment can be discussed and agreed. Successful treatment depends on the creation of a therapeutic relationship with both the young person and their family or carers. Young people with bulimia nervosa are commonly more motivated to get help than those with anorexia nervosa, due to the strength of fear and denial that is present within this group of young people. An alliance must be formed both with the young person and their parents or carers. If young people sense that the adults around them can trust the professional, so too might they be able to develop this trust. Where parents and professionals do not work together, progress can often be lacking (Bryant-Waugh & Lask 2004). Forming a therapeutic relationship may be challenging, due to the high levels of anxiety, blame, shame and guilt that are part of any eating disorder. However, forming a basis of trust is crucial if nurses are to successfully help young people and their families progress into treatment. There are a number of issues to be considered during the process of engagement.

Shared expertise, collaboration and not knowing

It must be acknowledged from the start that the young person, their parents or carers, and siblings are the experts on their family. Parents know their children much better than professionals can ever know them. It is likely to be parental support and determination that are crucial in making the journey to health successful. However, it is the treatment team that have expertise in health and eating disorders. Collaborative treatment starts from the position that this expertise should be shared, and that the family and professionals each have things that the other needs, and there are also things that each does not know. All views and possibilities must be considered if 'good enough' decisions are to be made in the interests of the young person. There will be many times during the course of treatment when those concerned find themselves tempted to do something without considering all the possibilities. This is illustrated in the following reflection by a nurse working with Susan, a 14 year-old girl with anorexia nervosa:

Susan

During the assessment with Susan, her parents said 'it would be nice if she were able to be at home for her birthday next weekend'. I felt excited about her birthday, and felt tempted to make plans with them as if everything were normal. I looked at Susan, emaciated and sad in front of me, whose reality was that she might not see any more birthdays if we didn't help her with her eating disorder. I said, 'It would be nice, but at this point is it helpful?' Susan and her mother began to cry as if I had spoiled all their good feelings. I felt mean. Managing to ask this question however opened up all the possibilities, and we had a positive discussion. The family eventually agreed that it would be better to visit Susan in hospital this year in the hope that next year's birthday would be different.

When establishing the boundaries necessary for successful treatment there is always the potential risk of forming polarised views. When one position is firmly held, there may be a tendency to simply take up an opposing view. Using the example above, the nurse could have said:

'You can't do anything on your birthday, you are too ill.'

Not only might Susan's birthday have been unnecessarily miserable, but this approach may have resulted in the family feeling pushed out, disregarded and misunderstood. If the nurse succumbs to the temptation to always 'know' what to do, the possibilities for creative thinking which are needed when working with such rigid difficulties are closed down. Asking a question that opens up the different possibilities to be considered is likely to facilitate a good enough solution and a partnership approach to the work. An important aspect of work with young people who have eating disorders is that of using motivational approaches (Geller et al. 2001; Geller 2002) to facilitate change. This style of working facilitates the collaborative approach, as it works solely on what the young person feels motivated to do. Using such questions as 'what do you want?', 'what would be most manageable?' and 'how can we help you settle in here?' help establish a therapeutic alliance and reinforce the message that the young person will be accepted. This approach is helpful to use with both young people and also their parents or carers.

It has already been stated that young people with eating disorders often have very low self-worth and feel that they are 'unlovable'. In part, this is due to the strength of the uncomfortable feelings that they are experiencing, including distaste, disgust, guilt, shame and hostility. The nurse should expect to be rejected, and so resilience and persistence are key to the success of forming and sustaining positive relationships in these circumstances. It is important that the nurse simply spends time being with the young person. This helps provide a therapeutic opportunity for the young person to experience things within themselves other than their eating disorder. The following is an excerpt from a nurse's reflective diary:

> *'Susan was a skilled mimic and enjoyed reading aloud. One session a week was spent reading to the nurse, and developing voices for all the characters in a particular story. This allowed her the opportunity to laugh, use her strengths and also to have a break from thoughts about eating.'*

Trust and getting to know one another can be built in this way. The nurse needs to spend as much time as possible talking with the young person and in getting to know them as a whole person. This is crucial in terms of validating the young person's sense of self and in the forming of a relationship in which some of the negative feelings can then be explored (Crouch 1998). Simple ideas such as watering the plants together, discussing a book or TV, doing a crossword together, or simply working at different tasks in the same room are all invaluable in forging links. Skills for nurses to manage silence will also be important as periods of silence are almost universal in working with patients with eating disorders, particularly during the painful process of eating itself (Magagna 2000).

Containment

Another key factor in building relationships with young people who have eating disorders is that of emotional containment. In simple terms, containment is a process which involves parental figures (the nurse in this case) having the capacity to be able to be in touch with, tolerate and connect with intense emotions, think about them, attempt to understand them and respond to them. It is a cycle of projection, introjection, reverie and communication (Seinfeld 1996).

We now examine the development of this process. An eating disorder provides the sufferer protection against the world, so it is no surprise that young people are often extremely ambivalent about treatment and nursing interventions. This is because such interventions pose a threat to their tightly held-together selves, achieved through anorectic or bulimic control. Help is therefore commonly refused, due to the young person's fear and anxiety, both of which are masked by the external symptoms. Refusal must be accepted and tolerated by the nurse, and should not be personalised. It can be helpful to remember,

'This is not about me, but something is being communicated which I have to try to understand.'

In the face of such rejection, it may be important to accept that until the young person has a sense of the nurse, the focus should be upon engaging the parents.

The nurse's task of emotional containment is a privileged but challenging one. It requires the nurse to fully engage with the young person's anxiety and distress. Feeling the feelings provides an insight into what the young person might be experiencing, and subsequently what they feel and therefore need. Due to the strength and nature of the feelings, the process of containment can often feel very frightening. However, it is a necessary part of the treatment if the nurse is to be effective. In order to be an effective container, the nurse must be aware of their own feelings in relation to the young person, and to be able to manage these in a balanced and sensitive way (Salzberger-Wittenberg 2003). Factors to be weighed include acknowledging the young person's reality, offering appropriate reassurance that their eating disorder is manageable, and retaining the ability to think independently. This process is similar to that which a mother goes through with her new baby: she tunes in to its communications to understand what it needs. The following account from the nurse's reflective diary illustrates some of the factors involved in the process of containment:

'Esme was found stealing loaves of bread from the kitchen. When her bag was searched, a plastic bag full of vomit was found. I felt angry with her. We had met an hour before and agreed a plan to help her with this behaviour. I told her to come and meet with me and I went to discard the vomit. On my way back to the room, I felt ashamed of my anger, and felt like crying. My anger subsided as I recognised that these might be Esme's feelings. As I entered, Esme's eyes filled with tears and she spoke of feeling useless, disgusted and angry that she had not been able to stick with the plan. My feelings had been a reflection of how Esme herself was feeling.'

In providing effective containment for young people who have eating disorders, it can be helpful to think of an 'internal supervisor'. This serves to remind us that strong emotions that we might be experiencing may be being projected by the young person. If we successfully manage the anxiety that the young person evokes in us, we will signal to them that we can also manage theirs, and trust and development can take place. If anxiety is not managed, nurses may find themselves tempted to 'do' rather than simply 'be with'. This can be a significant challenge to the nurse if the young person states that they do not want or need anything from us. If the nurse is able to successfully contain strong feelings, the young person is likely to have an experience of being accepted and understood, which builds self-esteem. Young people with eating disorders are extremely sensitive to the appraisal that others may have of them. For this reason, it is important that nurses are genuine and sincere in their interactions, saying what they mean and meaning what they say. This is illustrated in the following reflective diary entry:

> *'On an occasion when Susan refused her supper, I felt disappointed and useless. Susan asked if I was angry with her. I said that whilst I did feel angry, this was with the eating disorder not her. Susan had picked up my angry feelings.'*

Managing the process of emotional containment is one of the greatest challenges for the nurse. Given that these young people suffer from feelings of uselessness, guilt, hopelessness and unworthiness amongst others, it can be frightening to suddenly find oneself feeling the same. As a result of feeling these types of feelings, it is not uncommon to feel shame or humiliation, which can make one want to run away or disappear. The nurse needs supervision to be able to remain vigilant and self-aware to the feelings as they can creep up on them and paralyse them. Self-awareness on the part of the nurse allows a differentiation of the feelings and helps separate whose feelings are whose, and to understand them as a communication from the young person which is to be understood in the absence of words.

Boundaries

Young people with eating disorders sometimes feel out of control or chaotic and have difficulties with separation. Susan described her life and internal world as 'a mess' and needed the nurse to help her 'tidy things up'. Tidying up demands orderliness, clarity, predictability and consistency, and so clear use of boundaries is one of the most important aspects of treatment with young people who may be feeling fragmented, uncontained and worthless. In the first instance, structure is crucial. When external structures are clear and dependable, it becomes possible to work on an internal structure, a little like developing a filing system in the mind. Young people need help to create a timetable that offers as much predictability and reliability as possible. This is so that they can emotionally pace themselves and prepare for each aspect of the treatment process, rather than get 'caught out', as they have so often have been by their eating disorder.

Young people with eating disorders may find change extremely disturbing. It can completely throw them off balance, and they become tempted to turn once again to their eating disorder, which can offer them stability and certainty. Consequently, appointments with the nurse should be scheduled regularly and not changed unless this is absolutely necessary. Time-limits for therapeutic sessions must be established and maintained, and responses to particular behaviours should be consistent. Conveying these simple but crucial aspects of the therapeutic relationship also conveys a basic level of respect to the young person. Clear boundaries are also of value for the nurse, as they enable the nurse to pace and appropriately structure the session. Typically, young people need to understand, accept and feel comfortable with the external structures before they can depend on a person. This is crucial in the context of a dependant therapeutic relationship where recovery occurs. The nurse must demonstrate that they can be reliable and consistent towards the young person.

It is helpful in in-patient settings to have the week's staff rota posted. This is so that young people as well as their families or carers can see when their key nurse and other professionals are on duty. When a key worker is away, it is important to arrange cover so that the young person can still access support and so that continuity is maintained (National Health Service Executive 1999). It is important to give adequate notice for times when the nurse will be away. This allows mental preparation to occur and gives a message that the nurse and organisation is dependable even when there may be changes in personnel.

Treatment stage 2: working towards recovery

Working towards recovery commences at the point of initial assessment. Recovery from an eating disorder is not easy. The ambivalence that a young person feels about giving up the protection that their eating disorder provides can be very strong and therefore resistance to being treated can be fierce. The nurse should expect such resistance to continue until the young person can depend on the nurse or a parent to contain their feelings adequately. During the assessment stage, the young person's story will have been outlined. The nurse should have identified predisposing, precipitating and perpetuating factors, and plans towards recovery should have been set with the young person and their family or carers. It is important to note that evidence-based, specific and recommended treatments for eating disorder patients, such as cognitive behaviour therapy, family therapy, and individual psychotherapy, may all take place in addition to the treatment approach that is outlined below.

Taking charge of physical symptoms

As well as helping young people with eating disorders develop their identity and find a voice for feelings, it is important to take charge of physical symptoms and help young people towards physical recovery. Weight restoration and normalising eating patterns are at the core of the treatment process. Before anything else can happen, physical health has to be stabilised and parents have to be able to feed their child again. This is particularly significant in anorexia nervosa. Critical physical symptoms require immediate medical treatment, particularly where preservation of life is an issue as in life-threatening anorexia nervosa. The process of helping a young person to gain weight or to stop vomiting, when this is their biggest dread, can be incredibly challenging. It requires skills of sensitivity to the young person's fear, and firmness to manage the resistance. When young people reach the stage in treatment where reflection is possible, they often report a sense of relief that adults work hard to help them resist their eating disorder and protect them from their addictive behaviours. During the early stages of treatment however, the nurse should expect this experience to feel something like dragging a hibernating bear into a blizzard when it is still winter. Susan insisted:

> *'All my friends are thinner than me, I feel so fat, like a great big pig – disgusting, look at my thighs, why are you trying to make me so enormous, you feed people up like turkeys in here.'*

However, it is crucial that the resistance is weathered. At first, the young person can feel helpless in the face of giving up the control provided by their eating disorder. It is extremely important for the nurse to strike the right balance in sharing control with the young person. Until the young person develops the motivation to look after themselves again, the adults must be in control, taking charge using as much collaboration as possible. However, it is also important that as the young person progresses, control is gradually taken back. Achieving the right balance reduces the potential for young people to feel overwhelmed by guilt at siding with the nurse over and above their eating disorder.

When developing an eating plan, the nurse should make a statement about the feat that is to be tackled. They may suggest to the young people that it can feel like hiking up a mountain but that they will be supported, step by step. After taking a history of a typical day's eating, a balanced daily meal plan is devised. This is developed in consultation with parents or carers and the day is divided into small meals and snacks. The calorie content should be tailored in relation to what the young person has previously been eating, but should start at around 1000 calories, building up to an average of 2500 through increases of 250 calories each time depending on the amount of weight gained. Expected weight gain should be between 0.5–1kg per week for patients with anorexia nervosa (NICE 2004). Some professionals believe that setting target weights should be avoided. This is because they are not statistically derived, do not account for differences in frame and shape and young people may become fixated on numbers instead of their overall progress. Instead, it may be helpful to talk about the need for the body to develop as it should do, and that this is the goal of weight gain.

It is not only in anorexia nervosa that nurses may need to take control of physical symptoms. Until they develop a sense of internal control, young people with bulimia nervosa will also need support to control their binge eating. Nurses can help young people to control their bingeing by supporting them to be occupied, and by restricting access to the foods that they binge on at the times that they usually turn to these behaviours. With bulimia nervosa, it is much more helpful to support young people through a programme of increased normal activity and exercise rather than through dieting behaviours, though these will need careful monitoring to ensure they do not become excessive. Binges often happen in the evening, a time when comfort is commonly sought.

In cases where physical wellbeing is at serious risk, such as with dehydration, circulatory failure or significant growth delay, a programme of refeeding via nasogastric tube performed as an in-patient may be necessary. Refeeding should only be performed under medical supervision. The nasogastric tube usually remains in place until the young person can manage without its support. Small feeds in bolus form are given throughout the day so as to mimic normal eating patterns, and the content should be reviewed regularly. Total parenteral nutrition should not be used for young people with anorexia nervosa, unless there is significant gastrointestinal dysfunction (NICE 2004). Physical monitoring during refeeding is crucial as a young person who has starved themselves for some time is at risk of developing refeeding syndrome. This occurs when a young person who has been previously malnourished is fed with high carbohydrate meals. A range of medical complications can arise due to changes in phosphate, magnesium and potassium levels. A young person who is undergoing nasogastric refeeding should still attend mealtimes and have a small meal placed in front of them so that the expectation of eating normally remains consistent. This also communicates that the nurses are hopeful despite the young person's despair. Sitting at the table rather than taking food alone also provides the benefit of social intercourse and peer support, both of which are very powerful in terms of validating the young person's individuality.

Managing mealtimes

Susan would often say:

> 'I won't eat it if my dad goes near it! I have always been allowed to serve my own food at home. Mum – you serve it! You know how to put it on the plate so it doesn't all touch.'

The aim of a mealtime is to ensure that the young person both eats enough and also has an experience of being understood. Regular meals with families are therefore very important as this demonstrates the adults working together to support the young person on both of these tasks. Nurses should encourage family members to adopt styles of interaction that facilitate eating, as well as support parents to try different methods of supporting their child. Supporting a young person to eat when they experience food as an indigestible poison is an intensely distressing experience, and can make the parent feel like a bully. Again, attention must be paid to the feelings that are evoked, as this is commonly a signal as to how the young person feels. In this case, they are bullied by their eating disorder and the nurse must take care to ensure these feelings are not acted out, or treatment will become punishing. Subsequently, young people who feel 'bad' will believe they got what they deserved. It is vital that nurse and parents develop a balance between being firm and clear, at the same time as remaining nurturing and flexible. They can acknowledge the young person's difficult feelings and recognise that eating must seem unbearable, but it is important that the adults are clear that this step has to be taken on the young person's journey to recovery. Not only can the young person become exhausted during mealtime management, but the nurse and parents who support them require patience and need to set firm limits. Encouraging the young person to continue eating until their meal is finished can be a demanding task for all and support for the parents and supervision for the nurse can be beneficial.

Like all other activities, supervised mealtimes should have boundaries around them. Initially, young people should not be involved in food preparation and should have very limited choices about the food they eat. It is reasonable to agree some dislikes in advance, but nutritional and calorific value should be maintained. Young people in in-patient settings will need close supervision during mealtimes and meals should be time-limited (50 minutes for meals and 20 minutes for snacks). Meals should take equal importance during the day with everything else, and should not overrun despite what has been eaten. Completing meals demands an enormous amount of energy from the young person, and so they will need a break to clear their minds, and gather their strength ready for the next meal. The young person should be informed that the nurse understands how painful eating is so they do not have to engage in behaviours that demonstrate their pain. Reassurance from the nurse that they will be understood and supported can make the young person feel protected from their eating disorder and freed from succumbing to its demands.

Feelings that are expressed at the table can be acknowledged but the focus has to remain on eating rather than exploration during the meal. Separating food from feelings is very important, as it is these two in an eating disorder that have become inextricably linked. Exploration can take place during debriefing or in a prearranged session with the nurse. The form of support and encouragement that each young person finds helpful will be individual and may change. Some young people gather strength from being given positive praise. Others feel overwhelmingly guilty and would rather a statement was made that acknowledges they worked hard (Wood & Lewer 2004). It can be useful to talk to the young person about them being full with feelings that have not yet been digested. Until they can be digested in the relationship with the nurse and team members, the space inside for food feels limited. Working on feelings at the same time as increasing food intake is therefore necessary. This is why it is so important that the nurses take notice of the feelings that young people express, as they are messages and signals about the problems that need to be worked on. Time to talk through feelings before meals, and debriefing afterwards, even for five minutes, is often helpful for young people with eating disorders. By talking about just one thing they may be worried about, a space may be created which may make the next mealtime a tiny bit easier.

Susan described her eating disorder as a loud voice in her head telling her what to do. She felt compelled to listen to it even if she didn't want to. This should not be understood as a hallucination, characteristic of a psychotic disorder, but is a common phenomenon. It serves to create an identity for the illness as something that is separate from but a part of the young person, which can be taken charge of with the support from others. Exploring the young person's insights in these terms can feel supportive for the young person, as it allows them to appreciate being the victim of the illness rather than the creator of it. In key sessions with the nurse, the young person can be asked to draw what they imagine their eating disorder looks like, and to give it a name and describe its personality traits. When at the table, this gives a clearer image to what it is that they are working hard to fight against. The nurse's role during mealtime management is to model how she manages anxiety through the use of clear, firm, gentle and soothing expectations and limits. For parents, it can be useful for one adult to take charge of the social side of the meal and for the other to support the young person and challenge issues related to eating. Parents often take turns in taking on these roles and responsibilities.

Developing identity

An anxiety of Susan's was:

'The thing is, what if once its gone there's nothing there underneath?'

Difficulties related to growing up, separation and individuation are usual to most young people with eating disorders. It is no coincidence that they commonly arise in adolescence, the time when separating from parents begins (Nelson et al. 2005). For successful separation to occur, a sense of self is necessary so that reliance on parental figures is not so necessary. A sense of self arises from secure and dependent relationships with adults. In attachment theory, it is stated that identity and personality develop through the infant being engaged in a 'holding' secure relationship with the caregiver. The task of the nurse is to provide this holding relationship that parallels that of a parent and infant and brings about emotional containment (Williams 1997). This delicate process is achieved through the nurse tuning into the young person and allowing him or herself to feel the feelings that the young person feels. This gives a sense to the young person that they have got their message across and can now be understood without words (Briggs 2002). The nurse then uses her voice to represent the feelings in a reassuring and calm way even if what she felt was fear, anger or uncertainty. In doing this, she regulates and calms the young person's emotional state, so they do not feel that things are spiralling out of control. Over time, this protective regulation by the nurse or parent will be internalised by the young person and act like an internal protective muscle, which soothes and regulates at times of anxiety and uncertainty. In this way, it becomes possible for uncomfortable feelings to be experienced, tolerated and managed. This results in a sense of self developing and the need for the eating disorder becomes less.

Finding a voice for feelings

Susan tried to explain:

> 'It sounds stupid, but the most important thing is that you have taught me is how to feel. I never really understood that when I felt hot and tight inside, that I was angry. Those were the times when I used to decide I won't eat today.'

Eating disorders represent an internal difficulty in communication. There is commonly a struggle to recognise and describe emotions and feelings, and to differentiate between emotional states and bodily sensations. A secure relationship allows the young person's emotional state to be regulated by another, leading to a sense of safety that allows feelings to be felt. This may be a new experience for the young person. Feelings will be able to be expressed much more as the relationship with the nurse develops, and this has been described as stage 2 in the management of eating disorders (Lask & Bryant-Waugh 2000). Tolerating the expression of feelings is an essential part of the recovery process and all expressions of feelings should be positively affirmed, and encouraged by the nurse. In the absence of language, other forms of expression can be utilised. These include drawing, writing a feelings diary, making music and playing, which are all ways to support this process. This is illustrated in the following excerpt:

> 'Esme used a traffic-light system to communicate to her parents what she needed from them. Wearing a green hair clip signalled she felt ok. A yellow one meant that she was feeling uncertain and needed her Mum's reassurance, and a red one meant she needed time in the garden with her Mum as she felt like she might explode.'

Anger management sessions can be useful at this stage, in which physiological signs of anger are taught in order to help connect bodily sensations to feelings. However, it is important for the young person to explore other ways of expressing anger, until the voice is found and language is developed. Young people have found ripping up newspapers, punch bag sessions, and hitting pillows all useful ways of getting their feelings out. A further reason why emotional language needs to be developed is that feelings can be named rather than simply expressed. Words can digest, describe and contain the feelings that have got stuck inside, and prevent highly charged emotional releases from bursting out through the body as they have done so with the eating behaviours. The use of stories and metaphor can be very helpful in developing language (Dwivedi 1997). It can be very frightening and overwhelming for young people with eating disorders to find that they have a voice after repressing it for so long. They may benefit from practice time to develop their voice. Shouting in the garden, singing and talking to others allow the voice to be used and heard. It is important that adults support the new assertive adolescent whilst also managing them as one normally would, with limit setting and clear expectations.

Treatment stage 3: recovery

Recovery comes about after considerable emotional development within the young person. Many aspects of the process are completely new and recovery is therefore a path that must be tentatively and thoughtfully trodden. It may be helpful to define recovery more as 'a capacity to cope' rather than a belief that everything is completely 'better'. This capacity involves an ability to acknowledge and name difficulties rather than being in the throes of the eating disorder where difficulties are denied or minimised. Recovery also involves a capacity to tolerate grey areas and times of uncertainty, rather than having to have things black and white. Whilst it is change that is hoped for, it is also precisely when change begins to occur that things can often seem to go backwards. This is often a result of the young person testing out the security of the relationships that they are learning to depend on. Young people should be reminded that change can happen when we least expect it, and it can come about in the most difficult of times.

Hopefulness and a belief that things can and will get better are crucial aspects in the recovery stage during the treatment of eating disorders. At this stage, it is not unusual for some pain and areas of difficulty to persist. However, emergency responses are no longer demanded. The journey that has been travelled so far has involved the young person and their family making considerable changes to the ways in which they relate to one another. At this stage, coping should involve the whole family finding ways to live with some of the feelings and issues that the eating disorder has raised. By the time the young person has reached the recovery stage, the goals of treatment that were outlined at the beginning of the journey will be partly met. The young person, family, nurse and multidisciplinary team will have developed a much better understanding of the young person's eating disorder and should be able to communicate with openness, honesty and sincerity.

Developing networks and managing transitions

People with eating disorders can be seen to have temporarily retreated into their safe, internal world (Emanuel 2001). As such, a major part of recovery is of rejoining the outer world, a little like a butterfly emerging from its safe cocoon. The transition requires gentle, firm and sensitive coaxing and management on the part of the nurse. To follow the butterfly analogy, the cocoon may have felt protective enough for the young person to be able to develop and grow, but shouldn't have been so protective that the realities of life have been lost. Encouraging the young person to shed their cocoon can be facilitated by discussion about daily newspapers, discussions about the news and trips out of hospital for young people who are receiving in-patient treatment. Letter-writing and e-mail contact with friends is invaluable as it keeps the young person in touch with aspects of their life that were pleasurable and unaffected by the illness. It is helpful if the young person continues to remain in contact with as many aspects of their educational and social life as it is safe to do during the course of their treatment. This serves to affirm that their place in society, at school, or with friends is still there for them. As time progresses, more and more contact with the outside world can take place whilst they and their family continue to have the support of the treatment team who can continue to work with them on any difficulties that may arise. A consistently useful exercise for the nurse to plan with the young person involves how they might respond to questions from others about where they have been during the course of their treatment. Again, planning as much as possible offers a sense of predictability and safety.

Young people who are recovering from eating disorders often struggle with moving on. The young person will need to be supported to hold a balance in their mind of all of the experiences that they have had, both difficult and helpful and to take stock of the progress that they have made. They will often require a lot of notice about a change to their treatment status, or of ending, just as they need notice about their schedules in the context of boundaries earlier in the chapter. Ending is a decision that should be ideally taken in collaboration with the patient and the family, so it should come as no surprise as the goals and progress will have been regularly reviewed. Young people who are recovering from anorexia nervosa sometimes worry about returning to 'normal' life again. They may need a lot of reassurance that they will not be forgotten about just because they are no longer the emaciated, vomiting person with the eating disorder. During the recovery process, they have to be able to trust that even if they look better on the outside, adults will know that on the inside things remain difficult for them and for this they will need ongoing support.

Conclusion

This chapter has focused on the task of nursing children and young people with eating disorders. This task is complex and challenging, and involves the process of emotional containment throughout the young person's treatment journey. This process is necessary to allow emotional development and physical changes to be supported. It is hoped that this chapter has provided some useful insights and interesting ideas that can be utilised in nursing interventions with young people with eating disorders. The skills necessary for a nurse to work successfully with young people with eating disorders include: resilience; persistence; sensitivity; firmness; genuineness; and humour.

Young people with eating disorders invest a lot of their emotional energy and focus on controlling weight and maladaptive behaviours. It has been demonstrated that the nurse, the multidisciplinary team and young person's family or carers must understand these behaviours if they are to be successfully addressed. Space for regular reflection in groups and individually is necessary to enable reflection and understanding of the issues that are aroused from being ill. A crucial aspect of nursing young people with eating disorders is managing the overwhelming anxiety arising from the serious physical state and psychological complications that are present. In doing so, experiences and feelings can be understood and the contribution of the nurse will be optimised.

References

Bion, W. (1974). *Experiences in Groups and Other Papers*. New York: Basic Books.

Briggs, A. (2002). *Surviving Space: papers on infant observation*. New York: Karnac Books.

Bryant-Waugh, R. & Lask, B. (1995). Annotation: eating disorders in children. *Journal of Child Psychology and Psychiatry*, (36), 191–202.

Bryant-Waugh, R. & Lask, B. (2004). *Eating Disorders: a parent's guide*. New York: Brunner-Routledge.

Childline (2003). *I'm in Control: calls to Childline about eating disorders*. London: Childline.

Crouch, W. (1998). The therapeutic milieu and treatment of emotionally disturbed children: clinical application. *Clinical Child Psychology and Psychiatry*, (3), 115–29.

Dare, C., Le Grange, D., Eisler, I. & Rutherford, J. (1994). Redefining the psychosomatic family: family process of 26 eating disorder families. *International Journal of Eating Disorders*, (16), 211–26.

Dwivedi, K. (1997). *The therapeutic use of stories*. London: Routledge.

Emanuel, R. (2001). A void: an exploration of defences against sensing nothingness. *International Journal of Psychoanalysis*, (82), 1069–84.

Farrell, E. (2000). *Lost for Words: the psychoanalysis of anorexia and bulimia*. New York: Other Press.

Fombonne, E. (1995). Anorexia nervosa: no evidence of an increase. *British Journal of Psychiatry*, (166), 462–71.

Fosson, A., Knibbs, J., Bryant-Waugh, R. & Lask, B. (1987). Early onset anorexia nervosa. *Archives of Disease in Childhood*, (62), 114–18.

Geller, J. (2002). What a motivational approach is and what a motivational approach isn't: reflections and responses. *European Eating Disorders Review*, (10), 155–60.

Geller, J., Cockell, S. & Drab, D. (2001). Assessing readiness for change in the eating disorders: the psychometric properties of the readiness and motivation interview. *Psychological Assessment*, (13), 189–98.

Geller, J., Williams, K. & Srikameswaran, S. (2001). Clinician stance in the treatment of chronic eating disorders. *European Eating Disorders Review*, (9), 365–73.

Gowers, S. (2002). Eating disorders in childhood and adolescence. *Psychiatry*, **1** (2), 21–25.

Herpertz-Dahlmann, B. & Remschmidt, H. (1993). Depression and psychosocial adjustment in adolescent anorexia nervosa: a controlled 3-year follow-up study. *European Child and Adolescent Psychiatry*, (2), 146–54.

Honig, P. (2000). Family work. In: Lask, B. & Bryant-Waugh, R. (Eds). *Anorexia Nervosa and Related Eating Disorders in Childhood and Adolescence*. Brighton: Psychology Press.

Krautter, T. & Lock, J. (2004). Treatment of adolescent anorexia nervosa using manualized family based treatment. *Clinical Case Studies*, 107–23.

Lask, B. & Bryant-Waugh, R. (2000). *Anorexia Nervosa and Related Eating Disorders in Childhood and Adolescence*. (2nd edn). Brighton: Psychology Press.

Magagna, J. (2000). Individual psychotherapy. In: Lask, B. & Bryant-Waugh, R. (Eds). *Anorexia Nervosa and Related Eating Disorders in Childhood and Adolescence*. Brighton: Psychology Press.

National Health Service Executive (1999). *Effective Care Coordination in Mental Health Services: modernising the care programme approach*. London: NHSE.

National Institute for Clinical Excellence (2004). *Core Interventions in the Treatment and Management of Anorexia Nervosa, Bulimia Nervosa and Related Eating Disorders*. London: NICE.

Nelson, E., Leibenluft, E., McClure, E. & Pine, D. (2005). The social reorientation of adolescence: a neuroscience perspective on the process and its relation to psychopathology. *Psychological Medicine*, **35** (2), 163–74.

Nicholls, D., De Bruyn, R. & Gordon, I. (2000). *Physical assessment and complications in anorexia nervosa and related eating disorders in childhood and adolescence*. Brighton: Psychology Press.

North, C. & Gowers, S. (1999). Anorexia nervosa, psychopathology and outcome. *International Journal of Eating Disorders*, (26), 386–91.

Robinson, P. & McHugh, P. (1995). A physiology of starvation that sustains eating disorders. In: Szmukler, G., Dare, C. & Treasure, J. (Eds). *Handbook of Eating Disorders: theory, treatment and research*. New York: John Wiley.

Salzberger-Wittenberg, I. *Psychoanalytical insight and relationships*. London: Whurr Publishers.

Schmidt, U. & Treasure, J. (1997). *Clinician's Guide to Getting Better Bit(e) by Bit(e): a survival kit for sufferers of bulimia nervosa and binge eating disorders*. Brighton: Psychology Press.

Seinfeld, J. (1996). *Containing rage, terror and despair: an object relations approach to psychotherapy*. London: Aronson.

Williams, G. (1997). *Internal Landscapes and Foreign Bodies: eating disorders and other pathologies*. New York: Routledge.

Williams, G., Williams, P., Desmarais, J. & Ravenscroft, K. (2003). *Exploring Eating Disorders in Adolescents: the generosity of acceptance*. London: Karnac.

Wood, D. & Lewer, L. (2004). *Affect Regulation, Mentalisation and the Therapeutic Milieu*. Edinburgh: Royal College of Psychiatrists Child Faculty Annual Meeting.

Chapter 7

Young People and Early Onset Psychosis: a nursing perspective

Sally Sanderson

Key points

- Schizophrenia is the most persistent and disabling of the major mental illnesses. Although childhood onset schizophrenia is rare, the rate of onset for all psychotic disorders rises sharply during adolescence, particularly between the ages of 15 and 19.

- With an increased risk of relapse and disproportionate suicide rates occurring within the first five years of a psychotic disorder, early intervention has the potential to create real and meaningful differences to a young person's outcomes.

- Assessing all young people with first episode psychosis as soon as possible, and preferably within 24 hours, may have a positive impact on the course and prognosis of their illness.

- Treatment for psychosis involves the use of antipsychotic medication, individual psychological support and a range of psychosocial and family interventions.

- Strong links with schools and educational institutions are vital to promote and maintain recovery, to encourage social inclusion and to reduce the stigma associated with serious mental illness. Nurses in hospital, community settings and schools are well placed to form effective networks.

- Nurses are in key positions to provide psychological interventions for young people, their families and carers, across a range of practice settings. Nurses who have been trained to use cognitive behaviour therapy (CBT) for psychosis can apply this approach to assess individual symptoms such as auditory hallucinations, delusions and paranoia.

Introduction

Psychosis is a term used to describe a range of conditions, including schizophrenia, which are characterised by a loss of contact with reality, typically including delusions (false ideas about what is taking place or who one is) and hallucinations (seeing or hearing things which aren't there) (Medline 2005). With a lifetime incidence of below 1% (World Health Organization 2001), psychosis remains a relatively uncommon disorder. However, it is ranked as the third most disabling condition, behind only quadriplegia and dementia (WHO 2001), due to its disproportionate impact upon the individual, their family and the wider society (Weiden & Olfson 1995). During the early 1990s the annual cost of schizophrenia in the UK reached £397 million (Frith & Johnstone 2003), a figure that demonstrates the huge financial cost and burden to the state. However the human costs to the individual and their family are less well understood. Although clearly immense, the needs of the individual suffering from a psychotic disorder are complex and heterogeneous. When this is more closely examined within the context of adolescent development, the needs of the individual and their family become amplified (Yung & McGorry 1996). This chapter will explore some of the issues raised in caring for the young person who is experiencing a psychotic disorder and their family from a nursing perspective. It will focus upon:

- The prevalence of psychotic disorders.
- The course and prognosis of psychotic disorders.
- The early intervention in psychosis agenda, with reference to the national and international driving forces.
- The specific issues of engagement and assessment together with an examination of evidence-based interventions for both the young person and their family.
- Some of the specific challenges raised whilst nursing children and young people, illustrated through the use of case studies.

Prevalence

Affecting approximately 1% of the population worldwide, schizophrenia is the most persistent and disabling of the major mental illnesses (McGlashan 1998). Childhood or pre-adolescent onset schizophrenia (below the age of 12) is very rare, with an estimated incidence of between 0.14 and 1.0 per 10 000 (Hafner et al. 1998; Hollis 2000). It is acknowledged, however, that the rate of onset for all psychotic disorders rises sharply during adolescence, particularly between the ages of 15 and 19 (Hafner et al. 1998). Within this younger age range schizophrenia is more common within males by a factor of approximately 2:1, although this difference becomes less marked with a later age of onset (Russell et al. 1998). Adolescence is a crucial life-stage which involves the consolidation of identity, the quest for independence, educational and vocational endeavours and the development of important peer relationships (McGorry & Edwards 1997). It also represents a time of development and change, just as individuals begin to realise their potential (Parlato et al. 1999). Thus, when the development of a psychotic illness occurs during adolescence or young adulthood, the effects can be devastating (Yung & McGorry 1996; McGorry & Edwards 1997; Hollis 2000); and the associated needs of the individuals and their family or carers may be many and varied (Parlato et al. 1999).

Course and prognosis

Kaepelin & Bleuler believed schizophrenia to be evident, albeit more rarely than in adulthood, during childhood and adolescence (Hollis 2000). In the years following Kraepelin's & Bleuler's initial work on this 'dementia praecox' in the early 1900s (see Bleuler 1911), there was often heavy pessimism associated with schizophrenia and the diagnosis was often viewed as a life sentence (Albiston et al. 1998; McGorry 1998). There was thought to be little hope for improvement, let alone recovery (Edwards et al. 1994: Albiston et al. 1998). However, the deteriorating course proposed by Kraepelin has since been brought into question. Ciompi (1980) noted a high degree of variability in the course of schizophrenia, with only one-third of individuals displaying the chronic course assumed by Kraepelin to be a defining feature of the disorder. In their book on early onset psychosis, Birchwood et al. (1998) cite Bleuler (1978), noting that a 'plateau of psychopathology and disability' is reached early in the illness, a finding subsequently replicated by numerous studies (Dube et al. 1984; Carpenter & Strauss 1991). This finding has been further refined, with the suggestion that deterioration, though variable, occurs early in the course of schizophrenia, often stabilising within two to five years from onset (Birchwood et al. 1998).

With the growing interest in the early years of psychosis, also came increasing recognition of the risks associated with that period. These risks include: increased relapse rates; increased rates of decline in cognitive ability and social functioning; the development of traumatic symptoms resulting from both the experiences associated with the illness and also its treatments; and the increased risk of suicide. Coining the phrase 'the critical period' Birchwood et al. (1998) proposed that focused interventions within the early years following onset had a disproportionate impact relative to interventions later in the course of the disorder. This was found to result in a substantial reduction in morbidity, together with a better quality of life for individuals and their families. The 1990s witnessed a growing optimism regarding improved outcomes for individuals experiencing a psychotic episode, together with a drive to reform the access to, and the quality of, treatments and services available. This was partly due to the development of novel antipsychotic medicines which reported improved efficacy while inducing fewer side-effects; however, there was also a renewed interest in the psychological and psychosocial management of psychotic symptoms.

Early intervention

Whilst the significance of intervening early in the course of psychosis has been acknowledged now for over 50 years (Cameron 1938; McGorry 1998), a developing body of research evidence has continued to demonstrate the efficacy of early detection and intervention in achieving a measurable reduction in such areas as treatment resistance, outcome and recovery (Edwards et al. 1994; Falloon et al. 1998; McGlashan 1998).

With the increased risk of relapse, and disproportionate suicide rates within the first five years of a psychotic disorder, early intervention has the potential to create real and meaningful differences to a young person's outcomes. Throughout the past two decades in Australia the increasing awareness and understanding of the significance of the early course of psychosis has been led by the work of the Early Psychosis Prevention and Intervention Centre (EPPIC) (www.eppic.org.au). Focusing upon the unique needs of young people with psychosis while being mindful of the problems created as a result of standard care, the development of a comprehensive evidence base has resulted in a new era in early psychosis services. Adopting a recovery focus, significant emphasis has been placed upon not only the effective management of symptoms, but also on the development of life-skills within a social inclusion framework. The early stage of psychosis is now a subject of wide international interest, with a project called the Initiative to Reduce the Impact of Schizophrenia (IRIS) leading the way in the UK (www.iris-initiative.org.uk). In response to the overwhelming evidence supporting early intervention in psychosis, the British government announced the development of 50 early psychosis services (Department of Health 2000). The report *Improvement, Expansion and Reform* set the expectation that all children and adolescents who develop a first episode of psychosis wait no longer than three months for a service and have support for a minimum of three years (DoH 2002). Key requirements of these services are to:

- Reduce the length of time that young people remain undiagnosed and untreated.
- Provide a seamless service available for those from age 14 to 35 that effectively integrates child, adolescent and adult mental health services and works in partnership with primary care, education, social services, and youth and other services.
- Develop meaningful engagement, provide evidence-based interventions and promote recovery during the early phase of illness.
- Increase stability in the lives of service users, facilitate development and provide opportunities for personal fulfilment.
- Ensure that the care is transferred thoughtfully and effectively at the end of the treatment period.
- Reduce the stigma associated with psychosis and improve professional and lay awareness of the symptoms of psychosis and the need for early intervention.

In addition, the *Newcastle Early Psychosis Declaration*, supported by the World Health Organization was launched in 2002. This sets out core values, a clear vision and the action required to achieve early intervention and recovery for all young people experiencing psychosis. Although the declaration is not a service or performance-monitoring tool, a number of research-based areas for action are identified in which nurses play a central role. These are: access and engagement; promoting recovery and re-engagement with everyday life; family engagement and support; provision of practitioner learning; and raising community awareness and health promotion.

The cost of untreated psychosis

Adolescent schizophrenia often presents with an insidious rather than acute onset. For this reason, early recognition of the disorder can be problematic, as premorbid cognitive and social impairments gradually shade into prodromal symptoms before the onset of positive psychotic symptoms (Hollis 2000). Effective treatments are readily available for young people with psychosis. Generally speaking, the earlier treatment is started, the quicker and better the recovery. A number of studies have identified the occurrence of delays of up to two years in accessing effective treatment (Keshevan & Schooler 1992). This is not only distressing for the young person concerned, but the duration of untreated psychosis has been closely linked inversely to the time and quality of remission (Loebel et al. 1992). Increased understanding of the role that duration of untreated psychosis plays in the course of the disorder has led to its recognition as a key measure and indicator of outcome and prognosis for sufferers (Larsen et al. 1996). It has been suggested that the longer the psychosis remains untreated, the more severe symptoms become (Drake et al. 2000). This study modelled the duration of untreated psychosis against short-term outcomes. The biggest gains, in terms of improvements in outcome, were found by bringing treatment forward by a period of one to two weeks in cases where the psychosis had remained untreated for a relatively short period of time. This produced better outcomes than bringing the treatment forward by one to two *months* for those people who had remained untreated for a long time. The implication for service delivery is that assessing all young people with first-episode psychosis as soon as possible, and preferably within 24 hours, may have an ameliorating impact on outcomes.

It has also been proposed that delay in gaining access to appropriate services may be a direct consequence of the stigma associated with schizophrenia and mental illness (Sayce 2000). It has been estimated that up to one-third of individuals with a diagnosable mental illness avoid seeking the appropriate help and treatment as a direct consequence of the stigma associated with mental illness (Surgeon General 1999; Gaebel et al. 2002). Though widely acknowledged, this should not be accepted as the sole cause for an extended duration of untreated psychosis. Other reasons for such untreated psychosis may include the difficulties in establishing a clear diagnosis in the early stages of psychosis, due the insidious nature and relative rareness of these disorders (McGorry et al. 1995; Hafner et al. 1998). There is however, evidence of service users making repeated attempts to seek help. It has been suggested that some individuals who present for help, would and could have provided sufficient information to produce a clinical diagnosis and commence effective treatment. However, it was discovered that the mental health professionals conducting interviews often failed to persist in their questioning or failed to ask sufficiently in-depth questions to elicit this revealing information (De Haan et al. 2002).

In order to address the extended periods of waiting for treatment that young people with psychotic symptoms currently experience, there is a need to attempt to eradicate some of the myths surrounding mental illness and improve general awareness of the value of seeking early help. Comprehensive education packages aimed at improving the mental health literacy of communities have proved to produce a significant reduction in treatment delay. The TIPS (see glossary) project from Norway (www.tips-info.com) demonstrated that a substantial reduction in treatment delay could be achieved through a widely reaching awareness-raising programme. This project has also demonstrated a reduction in the stigma surrounding serious mental health problems. Given that all UK students in secondary education now have time dedicated to look at health and welfare issues, through the personal health and social education (PHSE) agenda and with the recent emphasis on developing 'healthy' schools, it is not unreasonable to suggest that all students should be exposed to mental health literacy programmes. Such programmes should not only focus on increasing understanding of mental health problems, but should also incorporate the development of healthy coping strategies and information about how and where to access help if a family member shows signs of such a problem.

Psychological interventions

The argument for antipsychotic medication as the mainstay of intervention for psychotic disorders is widely acknowledged, but additional benefits may be gained from the use of complimentary psychological approaches (Falloon et al. 1996; Penn & Mueser 1996). The late twentieth century saw a growing body of research evidence which advocated the use of individualised CBT interventions to reduce the distress associated with the experience of residual psychotic symptoms (Haddock et al. 1998). Nurses who have been trained to use CBT for psychosis can apply this approach to assess individual symptoms such as auditory hallucinations, delusions and paranoia. Recognition of the potential benefits of CBT for people suffering from schizophrenia has led to the development of clinical standards and guidelines by the National Institute for Clinical Excellence (NICE). The use of CBT is advocated for all people suffering from this disorder and for their families (NICE 2002).

Psychological interventions with young people with psychotic disorders involve a combination of methods, including distraction from persistent voices, focusing on the auditory hallucinations, and techniques where the primary aim of intervention is anxiety reduction (Bentall et al. 1994). These interventions are based on assessments, questionnaires and self-rating scales. The Cognitive Assessment Schedule (CAS) (Chadwick et al. 1996) can be used to assess the nature of auditory hallucinations, the evidence young people attribute to their beliefs, and their emotional and behavioural responses to delusions, voices and paranoia. Similarly, the Beliefs About Voices Questionnaire (BAVQ) (Birchwood & Chadwick 1997) is a psychometrically validated measure of key beliefs about auditory hallucinations. This enables the nurse or other mental health professional to evaluate the malevolence, or benevolence of voices, as well as aspects of coping such as resistance and engagement. In addition, an adapted Topograhpy of Voices Rating Scale (Hustig & Hafner 1990) can be used to measure the frequency, audibility and intrusiveness of voices reported by young people. The primary aim of CBT for psychosis is to enable the young person to cope with their psychotic symptoms, reappraise their meaning and make them less distressing. Positive psychotic symptoms such as command auditory hallucinations can be assessed and managed within a CBT frame-work. Close attention is paid to the voices themselves, the meaning a young person attaches to their voices, and how they subsequently feel and behave as a consequence. Coping strategy enhancement (CSE) is formulated from the work of Yusupoff and Tarrier (1996), and involves ways of empowering young people to cope with symptoms that may be distressing or upsetting. Altern-ative ways of thinking and behaving are explored. In order to use CBT with young people with psychosis it is necessary first to perform a thorough assess-ment. This should include: exploration of activating events occurring prior to the onset of psychotic symptoms; assessment of the levels of conviction, control and distress associated with the psychotic symptoms; assessment of the meaning that the young person attributes to their psychotic symptoms; assessment of dysfunctional assumptions and beliefs about others; assessment of adaptive and maladaptive coping strategies; and an assessment of any con-current risk of violence to self or others arising from the psychotic symptoms (McDougall 1999).

It has been suggested that the styles and patterns of intervention for the early phase of a psychotic disorder differ from those required later in the course of the illness. This indicates the need for a staged approach, however it is recognised that the timing and quality of intervention are crucial. Active supportive psychological intervention, together with strong emotional support, is essential in the early stages of psychosis. It is acknowledged that this can be difficult to provide when engagement is undermined by an array of issues, not least by the obstacles raised by the disorder itself. During the later stages

---

Charlotte

Charlotte, aged 14, is detained within Section 3 of the Mental Health Act 1983, following attempts to abduct a baby from a local nursery. Charlotte is an only child who has grown up in care and experienced numerous and disrupted foster placements. Charlotte has no close friends of her own age and is described by her teacher as being quiet, thoughtful and considerate. Charlotte had recently told both her social worker and teacher that she was going to 'pinch' a baby.

Charlotte was first assessed by an adolescent forensic mental health nurse in police custody. She stated that she believed the baby's mother was about to sacrifice him and so she attempted to take him to save his life. Charlotte believed that the baby was special and now belonged to her. Charlotte was assessed by a police surgeon and released from custody without charge. She was then sectioned and admitted to the local adolescent unit, where, on admission, it was clear that she was floridly psychotic. She agreed to take atypical antipsychotic medication. Charlotte described an elaborate delusional system and said that voices were talking about her in whispers. She believed that nurses could place 'wishes' in her head. During the initial stages of her admission Charlotte was guarded, reticent about her thoughts and feelings, and difficult to engage. With close support from her primary nurse, and with involvement by her social worker, Charlotte was eventually able to complete a BAVQ and a self-rating scale which measured the conviction, control and distress associated with her beliefs about the 'wishes' and voices she was hearing.

During an eight-month period of treatment Charlotte was diagnosed as having paranoid schizophrenia and was stabilised on antipsychotic medication. While her delusional system remained largely intact, her voices almost completely disappeared. Using a CBT approach, Charlotte became able to recognise that her psychotic symptoms were triggered by strong feelings of loneliness and sadness. Associated levels of distress were low and Charlotte developed coping strategies such as distracting herself by listening to music on her Walkman. The CAMHS multidisciplinary team paid close attention to Charlotte's beliefs and the potential risks to others arising from these. Charlotte was able to resume education in mainstream school, completed a programme of social skills-building and was successfully discharged to a specialist foster placement. She remains under the care and treatment of the local specialist CAMHS.

---

of the recovery process, specific strategies to prevent psychotic symptoms and increase social inclusions become increasingly important. Perhaps the most important aspect of individual psychological work is the process of enabling the young person to make sense of their experiences and the promotion of psychological and social recovery.

One further key aspect of working with young people who have experienced a first episode of psychosis is concentrating on the prevention of subsequent episodes. The identification of idiosyncratic relapse signatures through the recognition of early warning signs (Birchwood et al. 2000) enables individuals to access support at the earliest sign of symptoms reemerging. It is then possible to manage problems early and a relapse of psychotic symptoms may be averted. This approach also serves to enhance the young person's autonomy, leading to a reduction in the feelings of powerlessness that psychotic disorders can often create.

Peter

Peter, now 17, first experienced a psychotic episode at the age of 15. Over the past two years he has been taking large doses of antipsychotic medication and has become significantly dependent upon his community mental health nurse. Whilst repeated attempts have been made to enable Peter to become more independent and function autonomously, he has remained reluctant to do so. On closer investigation by the nurse, it became evident that Peter was afraid that he would relapse and become unable to cope. The nurse spent time with Peter exploring his high-risk periods and also attempting to identify his early warning signs. Coincidentally, a period of stressful life-events led to the breakthrough of some previously well-controlled positive psychotic symptoms. Supported by using a relapse-prevention approach by the nurse, Peter was able to manage this period with limited disruption to his normal activities. This experience eventually helped Peter develop a degree of confidence and he later undertook a part-time training course in order to obtain work. Peter is currently managing well and has developed a greater social network and renewed social life.

Family interventions

The early stage of a psychotic illness is often a frightening and bewildering time. The presence of unusual behaviour can generate a range of emotions such as fear, sadness, anger and guilt. Whilst family members play an invaluable role in the recovery process, the unfamiliar territory that the development of a psychotic illness presents can often feel overwhelming to the family. Like any serious illness, the development of psychosis during childhood or adolescence can result in extending the caregiver's role. Thus as the impact of psychosis continues to affect the functioning of the young person, the family members become critically important caregivers (Jackson & Edwards 1992). The development of the vulnerability–stress model (Zubin & Spring 1977) reinforced the concept of the sustaining role of social, familial and environmental stressors upon the course of serious mental illness, attributing causation to an inherent vulnerability, and these have all had a great influence on the development of family intervention (Tarrier 1996). Psychosocial family interventions based upon the vulnerability–stress model have been demonstrated to be of value not only to the family (Hogarty et al. 1986; Brooker et al. 1994), but also to the sufferer, by reducing cognitive and emotional problems (Falloon et al. 1985) and improving social functioning (Falloon et al. 1985; Brooker et al. 1994).

Of all of the psychological interventions advocated for the treatment of psychosis, family interventions have perhaps the greatest evidence base. However, the interventions to date have been examined largely within the context of longer-term disorders, particularly during the post-hospitalisation period; the needs of family members in early psychosis have not been adequately addressed in research. Traditionally, family interventions have mainly focused upon the provision of psychological educational packages, reducing tensions within the household through goal-setting, problem-solving and stress-management, and the improvement of communication patterns within the family. However, it has been suggested that psycho-education packages are only necessary for individuals experiencing a first psychotic episode and their families (Kottgen et al. 1984). With this fact in mind the IMPACT early psychosis team based at Bolton, Salford and Trafford NHS Trust have developed a family psycho-education group focusing upon key aspects of the illness, its treatment and management together with touching upon comorbidity issues that commonly occur within the target population.

One commonly occurring but often overlooked area of concern is the ongoing parenting of young people who have developed a psychotic disorder. This is particularly evident if the young person has spent a period of time away from home in hospital. Parents may experience a general reluctance to impose boundaries, particularly in relation to the challenging behaviours presented during the adolescent period. One commonly cited reason for this tendency is the desire to avoid a potentially distressing or stress-provoking confrontation. This may partially arise from an incomplete explanation of the stress–vulnerability model, with emphasis placed upon the avoidance of stress-provoking situations rather than encouraging stress-management strategies. The development of a framework such as the stress–vulnerability model to explain the development of psychotic experiences has been beneficial in terms of aiding greater understanding of the disorder. However if the model is not properly understood it can lead to the adoption of unhealthy behaviours, which may further compound social isolation, exclusion and the maintenance of psychotic symptoms. This suggests that even for young people who experience a first episode of psychosis, stress-management and goal-setting is crucially important. This is in order to provide families with the confidence and abilities to parent effectively their psychotic youngster.

Jill

Jill, aged 16, has a three-year history of psychosis, resulting in her admission to an adolescent unit for several months. Following her discharge, Jill's parents displayed considerable anxiety about her mental state, becoming over-sensitive to any indication that her illness might be returning. After leaving hospital, Jill felt very aggrieved at having missed out on being with her friends and going out. She began drinking heavily and smoking cannabis. Jill's parents interpreted this as being a sign of her illness and persistently contacted services about her behaviour, requesting that she be readmitted to hospital.

However, throughout there was no evidence of psychotic symptoms reemerging and Jill continued to engage fully with services and the treatment programme. Discussion between the community mental health nurse and Jill's parents revealed a lack of understanding about her illness and a fear of creating a stressful environment. This was addressed through a package of education, and a normalising approach in relation to Jill's behaviours. During goal-setting sessions, Jill's parents were encouraged to set ground rules and appropriate sanctions in an attempt to resume their parenting role. This has been largely positive and Jill's parents have come to understand her behaviour is a result of the pressures facing young people rather than the result of her psychotic illness.

Social inclusion

As psychotic symptoms often emerge during the crucial developmental period of adolescence, young people often experience considerable disruption to their academic, vocational and social development. In a large study of adolescent schizophrenia, one-third of young people had significant difficulties in social development, affecting their ability to make and keep friends (Hollis 2000). Due to the value that western society places upon autonomy and social validation (Littlewood 1998), this can lead to negative outcomes for the young person, both in terms of their contribution to and burden upon society, but also in terms of how they are understood and viewed by society. Concurrently, these factors may impact negatively and lead to the loss of self-esteem. This may in turn threaten the ability of the young person to cope with their illness (Link et al. 2001). With evidence to suggest that increased social networks and improved occupational functioning improve outcomes for individuals with serious mental health problems, the social-inclusion agenda forms a crucial aspect of the intervention process for young people with a psychotic disorder. Links with schools and educational settings are crucially important. Given that the development of a psychotic disorder may well result in disruption to the educational process, which in turn reduces future career options, working with schools, educational institutions and employment services is therefore essential.

However, with widely documented reluctance to fully accept individuals with psychosis due to fears about violence and unpredictability (Link et al. 2001), educational staff are often hesitant to maintain young people within school. This reduces the opportunity for the maintenance of recovery, social inclusion and the normalisation of mental health. Engagement of school nurses and key individuals within the education system are vital links in the initiation of this process, allowing the development of interagency working to allow increased confidence through the development of a liaison and advisory process. This process of engaging individuals and raising awareness of individual's needs

---

Tim

Tim developed mental health problems at the age of 14. This seriously disrupted his education and resulted in him finding it increasingly difficult to attend school in general. He was finally taken off the register during his GCSE year due to an exacerbation of his health problems and the emergence of acute psychotic symptoms. Although academically gifted, Tim only achieved one GCSE, in maths, an exam he sat whilst in hospital. He was unable to complete his other studies due to the process of continual assessment and the amount of coursework he had missed. Now 16, Tim has tried to gain further education through the local college but has been unable to complete any programmes due to the length of time they take to complete. Tim feels trapped – unable to access meaningful employment due to his lack of qualifications and unable to complete formal academic courses due to the length of time involved. His main regret is that he was unable to attend school on a more flexible basis in order to complete his education in key areas that he enjoyed, which may have led to him gaining a range of formal qualifications.

in a managed way is one that is required across a range of occupational and leisure agencies. Through the development of interagency cooperation with an appropriate range of liaison and support options, it is possible for young people to commence the process of recovery and personal fulfilment.

Integrated care pathways

Perhaps unlike many other health services, early psychosis services transgress all traditional barriers. Spanning primary and secondary mental health care, CAMHS and adult mental health services, these teams are required to interact with all agencies that have contact with young people within this age-range. This includes education, employment, legal, youth and social services. With such a wide field there exists the potential for inconsistency and miscommunication. It is therefore essential that communication pathways are maintained with all agencies to ensure that care programmes are delivered in a seamless and timely manner.

Throughout this process it is essential to keep the young person, and their family or carers at the centre of the service ensuring that their needs are met, and it is important that nurses remain mindful of where those needs are best met. With the role of early psychosis services encompassing liaison and advice, it is feasible for young people to be managed in one service, for example CAMHS, with additional support from early psychosis services. This pattern of partnership working allows a young person's individual needs to be addressed. This is particularly important when working with young people where there is no clear diagnosis but potential prodromal symptoms may be evident. Nursing is a profession developing in the area of caring for young people with a psychosis. Though historically within the remit of psychologists and psychiatrists, the rise in interest in psychosocial interventions has led to number of other professions being trained in their use, particularly nurses. With the wealth of training opportunities, together with the increased satisfaction that working in this manner can bring, the role of the nurse in caring for people experiencing a psychotic disorder is likely to grow and develop in the coming years.

References

Albiston, D., Francey, S. & Harrigan, S. (1998). Group programmes for recovery from early psychosis. *British Journal of Psychiatry*, **172** (33), 117–21.
Bentall, R., Haddock, G. & Slade, P. (1994). Psychological treatment for auditory hallucinations: from theory to therapy. *Behaviour Therapy*, (25), 51–66.
Birchwood, M. & Chadwick, P. (1997). The omnipotence of voices: testing the validity of a cognitive model. *Psychological Medicine*, (27), 1345–53.
Birchwood, M., Todd, P. & Jackson, C. (1998). Early intervention in psychosis: the critical period hypothesis. *British Journal of Psychiatry*, **172** (33), 53–59.

Birchwood, M., Spencer, E. & McGovern, D. (2000). Schizophrenia: early warning signs. *Advances in Psychiatric Treatment*, (6), 93–101.

Bleuler, E. (1911). *Dementia Praecox or the Group of Schizophrenias*, New York: International University Press.

Bleuler, M. (1978). The schizophrenic disorders: long-term patient and family studies. In: Birchwood, M., Todd, P. & Jackson, C. (Eds) (1998). Early intervention in psychosis: the critical period hypothesis. *British Journal of Psychiatry*, **172** (33), 53–59.

Brooker, C., Falloon, I., Butterworth, T., Goldberg, D., Graham-Hole, V. & Hillier, V. (1994). The outcome of training CPNs to deliver psychosocial interventions. *British Journal of Psychiatry*, (165), 122–30.

Cameron, D. (1938). Early schizophrenia. *American Journal of Psychiatry*, (95), 567–78.

Carpenter, W. & Strauss, J. (1991). The prediction of outcome in schizophrenia IV: eleven-year follow-up of the Washington IPSS cohort. *Journal of Nervous and Mental Disease*, **179** (9), 517–25.

Chadwick, P., Birchwood, M. & Trower, P. (1996). *Cognitive Therapy for Delusions, Voices and Paranoia*. Chichester: John Wiley.

Ciompi, L. (1980). Catamnestic long-term study of the course of life and aging of schizophrenics. *Schizophrenia Bulletin*, (6), 606–18.

De Haan, L., Peters, B., Dingemans, P., Wouters, L. & Linszen, D. (2002). Attitudes of patients toward the first psychotic episode and the start of treatment. *Schizophrenia Bulletin*, **28** (3), 431–42.

Department of Health (2000). *The National Plan: a plan for investment, a plan for reform*. London: HMSO.

Department of Health (2002). *Improvement, Expansion and Reform: priorities and planning framework*. London: HMSO.

Drake, R., Haley, J., Akhtar, S. & Lewis, S. (2000). Causes of duration of untreated psychosis in schizophrenia. *British Journal of Psychiatry*, (177), 511–15.

Dube, K., Kumar, N. & Dube, S. (1984). Long-term course and outcome of the Agra cases in the International Pilot Study of Schizophrenia. *Acta Psychiatrica Scandanavica*, (170), 170–79.

Edwards, J., Francey, S., McGorry, P. & Jackson, H. (1994). Early psychosis prevention and intervention: evolution of a comprehensive community-based specialised service. *Behaviour Change*, **11** (4), 223–33.

Falloon, I., Boyd, J., McGill, C., Williamson, M., Razani, J., Moss, H., Gilderman, A. & Simson, G. (1985). Family management in the prevention of morbidity of schizophrenia. *Archives of General Psychiatry*, (34), 171–84.

Falloon, I., Coverdale, J. & Brooker, C. (1996). Psychosocial interventions in schizophrenia: a review. *International Journal of Mental Health*, (25), 3–21.

Falloon, I., Coverdale, J., Laidlaw, T., Merry, S., Kydd, R. & Morosini, P. (1998). Early intervention for schizophrenic disorders: implementing optimal treatment strategies in routine clinical services. *British Journal of Psychiatry*, **172** (33), 33–38.

Frith, C. & Johnstone, E. (2003). *Schizophrenia*. Oxford: Oxford University Press.

Gaebel, W., Baumann, A., Witte, A. & Zaeske, H. (2002). Public attitudes towards people with mental illness in six German cities: results of a public survey under special consideration of schizophrenia. *European Archives of Psychiatry and Clinical Neuroscience*, **252** (6), 278–87.

Haddock, G., Tarrier, N., Spaulding, W., Yusupoff, L., Kinney, C. & McCarthy, E. (1998). Individual cognitive-behaviour therapy in the treatment of hallucinations and delusions: a review. *Clinical Psychology Review*, **18** (7), 821–38.

Hafner, H., Hambrecht, M., Loffler, W., Munk-Jorgensen, P. & Riecher-Rossler, A. (1998). Is schizophrenia a disorder of all ages?: a comparison of first episodes and early course across the life-cycle. *Psychological Medicine*, (28), 351–56.

Hogarty, G., Anderson, C., Reiss, D. & Kornblith, S. (1986). Family psycho-education, social skills training and maintenance chemotherapy in the aftercare of schizophrenia. *Archives of General Psychiatry*, (43), 633–42.

Hollis, C. (2000). Adolescent schizophrenia. *Advances in Psychiatric Treatment*, (6), 83–92.

Hustig, H. & Hafner, R. (1990). Persistent auditory hallucinations and their relationship to delusions of mood. *Journal of Nervous and Mental Disease*, (178), 264–67.

Jackson, H. & Edwards, J. (1992). Social networks and social support in schizophrenia: correlates and assessment. In: Kavanagh, D. (Ed.). *Schizophrenia: an overview and practical handbook*. London: Chapman & Hall.

Keshevan, S. & Schooler, N. (1992). First episode studies in schizophrenia: criteria and characterisation. *Schizophrenia Bulletin*, (18), 491–513.

Kottgen, C., Soinnichsen, I. & Mollenhauer, K. (1984). Results of the Hamburg Camberwell family interview study, I–III. *International Journal of Family Psychiatry*, (5), 61–94.

Kraepelin, E. (1986). Dementia praecox. In: Cutting, J. & Shepherd, M. (Eds). *The Clinical Roots of Schizophrenia* (translated into English 1987). Cambridge: Cambridge University Press.

Larsen, T., McGlashan, T., & Moe, L. (1996). First episode schizophrenia: early course parameters. *Schizophrenia Bulletin*, **22** (2), 241–56.

Link, B., Struening, E., Neese-Todd, S., Asmussen, S. & Phelan, J. (2001). The consequences of stigma for the self-esteem of people with mental illness. *Psychiatric Services*, **52** (12), 1621–26.

Littlewood, R. (1998). Cultural variation in the stigmatisation of mental illness. *The Lancet*, (352), 1056–57.

Loebel, A., Lieberman, J., Alvir, J., Mayerhoff, D., Geisler, S., & Szymanski, S. (1992). Duration of psychosis and outcome in first episode schizophrenia. *American Journal of Psychiatry*, (149), 1183–88.

McDougall, T. (1999). Adolescent forensic mental health nursing. In: Chaloner, C. & Coffey, M. (eds). *Forensic Mental Health Nursing: from principles to practice*. Oxford: Blackwell.

McGlashan, T. (1998). Early detection and intervention of schizophrenia: rationale and research. *British Journal of Psychiatry*, **172** (33), 3–6.

McGorry, P. (1998). Preventative strategies in early psychosis: verging on reality. *British Journal of Psychiatry*, **172** (33), 1–2.

McGorry, P., McFarlane, C., Patton, G., Bell, R., Jackson, H., Hibbert, M. & Bower, G. (1995). The prevalence of prodromal symptoms of schizophrenia in adolescence: a preliminary survey. *Acta Psychiatrica Scandinavica*, (92), 241–49.

McGorry, P. & Edwards, J. (1997). *Social Treatments the Early Psychosis Training Pack*. Macclesfield: Gardiner-Caldwell Communications.

Medline (2005). http://www.nlm.nih.gov/medlineplus/ency/article/ 001553.htm#Definition last accessed on 27.07.2005.

National Institute for Clinical Excellence (2002). *Schizophrenia: core interventions in the treatment and management of schizophrenia in primary and secondary care*. London: NICE.

Parlato, L., Lloyd, C. & Bassett, J. (1999). Young Occupations Unlimited: an early intervention programme for young people with psychosis. *British Journal of Occupational Therapy*, **62** (3), 113–16.

Penn, D.L. and Mueser, K.T. (1996). Research update on the psychosocial treatment of schizophrenia. *American Journal of Psychiatry*, (153), 607–17.

Russell, A., Bott, L. & Sammons, C. (1989). The phenomenology of schizophrenia occurring in childhood. *Journal of the American Academy of Child and Adolescent Psychiatry*, (28), 399–407.

Sayce, L. (2000). *From Psychiatric Patient to Citizen*. Hampshire: Palgrave Macmillan.

Surgeon General (1999). *Mental Health: a report of the surgeon general.* Washington DC: US Department of Health and Human Sciences.

Tarrier, N. (1996). Family interventions and schizophrenia, In: Haddock, G. & Slade, P. (Eds). *Cognitive-Behavioural Interventions with Psychotic Disorders*. London: Routledge.

Weiden, P. & Olfson, M. (1995). Cost of relapse in schizophrenia. *Schizophrenia Bulletin*, (21), 419–28.

World Health Organization (2001). *Mental Health: new understanding, new hope*. Geneva: WHO.

Yung, A. & McGorry, P. (1996). The prodromal phase of first episode psychosis: past and present conceptualisations. *Schizophrenia Bulletin*, (22), 353–70.

Yusupoff, I. & Tarrier, N. (1996). Coping strategy enhancement for persistent hallucinations and delusions. In: Haddock, G. & Slade, P. (Eds). *Cognitive Behavioural Interventions with Psychotic Disorders*. London: Routledge.

Zubin, J. & Spring, B. (1977). Vulnerability: a new view of schizophrenia. *Journal of Abnormal Psychology*, (86), 103–26.

Chapter 8

Nursing Children and Adolescents who are Aggressive or Violent: a psychological approach

Ian Higgins and Tim McDougall

Key points

- Working with children and young people who may use aggression and violence to communicate distress, solve problems or compete for adult attention is no easy task. Nurses working in residential settings need to achieve a careful balance of authority, responsibility and risk-taking.

- Strategies for the management of aggression and violence must always be underpinned by a thorough assessment undertaken with the young person, and their family or carers. This is to understand the scope, frequency, duration, severity and function of the aggressive or violent behaviour.

- Appropriate and effective limit-setting by nurses for young people with behaviour problems is rarely straightforward. However, fair and consistent rules and boundaries are important external controls that enable young people with behaviour problems to develop internal controls and learn alternative coping strategies.

- The ability of the nurse to remain calm and manage their own emotions is important. Young people with behaviour problems who are angry or aggressive may feel out of control and will not feel contained or reassured by highly emotional, frustrated or frightened staff.

- It is crucial that nurses are able to acknowledge that they find some young people more challenging and harder to work with than others. This is neither uncaring nor unprofessional if it is acknowledged with insight and understanding and explored and reflected on within supervision.

- The nursing contribution to working with young people who are aggressive or violent is unique. It is the nurse that provides the 24-hour support, care and treatment for the distressed, angry and frightened young person. This requires them to call upon a variety of skills and approaches whilst also considering other young people and the contribution of their multi-disciplinary team colleagues.

Introduction

Nurses in a range of hospital, custodial or school settings may be required to help children and adolescents with severe behaviour problems or those who are aggressive or violent. These young people often have a diagnosis of conduct disorder and may require high levels of support, supervision and guidance. This chapter focuses on a range of behaviour problems, as well as exploring psychological strategies for managing the most challenging or severe behaviour problems that may be associated with violent behaviour. Through the use of practice scenarios, a range of interpersonal skills and management strategies that enhance nursing practice will be discussed. The individual strategies that are described can be applied in all settings where young people with behaviour problems receive services. However, particular attention is paid to working with young people in residential health, care and education services; they may, for example, be in child and adolescent units, children's homes or residential schools. Physical interventions to contain violent behaviour will be only briefly discussed as part of the wider continuum of interventions.

Background

The needs of children and young people with behaviour problems, particularly those associated with aggressive or violent behaviour have long preoccupied policymakers, researchers and service providers. Research on behaviour problems and their association with aggression and violent behaviour is wide and varied. Psychosocial factors such as trauma, abuse and loss (Boswell 1995), early exposure to violence (Rutter et al. 1998), and harsh and inconsistent discipline as well as lack of reinforcement for positive, prosocial behaviour (Varma 1999), have all been strongly correlated with behaviour problems and violence displayed by children and young people. Nurses frequently encounter young people with behaviour problems and those who are aggressive or violent during their day-to-day work. Factors such as involuntary treatment in hospital, detention in security and separation from family or carers and friends all impact negatively on the therapeutic relationship. However, though the specific contribution that nurses make to supporting children and adolescents has not been well articulated in the literature, there is much that nurses can do which is effective.

What is meant by behaviour problems and conduct disorder terms in use?

The *Diagnostic and Statistical Manual of Mental Disorders* (DSM-IV) describes conduct disorder as a repetitive and persistent pattern of behaviour involving aggressive behaviour that causes or threatens physical harm to others; non-aggressive conduct that causes property damage; and deceitfulness or theft and serious rule-violation. Similarly, the ICD (international classification of diseases) classification of mental and behavioural disorders (ICD-10) focuses on repetitive and persistent patterns of antisocial, aggressive or defiant behaviour. Mental health professionals and researchers use a plethora of terms to describe conduct disorders. These include disobedient, aggressive, antisocial, challenging, oppositional, defiant and delinquent behaviour. Much more than mischief, rebelliousness or temporary behavioural change, persistent conduct disorder involves the violation of social norms, rule-breaking and a disregard for authority.

The prevalence of conduct disorders in the general population of 11 to 16 year-olds is 8.1% for boys and 5.1% for girls (Green et al. 2005). It is important to make a distinction between particular disruptive behaviours, and short-term adjustment difficulties which are usually a transient part of ordinary development, and more often than not, the child grows out of them. Challenging though these can be for parents and carers, they are not in the same category as the pervasive, long-standing conduct problems that often lead to referral to child and adolescent mental health services (CAMHS). Research tends to describe behaviour problems and a number of related terms such as anger and aggression in diagnostic terms. However, since nurses use a holistic, humanistic approach in their work, it is important that we consider behaviour problems (and related issues) from a number of different theoretical perspectives not just from a simple diagnostic perspective.

The first challenge is to try and define what is meant by (even the obvious) terms used in this chapter. In talking about behaviour problems, a number of words are used including anger, aggression, arousal and violence, and it is worth defining these. Whilst it is generally acknowledged that people become aggressive or violent because something has angered them, the interrelationship between anger, aggression and violence in young people with conduct disorders is complex. Anger is a normal healthy emotion with positive expressive qualities. It is neither necessary nor sufficient for aggression to follow or violence to occur after the expression of anger. Whilst arousal is not intrinsically associated with anger, there are strong links between arousal, aggression and violence (McDougall 2000a). Aggression may be either hostile or angry, or be instrumental and lack anger. For example, a child may use aggression instrumentally to achieve a particular goal such as robbery without being angry. By comparison, hostile aggression may erupt in response to provocation while a child is highly aroused and angry. Violence can be defined in a number of ways, but generally refers to behaviour which may cause physical or psychological harm (Gulbenkian Foundation 1995).

How can nurses help?

The goal of any individual nursing intervention with a child or young person who has behaviour problems, or who is aggressive or violent, is to help them make sense of their behaviour and understand why this may be problematic.

Any therapeutic approach can only be effective if it is delivered with knowledge, empathy and in a way that can be accessed by the young people involved. Very little has been written about the effect of direct nursing care on young people with behaviour problems. Treatment strategies that have been evaluated have tended to focus on psychosocial interventions, individual psychotherapies and multimodal treatment strategies (Fonagy et al. 2002), rather than the therapeutic relationship between the nurse and young person. Research about specific nursing interventions is sparse and much of the practice highlighted in this chapter is based on nursing interventions that have not been evaluated but have common currency across a range of practice settings.

Before attempting to embark on management strategies it is important for the nurse to undertake a thorough assessment that is appropriate to the young person's developmental level and understanding. This requires the collection of information from a number of sources in multiple settings using a variety of methods. The purpose of undertaking a thorough assessment with the young person, their family or carers is to understand the scope, frequency, duration and severity of the aggression, violence or behaviour problems. Many young people use challenging and oppositional behaviour to maintain control of their environment and the people around them. Introducing a particular treatment approach without this assessment and detailed planning and preparation may simply lead to a repetition or escalation of the oppositional and challenging behaviour (Higgins & Burke 1998).

In a book about mental health problems it is appropriate to briefly discuss the association between mental disorder and aggression, violence and behaviour problems. The large majority of children and young people with behaviour problems do not have significant mental health problems, and only a minority are aggressive or violent, and some will have coexisting mental disorders. Some mental health and developmental disorders are more closely associated than others with behaviour problems. These include conduct disorder (Fonagy & Kurtz 2002), ADHD (attention deficit hyperactivity disorder) (Gaub & Carlson 1997) and a range of other emotional disorders including anxiety and depression (Malmquist 1990; Biederman et al. 1991). Box 8.1 shows a number of assessment tools that may be used by nurses to form a thorough assessment of mental state and associated behaviour problems.

Box 8.1 Assessment tools.

- Health of the Nation Outcome Scale for Children and Adolescents (HoNOSCA) (Gowers et al. 1998).
- HoNOSCA-SR (Gowers et al. 2002).
- The Child Behaviour Checklist (CBC) (Achenbach & Edelbrock 1991).
- The Eyberg Child Behaviour Inventory (ECBI) (Eyberg & Pincus 1999).
- The Conners' Parent-Teacher Rating Scales (CPTRS) (Conners 1989).
- Strengths and Difficulties Questionnaire (SDQ) (Goodman 1997).
- Children's Global Assessment Scale (C-GAS) (Shaffer et al. 1983).

Engaging children and young people with behaviour problems

Behaviour problems cannot successfully be managed without first establishing the conditions for engagement in a therapeutic relationship between the nurse and child or adolescent. Young people in public services may often be suspicious of the motives of adults who are trying to help them. They may have been through a number of similar situations with other professionals and agencies and may well have experienced a sense of failure. This will inevitably shape their current responses and their motivation to change. The pressure across CAMHS and the NHS (National Health Service) in general is to get on with the work and not become too concerned about the process of engagement. However, if we attempt to embark on help or treatment without first laying the necessary foundations, the intervention is unlikely to be successful.

Jamal

Jamal is a 10 year-old boy who is meeting the nurse for the first time. He is angry, sitting with his feet on the coffee table and demands to know when he can leave the hospital.

Nursing staff need to be acutely aware that the young person will be closely observing the interactions that are taking place. If they already have a sense of ambivalence about getting help, they will be assessing how the nurse is reacting to their behaviour. In this practice scenario, the nurse is being invited to react either to the feet on the table or the question itself, and this could lead to the battle that Jamal is expecting. The following response from the nurse may be productive:

> *'I wonder how many times you have had to meet with people like me. You probably do want to get out of here.'*

Although this response may seem short and simple, it provides an opportunity to model an alternative way of responding. Children who are angry or aggressive often have difficulties in relation to appraisal, information-processing and attribution. This has a profound effect on their capacity to solve problems, consider alternative options and contain themselves through self-control. They often have difficulty in taking another person's perspective and may develop an 'all-or-nothing' stance to life. They see situations and people as either all good or all bad and consider all situations to have definitive outcomes. It has been said that children and adolescents with conduct disorder often jump to conclusions and think in terms of winning or losing (Bandura 1986).

Nurses should pay attention to what they say and how they say it. Young people are likely to find short, simple non-abstract sentences easier to process if they are angry. Therefore the nurse's voice should be lowered and sentences should be short, simple and lack abstract concepts. This simplifies information-processing and reduces cognitive workload. Responding in this way also lacks high expressed emotion and heightened arousal, and is likely to be appraised as non-threatening to the young person. Though many nurses might regard these strategies as very basic, they are essential communication skills that are often undervalued by nurses and go unnoticed by the wider multidisciplinary team. It is these core skills that enable nurses to manage and contain a range of complex challenges and difficulties within a busy, emotionally charged and demanding environment. Asking simpler questions involving 'when', 'how' or 'how often', suggests to the young person that you already have a degree of knowledge about them. These closed questions can be more useful than those that ask young people more open questions such as 'why' and 'what do you need to do about it?'. Cotton (1993) describes this process as 'helpful talking' and is a vital tool in the engagement process.

Containment

The most effective strategies for managing aggression or violence are not physical but psychological and the ability to provide a containing emotional (as well as physical) environment is crucial. This needs to be established if any therapeutic work is to be successfully developed. The aim of containment is to create an environment and therapeutic space where the young person becomes increasingly confident that the nurse can cope with their challenging behaviour and is not going to give up on them. Aggressive behaviour is often a strategy for coping by young people who have not developed other skills and resources for managing emotions, anxiety or conflict. It is important that nursing staff feel confident to raise issues around the management of aggression and violence, including the potential to be physically restrained, before they become an issue. Some nurses are uncertain about this preemptive approach and are concerned that talking to the young person about potential aggression could in itself precipitate an incident. This is possible but unlikely. Many young people will feel contained by experiencing a nurse who is not over-whelmed by their anxiety and is assured and confident enough to discuss an area that other professionals may have previously avoided.

The importance of limit-setting

Appropriate and effective limit-setting for young people with behaviour problems is an essential but rarely straightforward process. Fair and consistent rules and boundaries are important external controls that enable young people to link their own behaviour with predictable consequences and thus develop internal controls. When expectations are clearly stated and consequences for antisocial behaviour are known in advance, there is implied control and the organisational structure is safe, supportive and containing (Bailey 2002). Agreeing a plan with the young person about issues of power and control is better than waiting for a situation to arise that will test this out. This requires nurses to have a high level of self-awareness and an ability to stand back from the immediate situation.

The young person will often challenge the nurse's authority by testing them through angry words or non-compliant behaviour:

'You can't make me do that.'

This is a response often encountered by nurses and presents an immediate challenge. It is important for the nurse not to argue or get drawn into a debate. This is because presenting one side of an argument to a young person who is angry invites them to take up the counter-argument. This is not likely to be productive. The more a young person defends their position, the more committed they become to it, and the potential for attitudinal change is greatly reduced. Instead, if the nurse accepts that the young person is 'right', they can then find a way of using this dynamic to develop a therapeutic alliance. It is not unusual for a young person with behaviour problems to use denial, projection and anger as defence mechanisms when questioned about their behaviour and actions. They may well invite the nurse to become embroiled in verbal conflict and the response from the nurse to this initial 'test' is likely to have a significant impact on their ongoing relationship. If the nurse enters into the therapeutic relationship with the need to assert their authority and immediately gain control, this may well lead to an escalation of conflict. It is therefore crucial that the nurse is aware of the potential dynamics that may be played out during the therapeutic encounter and how they may respond to them.

One strategy is to allow the young person to take the lead and have some control rather than them having to wrestle with the nurse to gain it. This takes a high degree of self-confidence on the part of the nurse, but can be very effective in changing the dynamics that the young person has grown used to. This is often a difficult issue for nurses to accept, and some believe that it would require them to accept anything that the young person says or does, in order to enable the young person to engage. This approach may indeed at first lead to an escalation in oppositional behaviour, as the young person is uncertain where the limits of acceptable behaviour are, and is unable to set these themselves. Young people in this situation may become more anxious by the lack of containment, and such anxiety will often lead to reactive, challenging behaviour. Working through this stage requires patience, and confidence on the part of the nurse and also a support-system for the nurse. Developing an interpersonal style that is relaxed, confident and containing does not happen overnight, and the importance of providing modelling, support and supervision for nursing staff cannot be overstated. This provides a professional environment that is containing and collaborative and enables staff to reflect, interpret and learn from situations that occur during practice (Butterworth et al. 1998). The nurse should try:

> 'You're right, I can't make you, but it would be good if we can find a way of working together.'

As stated, nurses are often ambivalent about this approach as they are concerned that it gives the young person permission to misbehave or test the nurse. However, this is a necessary part of the process of engagement and developing a helping relationship. Nurses must take time to name the issues and explore them rather than attempt to set a rigid boundary that could constrain the development of any further change. Without this essential part of the therapeutic process, the child may overreact or refuse to engage as they may anticipate a repeat of previous negative experiences. By responding in this way, the nurse is trying to keep the dialogue going rather than becoming stuck in a battle of wills. This not only helps avoid a power struggle, but also enables the young person to express their views and make suggestions. By contrast if the nurse was to allow the young person to take control of what the nurse is able to say, they would be in a very powerful and uncontained situation. Such a lack of containment by a responsible adult would be likely to make the young person feel anxious and out of control.

This approach to working with young people who have behaviour problems takes account of the theory of arousal in young people with behaviour problems. This suggests that they have lower arousal levels than their peers and are unable to respond to reinforcement or to avoid antisocial behaviour (Raine et al. 1994). The response of the nurse will affect the level of arousal in the young person. If the nurse becomes competitive or over-focused on achieving compliance, there may be a subsequent increase in tension, and this in turn may lead to an increase in arousal in the young person. It is therefore important that the nurse is able to monitor their own responses. If they are angry or frustrated with the young person this is likely to be communicated non-verbally and the young person may respond defensively or aggressively. Angry nurses are at greater risk of being assaulted by young people (McDougall 2000a).

Limit-setting can often be a difficult line for the nurse to tread. It is important to be clear with the young person about the boundaries and limits that are expected, without this being a continuous focus. This means that the nurse may need to be able to tolerate a degree of challenging or indeed antisocial behaviour in order to set that limit. If the limit is set early and before the behaviour has occurred there may well be an invitation for the young person to test the limit. Providing therapeutic containment requires great skill and dexterity on the part of the nurse. There is a delicate balance to be struck between creating an environment where the young person feels contained enough to work on their difficulties and one where they understand and accept the limits that have been set in relation to their behaviour. This balance is particularly difficult to achieve in residential settings, where several nurses may be involved in setting limits and containing behaviour at the same time. Some nurses may have a fear of losing control and consequently apply a rigid, over-controlling approach to behaviour management. Others may meet unreasonable requests or ignore antisocial behaviour for fear of generating an angry or aggressive response. Young people who feel uncontained and out-of-control often want the adults around them to contain their behaviour for them. Setting no boundaries is as unhelpful as sticking to the boundaries very strictly without taking into account the individual child and their specific circumstances. Managing authority and responsibility with challenging young people in residential settings requires facilitative and authoritative skills, and is identified as an area for staff support, training and development (McDougall 2000b). A response to challenging behaviour might be phrased:

> *'If you swear during the session we will have to stop and you will have to take 5 minutes' time out.'*

Like any institutions, residential care, and treatment and education settings, depend on consistent rules, clear expectations and the application of reasonable sanctions to function effectively. Behavioural approaches are based on the hypothesis that much of a young person's behaviour is learned, maintained and regulated by the effects of environmental consequences. Accordingly, aggressive or violent behaviour by young people, like any other learned response, can be unlearnt and replaced with non-violent, prosocial behaviour. The maintenance of behaviour problems is largely dependent on consequences. Whereas aggressive behaviour that is rewarded will tend to recur, behaviour that is unrewarded is likely to diminish. Young people with behaviour problems will almost inevitably need to see if the nurse can carry through the consequences they have suggested. It also gives the child a way out from having to think about and work on their difficulties. A nurse might try responding:

> *'What do other adults do when you swear?'*

This response places the responsibility back with the child and also models to them that the nurse is not shocked or avoiding the issue. There is then an opportunity for the nurse to discuss their approach to this issue. Limit-setting requires a careful balance of authority and responsibility. It is important that the nurse is able to question themselves about the limits they are setting and what the basic aim of the intervention is. Limits are often set to make the life of the nurse easier and they provide a structure and routine that can appear to make the chaos that often surrounds these young people easier to manage. Indeed, the use of limit-setting and the application of sanctions have been found to reflect staff frustration with the behaviour rather than the behaviour *per se* (Hogg & Hall 1992). Without these insights and skills of self-reflection, there is a danger that nurses may begin to respond in the same way as the young person and get caught in the 'all-or-nothing' dynamic.

Nurses often experience aggressive responses from young people during the process of limit-setting. Violence towards nurses by adult mental health service users has been extensively reviewed in the literature (Fisher & Kane 1998), and frustration is probably the most widely investigated psychological precursor and elicitor of aggressive behaviour. Conflict surrounding the use of rules in residential settings for young people can sometimes lead to aggression and violence. This is often when nurses attempt to gain control through punitive and aversive measures. The practice example below illustrates the way in which interactions between nurses and young people in the context of limit-setting can spiral out of control.

Dan

Dan, an 11 year-old boy, has had a major upset in the lounge and has required physical holding to maintain safety. He is calming down and asks for a drink. It is after 9:00 p.m. and the unit rule is no food or drink in the lounge after this time. One of the nurses tells him he can have a drink but will have to go to the kitchen to drink it. Dan quickly becomes upset and agitated and the situation further escalates. Eventually Dan requires physical holding by the nurses.

In this instance the nurse is being consistent and maintaining the ward limits, but for what purpose? Dan was not testing the limit and the nurse's response reinforces Dan's belief that he cannot get it right and that the world is against him. On some occasions, over-zealous limit-setting and the use of physical interventions may further frustrate the young person and escalate the behaviour it is intended to contain. Some inexperienced or junior nurses struggle with knowing when to be flexible and when to be consistent. This can lead to internal tension when the more experienced nurse takes a different approach to manage the situation. Here, the other nurse may feel undermined and object that their colleague is being inconsistent. Ways in which nurses can address these issues are discussed later in the chapter.

Unfortunately, the practice example above is not unusual, and typically, such incidents begin with limit-setting. However, such situations can often escalate, with hostility, anger and aggression being directed towards the nurse who is attempting to set the limits. One explanation for this spiral effect is that the nurse may themselves feel out of control, may identify with the young person's angry feelings and may then physically intervene to regain a sense of control over their own tension or aggression. Children and adolescents with behaviour problems often assume that the intentions of others, particularly those in an authority position, are hostile (Crick & Dodge 1994). Indeed, their oppositional behaviour is often an attempt to defend their fragile ego. Nurses who witness this behaviour often regard it as intimidating and unjustified, and may respond accordingly. This provides the aggressive child with confirmation that their initial behaviour was warranted. Developing an approach where the nurse does not take the young person's behaviour personally is not only important but also professionally challenging.

Paradoxically, failure by nurses to set and maintain reasonable and consistent limits may lead to further aggression and violence on the part of the young person. Indeed, there will be occasions when psychological interventions and verbal de-escalation strategies are ineffective, and physical restraint is needed to maintain safety and contain risk. The physical management of aggression and violence has been well-researched and is an area of contention and concern by nurses who manage young people with behaviour problems (McDougall 1996). The effects of physical touch are wide and varied. Whilst most young people experience the use of physical intervention both intrusive and aversive (Smith & Cantrell 1998), some young people may find physical touch comforting and reassuring (Barlow 1989). Research suggests that children who have been abused and young people who self harm often exhibit extreme reactions to being touched or held when they are upset (Mayton 1991). Nurses are usually in the frontline for managing aggressive and violent young people in hospital settings (McDougall 2000b) and the focus of physical training is often on the practicalities of how to hold and contain young people safely. Nurses who may be required to use physical interventions as part of a wider behaviour management strategy may feel vulnerable to complaints and allegations. However, it is important that nurses do not become frozen and adopt an inflexible hands-off approach when physical intervention is essential to prevent harm or injury occurring.

Managing imminent aggression and violence

We have heard that the successful management of anger and aggression is based on psychological approaches and skills used to avoid and resolve conflict. These skills are preventative, and include verbal de-escalation strategies using a range of skills to distract and divert the young person from their anger or aggression. Skills required for effective verbal de-escalation include the ability to remain calm, communicate openly and assertively and provide young people with 'face-saving' alternatives. This means that the nurse should enable young people to find ways of maintaining dignity and respect in front of their peers. Nurses should be aware of their non-verbal communication through careful attention to their posture, intention movements and use of personal space: nurses should avoid sudden movements and allow a wide personal space. This is because sudden movements may be perceived as an attack, and young people who are highly aroused, angry or aggressive command an enlarged sense of personal space. Verbal de-escalation is a proactive approach to managing anger or aggression before the young person becomes physically aggressive or violent. It is an interactional process and, whilst the young person's anger is the focus, attention is also paid to the nurse's use of self through posture, intention movements and the use of space.

Physical training courses usually comprise physical intervention skills and verbal de-escalation techniques, but invariably the former are disproportionate to the latter. This is unfortunate since the most effective skills to manage anger successfully, aggression and violence in the context of behaviour problems, are likely to be psychological rather than physical (McDougall 1997). Physical interventions should only be used as a last resort, and should only be taught as part of a wider strategy for managing behaviour problems. The option for physical management of aggression and violence is an important part of the overall approach, but equally crucial is the culture of the professional workplace towards the management of antisocial or challenging behaviour:

> 'We talked about how we would help you if you became physically aggressive when you first came here. Was this what you expected to happen?'

This nurse maintains the dialogue, as there can be a temptation to avoid reviewing what has happened because it could raise difficult, challenging emotions and again may lead to an escalation. The nurse is in a position to model to the young person that what has occurred is not so overwhelming that it cannot be talked about and learnt from. This process is crucial if the nurse is to support the young person to learn from their experiences. By working through their behaviour problems, young people are given the opportunity to learn that the nurse is able to talk about and listen to the young person's views. This may well be a new experience, as often they will have been directly challenged, told what happened and told simply to change their behaviour.

Talking about aggression and violence

Many young people have strong views about the role of adults and particularly those they see as in authority. They will often regard activities such as social skills-building or anger management as something that they simply have to oppose and challenge because an adult in authority is initiating it. The unique role of nurses is to develop an environment and relationship that will enable the young person to avail themselves of what is on offer without losing credibility and without feeling that they have had to surrender all control. This requires knowledge, a high level of self-awareness, patience and an ability to focus on the young person themselves rather than their presenting behaviour. The ability to name problems and difficult issues before they evolve into challenging behaviour is one of the key skills needed when supporting young people to resolve difficulties without resorting to aggression or violence. This requires confidence and self-awareness to predict and preempt what might happen.

> Nurse: 'If I sit here and ask you a lot of questions about your behaviour I think I will probably just wind you up.'
>
> Child: 'Yes, everyone winds me up.'
>
> Nurse: 'How can we spend some time together that will not wind you up?'

The aim here is to establish dialogue and collaboration to break the negative cycle of communication. We have heard that many young people with behaviour problems are acutely sensitive to the reactions of others. They quickly pick up on vulnerabilities and will often keep probing a particular area in an attempt to provoke a response. This can have the effect of making the young person feel both powerful and uncontained at the same time. Unlike other young people who will often respond to another person's upset through remorse or by reducing their aggressive behaviour, young people with behaviour problems often push boundaries and attempt to intimidate others even further. This is not to suggest that nursing staff should be prepared to tolerate all levels of antisocial behaviour or abuse. Indeed, it is important for the nurse to be able to look beyond the presenting behaviour and endeavour to remain calm and not respond to all the potential provocation and boundary-testing. The ability of the nurse to remain calm is crucially important. Young people with behaviour problems who are angry or aggressive may feel out-of-control and will not feel contained or reassured by angry, frustrated or frightened staff. The ability of the nurse to remain calm provides containment and modelling for the young person who will often be experiencing a new situation. They will expect their challenging behaviour to achieve a particular purpose, either to help them get their own way or to keep the nurse at a distance. This approach also provides nurses with an opportunity to demonstrate that they can cope with the young person's behaviour, contain their anxiety and not take what the child says personally. This provides emotional containment and an environment that is thoughtful and calm rather than reactive and tense:

'What happens when you lose your temper?'

Asking this question directly may at first appear blunt. However, this is clearer to the young person than avoiding or skirting around the topic. The nurse is also in a prime position to discuss previous interventions, both successful and unsuccessful. Here, the key issue is to try and develop a dialogue in relation to a particularly emotive subject rather than hope that such an incident will not materialise. It is also important to ensure that the young person has been prepared for the approaches that the hospital, children's home or residential school may use. Again the aim is to encourage communication and avoid the use of interventions that have not been discussed with the young person. This should include explaining when physical holding is likely to be required, and how it may be carried out. However, simply informing young people that they may be held or restrained if they are aggressive or violent is not enough. The nurse needs to be confident enough to provide details and clear explanations. The young person may not remember all the details but this allows the nurse to return to the discussion if such an incident arises. It is however, good practice to inform the young person of the process and how decisions are made and ensure that, wherever possible, they are fully involved. Where expectations are clearly stated and consequences are known in advance, there is implied control and the organisational culture is safe, supporting and containing (McDougall 2000b):

> 'You know when you broke the window yesterday and we had to hold you, what helped you in that situation?'

This shows the nurse using a real situation as a learning opportunity for both the young person and the team. It is often assumed that young people with behaviour problems or those who become aggressive have been taught how to behave properly, and have simply chosen to disregard concern for others. This is a myth. On the contrary, many of these young people have not had positive role models nor been taught the skills to resolve conflict in a non-destructive or adaptive manner. Learning comes from knowledge and an understanding of what actually happened, and reflecting on such incidents is an opportunity for nurses to model prosocial behaviour and provides an opportunity for young people to link the theory with the event itself.

How important is self-awareness?

Various nurses have asserted that the most valuable tool when working with children and young people who have mental health problems is the 'self' (Leighton et al. 2001; Holyoake & Fitzgibbon 2002). Indeed, we have heard that the most effective skills for the management of aggression and violence are psychological and interpersonal. The strategies outlined so far require the nurse to have developed an exhaustive understanding of their own strengths, vulnerabilities and weaknesses. They also require an awareness of how these may affect their management of children and young people. This is dependent on the nurse having sufficient support and supervision in relation to their appraisal and management of what is often challenging, oppositional and highly emotive behaviour. This may lead nurses to explore their own experiences of parenting, limit-setting, authority, discipline and how they may respond to particular behaviours.

The ability to be self-reflective is central to the successful management of behaviour problems and aggressive or violent behaviour by young people. For example, if the nurse is aware that he or she holds strong views about bullying because they experienced this themselves, they can factor this into how they approach a young person who may be bullying others. Similarly, attitudes to limit-setting will be influenced by the nurse's own experiences of having limits set on their behaviour as children. Bedtime routines, for example, may lead some nurses to be inconsistent because they resented the approach their own parents took when they were a child. Developing and sharing self-awareness is part of effective team functioning and can directly impact on how a young person's behaviour problems are managed. If a nurse is able to share with colleagues those situations they find challenging, then support and understanding can be given. Self-awareness and sharing insights of this nature also helps remove the myth that all nurses can cope equally well with all young people in all situations. It is important that nurses are able to acknowledge that they may find some young people more challenging and harder to work with than others. This is neither uncaring nor unprofessional, if it is acknowledged with insight and understanding, and explored and reflected on within appropriate supervision. This is an area where nursing has yet to fully establish an appropriate professional culture as the emphasis is often on 'doing' and 'responding', rather than predicting, preempting and containing. It could be argued that other disciplines within CAMHS have a more reflective and psychodynamic approach, giving themselves time and space to think, plan and reflect.

The importance of support and supervision

Supervision can be defined as a formal process of professional support and learning which enables nurses to develop knowledge and competence, assume responsibility for their practice and enhance service user satisfaction and safety of care (Department of Health 1992). Nurses and managers in CAMHS need to develop supervision and reflection as core components of their practice and service improvement strategies. It is vital to have the opportunity to learn from personal experience and the practice of others. This requires time, commitment and the support of nursing colleagues and the wider multidisciplinary team. Support, supervision and opportunities for practice development are particularly important when managing the inevitable transference and counter-transference issues that arise in the context of working with young people who are aggressive or violent. Transference refers to the range of emotions and previous psychological experiences a young person brings to the current setting. Counter-transference refers to the nurse's own hopes, expectations, fears and emotions and their response to the transference issues (Maroda 1994). It is important that the opportunities to learn from experience and reflection are regarded as part of continuing professional development, in a similar way to that in which formal courses and qualifications are regarded. It is the view of the authors that the potential for learning through skilled and reflective supervision is not currently given a high enough profile in nurse education and training programmes.

It is the responsibility of nurse managers and leaders to establish a culture of sharing practice and concerns. Nurses need to feel confident that they can question each other's practice in an open and supportive manner. This can be a challenge in nursing, where questioning and constructive criticism are often seen as negative and even considered taboo. However, as well as formal theory, it is vital that reflective practice is seen as part of continuing professional development, where nurses learn through their day-to-day experiences. This can take place in individual supervision, where the nurse can explore their own responses and role in the situation. In addition, group supervision or practice development forums for nurses, facilitated by an experienced nurse, can also be a useful arena for discussing challenges and dilemmas in nursing practice. The facilitator needs to have an understanding of the day-to-day issues so that they can raise topics and encourage discussion and sharing without necessarily focusing on a particular individual. Most important however, is the establishment of a culture where discussion, dialogue and open debate are regarded as a key component of practical, professional and personal development.

Conclusion

The management of young people who are aggressive or violent is no easy task. Working with children and young people who may use aggression and violence to communicate distress, solve problems or compete for adult attention within residential settings requires nurses to achieve a careful balance of authority, responsibility and risk-taking. Most nurses who work with young people who are aggressive or violent work in services that have policies, protocols or procedures for managing potential or actual violent incidents. These may provide nurses with useful information about who should be contacted and what paperwork should be completed. However, guidance on the subtleties of de-escalating, defusing and managing aggressive or violent problems is rarely written down or explicitly shared amongst nurses and the wider team. Therapeutic opportunities and how to make best use of psychological strategies and interpersonal skills are not usually given the same weight as operational policies and procedures.

This chapter has highlighted the unique range of skills required by nurses working with young people who are aggressive or violent. The challenge for nurses is to develop skills, knowledge, self-awareness and attitudes that enable them to remain positive, nurturing and accepting of the young person as an individual whilst setting and maintaining fair boundaries and expectations. What is unique about the nurse's role is the opportunity they have to use a wide range of skills and approaches in highly diverse environments and time-frames. It is the nurse who provides 24-hour support, care and treatment for the distressed, angry and frightened young person. This requires them to call upon a variety of skills and approaches, while also remaining aware of other young people and the contribution of their multidisciplinary team colleagues.

Nursing young people with behaviour problems and those who are aggressive or violent requires the nurse to wear many hats. At different times they will need to act as a carer, therapist, friend or parent. The skills required to manage this role effectively are often underestimated and rarely highlighted or celebrated by nurses themselves. Managing an aggressive and potentially violent young person late at night or during a group session with their peers, requires a wide range of knowledge and skills and also considerable personal resilience. Unlike a planned therapy session or interview, the nurse managing a young person's behaviour problems does not usually have the luxury of a contained room or the opportunity to plan for a range of eventualities. The range of skills required to manage oppositional behaviour, whilst meeting the needs of a diverse group of other young people cannot be underestimated. The ultimate tool however, is the individual nurse. How they interact, model their behaviour and the degree to which they understand their responses to the young people in their charge will ultimately make the greatest difference. It is incumbent upon nurses to share their experiences, expertise and skills to ensure that they become an integral part of learning and development for the future. In this era of research-based practice, it is essential that nurses do not lose sight of some of the unique contributions they make to people's lives. This after all, is part of the essence of nursing.

References

Achenbach, T. & Edelbrock, C. (1991). *Manual for the Child Behavior Checklist and Revised Child Behavior Profile*. Texas: University Associates in Psychiatry.

American Psychiatric Association (1994). *Diagnostic and Statistical Manual of Mental Disorders*. 4th edn. Washington DC: American Psychiatric Association.

Bailey, S. (2002). Violent children: a framework for assessment. *Advances in Psychiatric Treatment*, (8), 97–106.

Bandura, A. (1986). *Social Foundations of Thoughts and Action: a social cognitive theory*. New Jersey: Prentice-Hall.

Barlow, D. (1989). Therapeutic holding: effective intervention with the aggressive child. *Journal of Psychosocial Nursing*, **27** (1), 10–14.

Biederman, J., Newcorn, J. & Sprich, S. (1991). Comorbidity of attention deficit hyperactivity disorder with conduct, depressive, anxiety and other disorders. *American Journal of Psychiatry*, (148), 564–77.

Boswell, G. (1995). *Violent Victims: the prevalence of abuse and loss in the lives of Section 53 offenders*. London: The Prince's Trust.

Butterworth, T., Faugier, J. & Burnard, J. (1998). *Clinical Supervision and Mentoring in Nursing*. 2nd edn. Cheltenham: Stanley Thornes.

Campbell, S. (1995). Behaviour problems in pre-school children: a review of recent research. *Journal of Child Psychology and Psychiatry*, (36), 113–49.

Chesson, R. & Chisolm, D. (1996). *Child Psychiatric Units at the Crossroads*. London: Jessica Kingsley.

Conners, C. (1989). *Conners' Rating Scales Manual*. New York: Multi-Health Systems.

Cotton, N. (1993). *Lessons from the Lion's Den*. San Francisco: Jossey-Bass Publications.

Crick, N. & Dodge, K. (1994). A review and reformulation of social information-processing mechanisms in children's social adjustment. *Psychological Bulletin*, (115), 74–101.

Department of Health (1992). *A Vision for the Future*. London: HMSO.

Eyberg, S. & Pincus, D. (1999). *Eyberg Child Behavior Inventory and Sutter-Eyberg Behavior Inventory-Revised: professional manual*. Florida: Psychological Assessment Resources.

Fonagy, P. & Kurtz, Z. (2002). Disturbances of conduct. In: Fonagy, P., Target, M., Cottrell, D., Phillips, J. & Kurtz, Z. (2002). *What Works for Whom?: a critical review of treatments for children and adolescents*. London: Guilford Press.

Fonagy, P., Target, M., Cottrell, D., Phillips, J. & Kurtz, Z. (2002). *What Works for Whom?: a critical review of treatments for children and adolescents*. London: Guilford Press.

Gaub, M. & Carlson, C. (1997). Gender differences in ADHD: a meta-analysis and critical review. *Journal of the American Academy of Child and Adolescent Psychiatry*, (36), 1036–145.

Goodman, R. (1997). The strengths and difficulties questionnaire: a research note. *Journal of Child Psychology and Psychiatry*, 38, 581–86.

Gowers, S., Harrington, R. & Whitton, A. (1998). *Health of the Nation Outcome Scales for Children and Adolescents (HoNOSCA)*. London: Royal College of Psychiatrists.

Gowers, S., Levine, W. & Bailey-Rogers, S. (2002). The use of a routine self report outcome measure (HoNOSCA-SR) in two adolescent mental health services. *British Journal of Psychiatry*, (180), 266–69.

Green, H., McGinnity, A., Meltzer, H., Ford, T. & Goodman, R. (2005). *Mental Health of Children and Young People in Great Britain*. London: Office of National Satistics.

Green, J. & Jacobs, B. (1998). *In-patient Child Psychiatry: modern practice, research and the future*. London: Routledge.

Gulbenkian Foundation (1995). *Children and Violence: report of the commission on children and violence convened by the Gulbenkian Foundation*. London: Calouste Gulbenkian Foundation.

Higgins, I. & Burke, M. (1998). Managing oppositional and aggressive behaviour. In: Green, J. & Jacobs, B. (Eds) (1998). *In-patient Child Psychiatry: modern practice, research and the future*. London: Routledge.

Hogg, L. & Hall, J. (1992). Long-term impairments and challenging behaviour. In: Birchwood, M., & Tarrier, N. (Eds). *Innovations in the Psychological Treatment of Schizophrenia*. London: John Wiley.

Holyoake, D. & Fitzgibbon, S. (2002). *Discussing Child and Adolescent Mental Health Nursing*. Wiltshire: APS.

Leighton, S., Smith, C., Minns, K. & Crawford, P. (2001). Specialist child and adolescent mental health nurses: a force to be reckoned with? *Mental Health Practice*, 5 (2), 8–13.

McDougall, T. (1995). An emancipatory approach: therapeutic management of violence and aggression. *Psychiatric Care*, 2 (5), 158–60.

McDougall, T. (1996). Physical restraint: a review of the literature. *Psychiatric Care*, 3 (4), 132–38.

McDougall, T. (1997). Coercive interventions: the notion of the 'last resort'. *Journal of Psychiatric Care*, 4 (1), 19–21.

McDougall. T. (2000a). Violent incidents in a forensic adolescent unit: a retrospective analysis. *Nursing Times Research*, 5 (2), 87–98.

McDougall. T. (2000b). Violent incidents in a forensic adolescent unit: a functional analysis. *Nursing Times Research*, 5 (5), 346–63.

Malmquist, C. (1990). Depression in homicidal adolescents. *Bulletin of the American Academy of Psychiatry and the Law*, (18), 23–36.

Maroda, K. (1994). *The Power of Counter-transference: innovations in analytic technique*. London: Aronson.

Mayton, K. (1991). What are the considerations of the use of seclusion and restraint with children and adolescents? *Journal of Psychosocial Nursing*, 29 (3), 33–35.

Pfeiffer, S. & Strzelecki, S. (1990). In-patient psychiatric treatment of children and adolescents; a review of outcome studies. *Journal of the American Academy of Child and adolescent Psychiatry*, (29), 847–53.

Raine, A., Brennan, P. & Mednick, S. (1994). Birth complications combined with early maternal rejection at age 1 year predispose to violent crime at 18 years. *Archives of General Psychiatry*, (1), 984–88.

Rutter, M., Giller, H. & Hagell, A. (1998). *Antisocial behaviour by children and young people*. Cambridge: Cambridge University Press.

Shaffer, D., Gould, M., & Brasic, J. (1983). Children's Global Assessment Scale (CGAS). *Archives of General Psychiatry*, (40), 1228–31

Sharman, W. (1997). *Children and Adolescents with Mental Health Problems*. London: Balliere Tindall.

Smith, B. & Cantrell, P. (1988). Distance in nurse–patient encounters. *Journal of Psychosocial Nursing and Mental Health Services*, (26), 22–26.

Varma, V. (1999). *Violence in Children and Adolescents*. 2nd edn. London: Jessica Kingsley.

Chapter 9

Nursing Children and Young People with Learning Disabilities and Mental Health Problems

Tim McDougall

Key points

- Reports suggest that around one-third of a million children and young people in the UK have learning disabilities and as many as half experience mental health problems.

- Perhaps more than any other group of children, those with learning disabilities and mental health problems require multiagency services. Despite this, interagency service cooperation is often problematic and the needs of the young people and their families or carers are often fragmented.

- The majority of children and young people with learning disabilities do not require specialist CAMHS (child and adolescent mental health service). Instead, they require primary services in health, education and social services as part of mainstream children's services or lifespan learning disability services.

- To improve mental health services for children and young people with learning disabilities, nurses need to get better at transferring skills and expertise across organisations and systems with the minimum of bureaucracy.

- By virtue of their holistic approach and commitment to multiagency working, nurses are well placed to act as care coordinators or key workers for children with learning disabilities.

- Nurses are in key clinical, strategic and management positions to help establish competent care and treatment pathways and local and regional networks to help ensure that children and young people with learning disabilities and mental health problems reach their fullest potential.

Introduction

Most commonly accepted definitions of learning disability relate to the following three criteria: significant impairment in intellectual functioning, with an intelligence quotient (IQ) of 70 or less; significant impairment in two or more areas of adaptive functioning; and with onset during childhood (Thomson & McKenzie 2005). For the purposes of this chapter, the definition of learning disabilities is taken from the national guidance for learning disabilities, *Valuing People: A New Strategy for Learning Disability in the 21st Century* (Department of Health 2001). This defines learning disability as the presence of a significantly reduced ability to understand new or complex information; or to learn new skills (impaired intelligence); with a reduced ability to cope independently (impaired social functioning) which started in childhood; and which has a lasting effect on development. The following chapter describes current and emerging mental health service provision for children and adolescents with learning disabilities, and explores nursing assessment, care and treatment interventions for this client group.

Background

The mental health needs of children and adolescents with both learning disabilities and mental health problems have previously been neglected (YoungMinds 2000). The young people concerned, as well as their families and carers have suffered from fragmented service provision and discrimination arising from their disability. Across the UK, children and adolescents with learning disabilities have historically faced both geographical inequities in terms of access to and quality of NHS (National Health Service) services, and inequalities in comparison to those without learning disabilities (DoH 2001; Brown 2002). Only one-third of specialist CAMHS in England currently provide assessment and treatment for children and adolescents with learning disabilities (DoH & University of Durham 2004); and lifespan learning disability services include mental health in less than half of all local areas (DoH 2004a). Even where services are provided, many staff have not received specific education or training and only about 6% of nurses working in specialist CAMHS hold a qualification in learning disability nursing, i.e. the RNLD or RNMH (Jones 2004).

The focus of this chapter is on the nursing contribution to mental health services for children and young people with learning disabilities. However, nursing takes place in an interagency context and the roles of nurses compliment those of other multidisciplinary and multiagency team members. Responsibility for the mental health needs of children and young people with learning disabilities rests only in part with those who have backgrounds in child or learning disability nursing. Instead, each and every nurse, along with other children's professionals and workers, shares a responsibility to help ensure that health inequalities and social inclusion levels are improved for this group. Nurses who work with children and young people with learning disabilities do so in a range of community, residential, school and prison settings. This includes respite care, in-patient child and adolescent units, community services and young offender institutions. Wherever children and young people with learning disabilities receive their mental health services, there are a range of issues that impact on the nursing care and treatment interventions with this group.

The strategic context

The *Health of the Nation Strategy* published in 1995 included a priority to reduce rates of mental illness in people with learning disabilities (DoH 1995). However, it was not until the Children's Charter was published in 1997 that provision of mental health services for children and young people with learning disabilities was identified as an area of unmet need (DoH 1996). Since then, a range of strategic documents, legislation and guidance have set the scene in which mental health services for children with learning disabilities are evolving. This has culminated in publication of the National Service Framework (NSF) for Children, Young People and Maternity Services (DoH 2004a), in which the needs of young people with learning disabilities have been given a high profile.

Prior to publication of the NSF, the Department of Health in England published *Valuing People*, a modernisation strategy for learning disabilities services (DoH 2001). This was based on the key principles of rights, independence, choice and inclusion and contains a number of key messages to those who commission and provide learning disability services. First, children with disabilities have exactly the same healthcare needs as any other children. These are in addition to those generated by their particular disabilities and the additional family and social stresses of everyday life. Second, children with learning disabilities are more vulnerable to the full range of mental health problems and disorders (DoH 2001). The *Valuing People Strategy* was followed by *Count Us In*, a report by the Foundation for People with Learning Disabilities (FPLD 2003). This made key recommendations in relation to the emotional wellbeing of young people with learning disabilities, to family support and to workforce training and development. The report emphasised that like all young people, those with learning disabilities value friendships and relationships, benefit from purposeful activity, and have hopes and aspirations for their future.

The NSF for Children, Young People and Maternity Services has signalled the mental health of children with learning disabilities as a priority for action in England as part of the provision of comprehensive CAMHS (DoH 2004a). In addition, an NSF for children, young people and maternity services has also recently been published in Wales (National Assembly for Wales 2005), which includes a module on learning disabilities. The NSF in England is divided into two parts. There are five core standards that apply to all children and young people including those with learning disabilities. These relate to: the promotion of health and wellbeing; supporting parents and carers; child and family-centred services; growing up into adulthood; and safeguarding and promoting the welfare of children and young people. In addition, there are six specific chapters concerned with children and young people in particular circumstances. All specific chapters can be cross-referenced to the core standards and have common currency in relation to children and young people with learning disabilities. Though chapters should not be read in isolation, the following standards of the NSF are particularly relevant for nurses who are working with children and young people with learning disabilities and mental health problems.

Standard 8: disabled children and young people and those with complex health needs

This standard relates to children and young people who are disabled and/or those with complex health needs, including children and young people with learning disabilities, autistic spectrum disorders, sensory impairments, physical impairments and emotional/behavioural disorders. Whilst many children and young people with learning disabilities have no need for ongoing health interventions, others require ongoing treatment and/or nursing care and help with everyday activities. Some children and young people with learning disabilities will also be children in special circumstances (DoH 2004).

Standard 9: the mental health and psychological wellbeing of children and young people

This standard addresses the mental health needs of all children and young people, including those with learning disabilities. All children and young people with mental health problems, from birth to their eighteenth birthday, should have access to timely, integrated, high-quality, multidisciplinary and comprehensive mental health services to ensure effective assessment, treatment and support, for them and their families. This means that services for mental health promotion, illness prevention, early intervention and crisis resolution must be available in all local areas. Primary care trusts and local authorities must ensure that children and young people with learning disabilities receive equal access to mental health services at all tiers of CAMHS (DoH 2004a).

What kind of services do children and young people need?

It is important to be clear from the outset that children and young people with learning disabilities are children and young people first. This means that they have health, developmental, social and family needs, within which their disabilities are only one set of variables (DoH 2004a). They are unique individuals, with differing abilities, likes and dislikes. Most children and young people with learning disabilities have ordinary healthcare needs. This means that, like all children and young people, they need regular health checks, dental appointments and visits to their GP (general practitioner). On the whole, children and young people with learning disabilities should enjoy the same rights of access to healthcare services entitled to the general population (Lindsey 2002). Indeed, most children and young people with learning disabilities are physically well (Moss & Turner 1995) and many are educated in mainstream schools. Children and young people with more severe learning disabilities may attend special schools and often have associated medical disorders and sensory impairments, either as a cause or correlate of their learning disabilities (Simonoff 2005). However, despite the principle that children and young people with learning disabilities are children and young people first, this group does not currently have good access to comprehensive CAMHS.

Like all children and young people, those with learning disabilities have mental health needs. Notwithstanding issues of capacity and developmental delay, this means that they should enjoy the right to enter into, and sustain, mutually satisfying social relationships, and access opportunities to develop self-esteem and the skills to cope in the face of stress and adversity. Children and young people with learning disabilities are more vulnerable to the full range of mental health disorders and are at greater risk of developing mental health problems than those without learning disabilities (Dykens 2000; DoH 2001; Emerson 2003). Approximately 2–3% of the general population has a learning disability (Roeleveld et al. 1997). This means that around one-third of a million children and young people in the United Kingdom have learning disabilities and up to half experience mental health problems (Chadwick et al. 1998; Royal College of Psychiatrists 1998; FPLD 2002). Although the range of mental disorders experienced by children and adolescents with learning disabilities is similar to those experienced by young people in general, some disorders occur more frequently. These include hyperactivity and ADHD (attention deficit hyperactivity disorder) (Biederman et al. 1991; Fox & Wade 1998); pervasive developmental disorders including autism and autistic spectrum disorders (Gillberg 1999; Dekker & Koot 2003; Le Couteur & Baird 2003; Simonoff 2005); and emotional disorders (Emerson 2003). However, psychiatric disorders in this population manifest differently and the process of assessment and diagnosis is different due to specific language and communication needs (Fraser 2005). For example, assessing schizophrenia in children and young people with learning disabilities is extremely difficult. This is because diagnosis is dependent on labelling abstract symptoms such as hallucinations, delusions and paranoia (Wilson 1997), and because children and young people with learning disabilities may have imaginary friends, an active fantasy world or speak out loud to themselves (Levitas 2001). The challenges that the accurate assessment of mental disorders in this group presents will be discussed later in the chapter.

A substantial number of children and young people with learning disabilities also have additional psychosocial, physical and general health problems. These include self-injurious behaviour (Williams 2003); significant behavioural difficulties (Prior et al. 1999; Fraser 2005); speech and language problems

(Barr 1997); and difficulties with sleep, eating and elimination (Royal College of Psychiatrists 2004). Physical and general health problems include epilepsy (Deb 2000); sensory impairments such as problems with sight and hearing (Lindsey 2002); cerebral palsy; and other physical disabilities and syndromes associated with particular health risks (Lindsey 2002). For example, children and young people with Down's syndrome are at greater risk of congenital heart disease, gastrointestinal problems (Strafford & Gunn 1996) and thyroid difficulties (London 1985; Chong et al. 1998).

Vulnerable children and young people

The vulnerability of children and young people with learning disabilities arises from a combination of biological, psychological and social factors (Hardy & Bouras 2002). Biological influences include brain damage, physical illness and sensory impairments (Gravestock & Bouras 1997). Psychological factors include the emotional effects of trauma and adjustment to change or loss (Stavrakaki 1999), and social factors that impact on vulnerability include inappropriate care, education and treatment settings and social exclusion (Hardy & Bouras 2002). Due to their vulnerability, this group is at greater risk of abuse, neglect, bullying and exploitation from other children, young people or adults. They may also have additional risk factors that contribute to their vulnerability, such as difficulties with communication and dependence on others for intimate care needs (Jenkins & Davies 2004). These factors can increase social isolation and lead to further problems with self-consciousness, confidence and low self-esteem.

Children and young people with learning disabilities can also be both victims and perpetrators of sexual abuse. This may arise from vulnerability to exploitation, or poor understanding of sexual behaviour and interpersonal boundaries. They are at risk of being bullied due to looking 'different' due to dysmorphic features, and being emotionally immature. School nurses, in particular, encounter children and young people in a range of settings who are being exploited or bullied. Here their role is to help develop whole-school approaches to prevent and tackle bullying, as well as support individual children and young people who are involved in bullying (Offler 2000). All nurses share a responsibility to safeguard and protect children and young people with learning disabilities (McDougall 2003). This is enshrined in their code of professional conduct, performance and ethics (Nursing and Midwifery Council 2004). In order to fulfil their professional obligations, they must recognise and respond to the signs and symptoms of abuse, neglect, exploitation and bullying and ensure that competent protocols to manage these issues are in place. Where nurses are concerned about abuse and neglect, they should report their concerns to designated child protection professionals. For nurses in strategic roles, strong links with local boards safeguarding children's welfare are essential to ensure that clear operational policies and procedures are in place to safeguard children and young people.

How can nurses support young people with learning disabilities?

There are very few publications dedicated to child and adolescent learning disability nursing in general, and even fewer specifically concerned with mental health nursing interventions for this group. In the first report of its kind, *Promoting Health, Supporting Inclusion* (Scottish Executive 2002) explored the contribution that nurses and midwives make to the care and support of children (and adults) with learning disabilities. The report recommended a 'life-course' approach to nursing care and examined a range of key issues to reduce health inequalities and improve social inclusion for children and young people with learning disabilities. The report addressed the scope and range of nursing and midwifery contributions; areas of innovative and best nursing practice; future nursing and midwifery contributions; the education and training needs of student nurses and midwives; and the continuing professional development (CPD) needs of nurses to ensure that services for people with learning disabilities are improved. Mental health received a high priority in the recommendations, and the nursing workforce was identified as crucial in improving care and treatment services for children and young people with learning disabilities (Scottish Executive 2002).

Nursing in non-specialist CAMHS (Tier 1)

The majority of children with mild, moderate or severe learning disabilities do not require specialist mental health services. Instead, they require primary services in health, education and social services as part of mainstream children's services. This is to ensure health promotion, illness prevention and early intervention services. Mental health services at Tier 1 include mental health promotion, illness prevention, and the early intervention and detection of mental health problems. A small but growing range of service provision currently exists for children with learning disabilities in primary settings. These are provided by nurses and other professionals in paediatric services, schools and lifespan-learning disability services, as well as by preschool special needs workers and other voluntary sector workers in children's residential and community settings.

Mental health promotion, illness prevention and early intervention

Promoting health has always been a key component of nursing practice. Despite knowledge that children and young people with learning disabilities are at greater risk of developing mental health problems, mental health promotion programmes for children and young people with learning disabilities are few and far between. It is clearly important that mental health problems should be prevented as well as treated (FPLD 2002). However, universal pro-grammes aimed at protecting children from mental illness have not addressed the specific needs of this population (Hardy et al. 2004). It has been suggested that more than the general population of children and young people, those with learning disabilities need additional support to develop the emotional resilience to sustain mental health and psychological wellbeing (Edwards 2003). This is in order to cope with change; modify their environment; make and sustain relationships with others; recognise, understand and communicate thoughts and feelings; deal with stress and adversity; and develop feelings of self-worth (Edwards 2003). In order to fill the gap in mental health pro-motion for children and young people with learning disabilities, a small number of nurse-led targeted projects have been developed. These include the Tuesday Group which has produced promising results in terms of improved self-awareness and positive coping strategies (Hardy et al. 2004).

Research suggests that people with learning disabilities have an unhealthy diet, low levels of exercise, and are generally in poor physical health (Moore 2000). There is no doubt that physical and mental health are inextricably linked, and that poor health in general can be directly related to mental health prob-lems (Bullock & Little 1999; National Assembly for Wales 2002; DoH 2004b). Dealing with learning disability *per se* at the primary level is the responsibility of professionals such as obstetricians and midwives, genetic counsellors and paediatricians. However, nurses have a key role to play in helping children with learning disabilities develop mental health and resilience and prevent mental disorder. Mental health problems in children and young people with learning disabilities often go undetected and untreated (Hardy & Bouras 2002). There are many things that nurses can do in their public health and preventive role to improve this situation. Through their work in schools and community settings, nurses are well-placed to help children and young people with learn-ing disabilities develop social and communication skills, good self-esteem and assist them to achieve independence and complete the tasks of everyday living. These are all protective factors that may help develop emotional resilience. School nurses have also been identified as crucial in terms of helping children and young people choose healthy lifestyles (DoH 2004b). This can be in rela-tion to diet and exercise, personal health and hygiene, healthy sexual behav-iour and the use of drugs and alcohol through life-skills teaching (Moore 2000). However, for children and young people with learning disabilities, making healthy lifestyle choices is not always straightforward. This group may not understand the significance of a healthy lifestyle, value the import-ance of health screening or recognise the signs and symptoms of mental or physical ill-health (Lindsey 2002). This does not mean that health promotion is not important with children and young people with learning disabilities. Indeed, it is lack of interest in overcoming the challenges of providing effective health promotion that has previously contributed to the neglect, ill-treatment and abuse of people with learning disabilities. To improve health promotion services for this client group, nurses should ensure that children and young people have access to information that is suited to their communication needs. Information should not be presented in a complex fashion; the use of pictures and 'total communication' strategies (Wyman 2000) can be helpful and may assist comprehension and understanding (Hollins & Downer 2000).

Community nurses and health visitors play a vital early intervention role. Parenting children with learning disabilities does not come naturally and many of the rules that apply to rearing children in general do not apply to those with learning disabilities (Fraser 2005). By monitoring attachment behaviours between babies or infants and their parents, developmental concerns which may be indicative of learning disabilities can be identified and monitored. Through early intervention, nurses at Tier 1 CAMHS are well-placed to support children and young people with learning disabilities who have minor mental health problems. Common problems which may require the support of primary mental health services include sleep disorders, behaviour problems and transitional support. Sleep disorders are common in about one-third of children with learning disabilities (Quine 1991; 1992; Stores et al. 2000), and are very stressful for parents or carers to cope with. Nurses commonly provide support to individual children and their parents or carers through the use of sleep diaries, behavioural approaches and management of diet and sleep routines (Thorpe 2005).

Transitions

There is well-documented evidence that children and young people themselves, as well as their families or carers struggle more than usual with life transitions (McIntosh & Whitaker 1998; Morris 1999; Pearson 1999; Ward et al. 2003). Whether this is leaving school or care, or transferring from paediatric to adult services, or going from college to training or employment, transitions for young people with learning disabilities are periods of vulnerability which may impact negatively on their mental health and emotional resilience. This is in addition to the wider transitional issues involved in partaking of supporting friendships and engaging in community activities that promote good mental health and emotional wellbeing. This need is so widespread that learning disability partnership boards are now required to identify a 'transitions champion' (DoH 2001). Often a nurse, this person is required to take responsibility for continuity of care issues. Although transition planning for children and young people with learning disabilities is supposed to be schools-led (Department for Education and Skills 2001a; 2001b), many young people with learning disabilities fail to receive adequate support during these periods of vulnerability. School nurses as well as Connexions workers have vital roles to play in helping school-leavers with learning disabilities bridge the gap between leaving school and starting vocational, training or employment activities. This can be achieved through effective care-planning, and communication and liaison, as well as support for individual children and young people. During transitions to adult services, nurses should be mindful that there is wide variation in the age when young people achieve independence, and this is particularly important when planning services for those with learning disabilities, some of whom will never live independently.

Nursing in specialist CAMHS (Tiers 2–4)

The two main elements of service provision for people with learning disabilities are the enhancement of access to mainstream health services; and the provision of specialist services only when the needs of individuals cannot be met by mainstream services (Lindsey 2002). It has already been stated that wherever possible, children and young people with learning disabilities should be treated in mainstream children's services in primary settings. However, due to their increased risk for developing complex, severe or persistent mental disorders, this client group will sometimes require highly specialised CAMHS which may include in-patient treatment. Historically, most specialist CAMHS at Tier 3 have not provided learning disability services for children and adolescents. Treatment for this group has previously been institutional and it was not until the 1980s that care began to move from residential into community settings (Lowe & de Paiva 1991). The 1990s saw an accelerating programme of institutional closures and the development of new community services (Foster & Roberts 1998), with very few residential hospital settings left remaining. Whilst clinicians with learning disability skills, expertise and experience have been lacking, many specialist CAMHS have previously excluded children or young people on the grounds of their disability. This group has subsequently failed to access a service and this is clearly unacceptable in the era of modern children's services. Based on the principles of non-discrimination, social inclusion and accessibility, no child or young person should be excluded from receiving a mental health service by virtue of having a learning disability. However, inclusion without sensitivity, flexibility and attention to the particular needs of children and young people with learning disabilities described earlier, is not likely to be advantageous and may be no better than exclusion.

Assessment

The process of assessing mental disorder in young people with learning disabilities can be complex. The traditional process of examining a child's mental state may be insufficient for use with this group. Impaired communication skills can make accurate understanding and labelling of psychotic symptoms difficult, particularly as the degree of learning disability increases. Since children and young people may find it difficult to label emotions and articulate subjective experiences in abstract language, getting information about thoughts, feelings and their internal world can be problematic. They may be suggestible or acquiesce, telling the nurse what they believe they want hear, or say they understand when they do not for fear of appearing incompetent (Hardy & Bouras 2002). The potential for misunderstanding is significant; for instance, behaviours such as talking loudly or calling out, flapping hands, pulling people to attract their attention and refusing to talk are all common in those with learning disabilities. It is important that nurses understand such behaviours in the context of the learning disability rather than presume that they are evidence of mental disorder. For example, it is not unusual for children with learning disabilities to have specific individual behaviour patterns (Barr 1997). Nurses and other professionals must not presume that repetitive behaviour is necessarily part of an obsessive compulsive disorder. Psychomotor abnormalities and stereotypical movements are often associated with mental health problems. However, nurses should be aware that these are more common in people with learning disabilities, due to brain damage and the need for sensory stimulation. However, these kinds of movements may increase or worsen if the child or young person is under stress or suffering from a mental health problem (Dykens 1995). Self-injurious behaviour, also common in children and young people with severe learning disability must not be misunderstood as self-harm, where unlike self-injurious behaviour, the intention is usually clear.

It has been suggested that nurses who work with children who have learning disabilities must learn to listen with all their senses (Jenkins & Davies 2004). This means that due to the challenges of accurately assessing thoughts and emotions, nurses and other professionals often have to rely more on recognising the behavioural signs than identifying the psychological symptoms of mental disorder. Changes in functioning in children and young people with learning disabilities that could be associated with mental health problems have been identified by Hardy & Bouras (2002) and are listed in Box 9.1. As well as the ordinary and special needs of children and young people with learning disabilities, nurses involved in the assessment process should have a basic understanding of the genetic, neurological and social predisposition of this client group to mental health problems. This is as well as a good understanding of developmental disorders, particularly ADHD and autistic-spectrum disorders due to their high comorbidity (Beiderman et al. 1991; Simonoff 2005).

Box 9.1 Changes in functioning in children and young people with learning disabilities that could be associated with mental health problems.

- Biological changes such as in sleep pattern, appetite and weight.
- Reduction or loss in skills.
- Onset or increase in challenging behaviour.
- Increase in stereotypical movements.
- Increase in minor physical complaints.
- Communication levels.
- Social withdrawal or disinhibition.
- Energy and activity levels.
- Difficulties with memory and adaptation to new environments and situations.
- Reduced concentration span.
- Conflict in relationships.

Source: Hardy & Bouras (2002).

To help overcome the challenges of effectively meeting mental health needs in children and young people with learning disabilities, nurses need to consider a range of strategies, relating to the preparation and delivery of the assessment process. Prior to the assessment meeting, nurses should be aware of any special needs, including those associated with vision, hearing and communication. Wherever possible, the child or young person should be assessed in a familiar environment such as their home or school. If this is not possible, the environment should be comfortable, welcoming and free from distraction. Like all children and young people, those with learning disabilities should always be informed about what the assessment is for and what they should expect will happen during the process. They are entitled to an explanation about what the information in the assessment will be used for and who might have access to it. The assessment itself should be paced according to level of understanding, the need for explanations or reminders, and the child or young person's attention span. Open-ended rather than closed questions should be used, and abstract language should be avoided as much as possible. This is particularly important when assessing children and young people with autism or Asperger's Syndrome, for whom concrete questions will be easier to answer (Atwood 1998). This is no easy task and nurses may want to plan some of their questions in advance of the assessment.

Treatment and management strategies

Some children and adolescents with learning disabilities and mental health problems require highly specialised services at Tier 4 CAMHS. Due to the complexity of associated mental health problems and the presence of challenging behaviour, their needs and associated problems will usually be beyond the capability, expertise and experience of specialist CAMHS at Tier 3. Highly specialised multidisciplinary or multiagency Tier 4 provision such as in-patient adolescent provision, adolescent forensic services and residential special schools able to cater for children with learning disabilities and severe, complex or persistent mental disorders are extremely rare. The estimated need for in-patient hospital beds is in the region of 4 beds per 100 000 head of population (Scottish Executive 2000).

A small but significant number of adolescents with learning disabilities and mental health problems require secure provision due to their challenging, high-risk or offending behaviour. There may also be associated risk management issues such as aggressive, violent or sexualised behaviour that requires an intensive or secure intervention that Tier 3 CAMHS are unable to provide safely in a community setting. However, intensive care and low-secure health provision is often inadequate, and dedicated services within medium and maximum secure mental health facilities do not exist. Young people who require secure services are presently inappropriately detained within mental health or learning disability units for adults or in prison settings. Placement for such children within both open and locked adult mental health facilities presents significant child-protection concerns. On the occasions that in-patient services are required, the child or young person concerned invariably has to travel 'out of area', away from home, family and friends to receive an appropriate service. Although the following list is not exhaustive, the following may be associated with mental health problems and disorders and require an in-patient or forensic CAMHS intervention:

- Aggressive, violent or challenging behaviour towards others.
- High-risk or antisocial behaviour such as sexually inappropriate or abusive behaviour or fire-setting.
- Offending behaviour.
- Severe self-harm or self-injurious behaviour.
- Severe mental disorder associated with significant risk-management issues.
- Complex, severe or persistent eating disorders.
- Substance misuse.
- Complex neuropsychiatric, pervasive developmental disorders or neurological complications such as intractable epilepsy.
- The need for formal detention in hospital within Mental Health Act provisions.

As many as half of all children and young people with learning disabilities have behaviour problems and many of these may be associated with communication difficulties (Fraser 2005). Nursing skills to understand, prevent and manage challenging or antisocial behaviour in this group are central to their effective care, and treatment interventions are part of the learning disability nurse's role and cannot be underestimated. However, mental health and children's nurses receive little in the way of education and training to recognise and manage challenging behaviour, and are likely to appraise, understand and respond to aggressive, antisocial and self-injurious behaviour in a variety of ways (McKenzie et al. 2004). Nurses working in specialist CAMHS often receive referrals for children with behaviour problems (McDougall & Crocker 2002). As well as mental health problems, many also have specific developmental disorders and learning disabilities. Unfortunately, many of these referrals have previously been declined due to rigid exclusion criteria that are often arbitrary and of no use to the child or young person, their family or carers.

Nurses working in specialist in-patient, forensic or residential settings with children and young people with learning disabilities may occasionally need to hold or restrain children and young people if their behaviour is aggressive or violent and verbal de-escalation strategies have been ineffective (McDougall 2000). However, the use of physical intervention is an area of contention and a catalogue of child protection failures has shone light on all that we do with vulnerable children and young people in public care. There has also been debate about the legal basis and permissibility of particular forms of treatment, restraint and detention of children and young people with learning disabilities (Lyon 1995). Restrictive physical interventions may sometimes be necessary to prevent children or young people with learning disabilities from hurting themselves or others (British Institute of Learning Disabilities 2004).

It is fair to say that specialist CAMHS at Tiers 2, 3 and 4 vary in terms of their capacity, capability and willingness to provide comprehensive assessment and treatment services for children with learning disabilities. Only one-third of specialist CAMHS currently provide assessment and treatment for this client group (DoH 2004). However, there is significant room for improvement in terms of the contribution that specialist CAMHS can make to multiagency careplans for children and young people with learning disabilities who develop mental disorders. Specialist CAMHS at Tier 3 should move from being a 'can't do' service to a 'can do' service when a local child or young person with learning disabilities has a mental disorder which requires specialist help. The NSF recognises that there are significant resource and training factors associated with improving CAMHS for children and young people with learning disabilities and their needs have been highlighted as a priority for NSF delivery (DoH 2004). Referral pathways to specialist CAMHS for all children and young people, including those with learning disabilities, is poorly defined and has been likened to a postcode lottery (Audit Commission 1999). Whether a child remains at home or is placed in a residential school, local authority secure unit or hospital is not informed by multiagency referral pathways but rather by local service availability, professional expertise or chance. This can generate significant cost to the children and families concerned. Their needs are invariably fragmented and both aftercare and follow-up treatment can be problematic to arrange. Not only do children themselves suffer, but inappropriate placement in services within health, local authority, and education or youth justice agencies generates high financial costs for service commissioners who have limited budgets to meet the needs of local populations.

The importance of multidisciplinary team-working

It is clear that no single agency, service or professional can meet the wide range of needs presented by children and young people with learning disabilities and mental health problems. Not surprisingly, this population usually requires multiagency services. Despite this, interagency service cooperation is frequently problematic and the needs of the young people and their families are often fragmented (DoH 2004). *Together from the Start* (DoH & DfES 2002) provides practical guidance for professionals working with disabled children. (DoH & DfES 2003). This report demonstrated that children and young people with disabilities, as well as their families and carers, want a single point of contact via a trusted and informed professional, and clear pathways to support. This message was repeated in *Making Us Count* published by the FPLD (2005). Nurses are in key positions to champion the needs of children with learning disabilities and help improve interagency working (McDougall 2004). By virtue of their holistic approach and commitment to multiagency working, nurses are well-placed to act as care coordinators or key workers for children with learning disabilities. Nurses are valued by service-users and their parents and carers (Jackson & Stevenson 2000; Callaghan et al. 2002; Healthcare Commission 2004). It has been suggested that they are pivotal in securing access to primary and secondary healthcare services for people with learning disabilities (Manthorpe et al. 2003). Where comprehensive services close to home are lacking, it is important that children with learning disabilities and their families and carers have access to a competent network of professionals who can collaborate to provide a comprehensive intervention. Advocacy is an integral part of the nurse's role and is part of their code of professional conduct (Nursing & Midwifery Council 2002). It involves speaking up for, or promoting the interests of vulnerable people who are unable to do so themselves. Advocacy is particularly relevant in learning disability services, where children and young people may have difficulties with communication and be the subject of prejudice (Jaydeokar & Piachaud 2004). Since many children and young people with learning disabilities have a diminished capacity to understand their rights and articulate their viewpoint, nurses must advocate on their behalf in order to promote their best interests at all times.

Education and social services as well as paediatric and mental health services must work together if services for children with learning disabilities are to be comprehensive and seamless. Nurses work in all these sectors and are in key positions to coordinate multiagency interventions and engage teachers, social workers, health professionals and youth justice workers. This involves giving, receiving and seeking advice and consultation, networking and coworking, and being creative and innovative in how they assess, plan and manage the multiprofessional intervention programme. The care programme approach (CPA) can be used to develop careplans and agree roles and responsibilities for interagency working. Although the CPA was specifically developed to provide a framework for effective mental healthcare (NHS Executive 1999), it can be adapted to include planning in relation to services such as education and Connexions.

To function as effective care coordinators for children and young people who have learning disabilities and mental health problems, nurses must establish a number of key relationships. As well as with learning disability nurses, these relationships must be with professionals and other staff in both statutory and voluntary service organisations in health, education, social services and youth justice settings. A range of health service providers will have a role to play in the interagency assessment and treatment plan formation. As well as health visitors, paediatric nurses and community matrons, these will include paediatricians, physiotherapists, speech and language therapists and occupational therapists. Adult learning disability teams, early onset psychosis teams and services for young people aged 16 to 19 may also have a role to play during the transition from adolescent to adult mental health services. In social services, disabled children's teams, child protection services and respite workers are often required to contribute to the multiagency careplan and links between nurses and this wider workforce are vital. In youth justice agencies, nurses work in youth offending teams and young offender institutions and often encounter young people with learning disabilities who are involved in offending behaviour, anti-social or high-risk behaviour.

Education and training

Successful delivery of the *Every Child Matters* outcomes and NSF priorities for children with learning disabilities depends crucially on a competent, capable and supported workforce. However, there is currently a lack of appropriately trained and skilled CAMHS professionals including nurses (DoH 2004a). Frontline professionals such as mental health nurses, school nurses and paediatric nurses must have access to the kind of education and training that enables the development of skills and competencies in relation to normal childhood development, developmental delay and learning disabilities. However, nurses do not emerge from preregistration programmes with the skills and competencies to work effectively with children and young people who have learning disabilities and mental health problems. Not surprisingly, most nurses are inexperienced since very few have had access to placements with this group of children and young people (Scottish Executive 2002). Nurses who work with children and adolescents with learning disabilities require a broad range of skills and competencies. As well as skills to work with children and adolescents, competencies in relation to learning disabilities and skills to work with a range of mental health problems and disorders are also needed. These are in addition to the appropriate care and communication skills that ensure than the holistic needs of the child or young person and their family or carers are met. If nurses are to provide effective mental health promotion and early intervention services, they must receive education and training in relation to attachment, parenting and resilience-building.

Whilst mainstream services for children and young people with learning disabilities must undoubtedly improve, there will always be a need for professionals with specialist expertise. As Brown (2002) states, this is not an 'either-or' issue, as both are necessary and both have their place. Nurses working in primary settings need skills to recognise and understand a range of learning disabilities and developmental disorders. They also need to recognise and understand the difference between mild and moderate, severe or profound learning disabilities, autism and autistic spectrum disorders. In addition, specialist learning disability nurses and other learning disability experts must be able to support mainstream children's services by providing support for frontline professionals and assessment and treatment for young people with the most complex needs. These include young people with epilepsy, autistic spectrum disorders, challenging behaviours and mental disorders. All are areas of practice in which nurses have pioneered new roles and innovative ways of working (Brown 2004). It is not possible for every nurse to possess the full range of skills and competencies required to work with children and young people who have learning disabilities. However, nor is it appropriate for them merely to access short courses or workshops. Getting the balance right by influencing the nurse education and training curricula, challenging traditional practice and forging strong links with nurses and other colleagues in specialist and lifespan learning disability services is the key to workforce development.

Following the move away from hospital or institution-based healthcare, many commentators have questioned the need to prepare a specific group of nurses to work exclusively with people who have learning disabilities (Brown 2005; Fraser 2005). However, it can also be argued that the current four-branch system of nurse education and training in the UK does not, individually or collectively, adequately prepare nurses to meet the mental health needs of children and young people with learning disabilities. Many nurses are still unable to tell the difference between mental health problems and learning disabilities (Scottish Executive 2002). This is completely unacceptable. Nurses who are involved in the planning, commissioning and delivery of nurse education and training must ensure that the needs of children and young people with learning disabilities are given a higher profile in current and future education and training programmes for nurses and other professionals. In a recent UK survey of over 800 CAMHS nurses, understanding and working with children and young people who have learning disabilities was cited as a priority training need (Jones 2004).

Conclusion

It is only ten years since a report showed that some GPs were refusing to accept people with learning disabilities (Singh 1997) and a survey of general nurses found that the majority were in favour of segregating people with learning disabilities from other patients in hospital (Slevin & Sines 1996). Mental health services for children and young people with learning disabilities are in their infancy and we clearly have a long way to go before achieving comprehensive CAMHS for this group. There is much that nurses and other professionals can do to help ensure that services for children and young people with learning disabilities and mental health problems are improved. To do this they must shed traditional ways of working that have previously failed this group. In their place, creative, innovative and 'can do' practice must evolve (McDougall 2004).

Services for children and adolescents with learning disabilities should be provided within mainstream CAMHS. This supports the social inclusion and child-first principles that should guide the commissioning and delivery of all specialist services for children. This means that all children and young people who require CAMHS should be able to access mental health services regardless of physical, mental or developmental ability. There is no single model of service design and delivery that can be applied in all local areas. It is important that nurses and other professionals do not pursue the 'perfect' solution or a one-size-fits-all approach. However, there are some fundamental principles that should underpin all service commissioning, design and delivery. The 'child-first' principle suggests that mental health services should be provided in mainstream settings and interventions should be supported by those with training in learning disabilities. Wherever possible, children with learning disabilities and mental health problems should be treated close to home and with minimum disruption to school and family life. This will usually require a well-coordinated multiagency careplan involving the combined skills, talents and expertise of a range of professionals and supported by specialist learning disability services.

Nurses are in key clinical, strategic and management positions to help establish competent care and treatment pathways and local and regional networks to help ensure that the children and young people they work with reach their fullest potential. In line with the government's strategy, nurses should actively seek to promote the mental health of children and young people with learning disabilities. This can be achieved through their work in schools, hospitals and community settings with individuals, groups and by supporting other children's professionals. There are undoubtedly significant capacity and capability issues in terms of achieving comprehensive CAMHS for children and young people with learning disabilities. However, whilst shortfalls in training and workforce are addressed, nurses and other professionals must help develop managed clinical networks, local pathways and creative solutions to ensure that children and young people receive the best service possible. This does not mean that all nurses need to become experts in learning disabilities. Rather, nurses need to get better at transferring skills and expertise across organisations and systems with the minimum of bureaucracy. This will require new ways of working across traditional professional and service boundaries and more effective liaison and consultation with nurses and other colleagues in learning disability services.

References

Atwood, T. (1998). *Asperger's Syndrome: a guide for parents and professionals*. London: Jessica Kingsley.

Audit Commission (1999). *Children in Mind: a report on child and adolescent mental health services*. London: Audit Commission.

Beiderman, J., Newcorn, J. & Sprich, S. (1991). Comorbidity of attention deficit hyperactivity disorder with conduct, depressive, anxiety and other disorders. *American Journal of Psychiatry*, (148), 564–77.

Bernard, S. (1999). Mental health services for children and adolescents with learning disabilities. *Tizard Learning Disability Review*, (4), 43–45.

British Institute of Learning Disabilities (2004). *Easy guide to being held safely for children and young people with learning difficulties and/or autism, their teachers and parents.* London: BILD.

Brown, M. (2002). Executive decision. *Learning Disability Practice*, **5** (7), 8–10.

Brown, M. (2004). Three of a kind. *Learning Disability Practice*, **7** (8), 39.

Bullock, R. & Little, M. (1999). The interface between social and health services for children and adolescent persons. *Current Opinion in Psychiatry*, (12), 421–24.

Callaghan, P., Eales, S., Coats, T., Bowers, L. & Bunker, J. (2002). Patient feedback on liaison mental health care in A&E. *Nursing Times*, **98** (21), 34–36.

Chadwick, O., Taylor, E. & Bernard, S. (1998). *The Prevention of Behaviour Disorders in Children with Severe Learning Disability. Final Report to the NHS Executive.* London: Institute of Psychiatry.

Chong, E., Dennis, J. & Archer, N. (1998). The effectiveness of screening for congenital F53 heart disease in a 14-year cohort of children with Down's syndrome. *Archives of Disease in Childhood*, (2), 63.

Deb, S. (2000). Epidemiology and treatment of epilepsy in patients who are mentally retarded. *CNS Drugs*, (13), 117–28.

Dekker, M. & Koot, H. (2003). DSM-IV disorders in children with borderline to moderate intellectual disability: prevalence and impact. *Journal of the American Academy of Child and Adolescent Psychiatry*, (42), 15–22.

Department of Health (1995). *Health of the Nation: a strategy for people with learning disabilities.* London: HMSO.

Department of Health (1996). *The Patient's Charter: services for children and young people.* London: HMSO.

Department of Health (2001). *Valuing People: a strategy for learning disabilities in the 21st century.* London: HMSO.

Department of Health (2004a). *National Service Framework for Children, Young People and Maternity Services.* London: HMSO.

Department of Health (2004b). *Choosing Health: making healthier choices easier.* London: HMSO.

Department of Health and Department for Education and Skills (2001a). *The Connexions Framework for Assessment, Planning, Implementation and Review: guidance for personal advisors.* London: HMSO.

Department of Health and Department for Education and Skills (2001b). *Special Educational Needs: code of practice.* London: HMSO.

Department of Health and Department for Education and Skills (2003). *Together from the Start: practical guidance for professionals working with disabled children and their families.* London: HMSO.

Department of Health & University of Durham. National Child and Adolescent Mental Health Services Mapping Exercise. London: HMSO.

Dykens, E. (1995). Measuring behavioural phenotypes: provocations from the new genetics. *American Journal on Mental Retardation*, **99** (5), 522–32.

Dykens, E. (2000). Psychopathology in children with intellectual disability. *Journal of Child Psychology & Psychiatry*, **41** (4), 407–17.

Edwards, N. (2003). Promoting mental health and well-being. In: Edwards, N. (Ed.). *Mental Health in Adult Developmental Disability.* Queensland: Queensland Centre for Intellectual and Developmental Disability.

Emerson, M. (2003). Prevalence of psychiatric disorders in children and adolescents with and without intellectual disability. *Journal of Intellectual Disability Research*, (47), 51–58.

Foundation for People with Learning Disabilities (2002). *Count Us In: inquiry into meeting the needs of young people with learning disabilities.* London: FPLD.

Foundation for People with Learning Disabilities (2005). *Making us Count: identifying and improving mental health support for young people with learning disabilities.* London: FPLD.

Fox, R. & Wade, E. (1998). Attention deficit hyperactivity disorders among adults with severe and profound mental retardation. *Research in Developmental Disabilities*, (19), 275–80.

Fraser, W. (2005). Children and adolescents who have a learning disability: the challenges to services. In: Williams, R. & Kerfoot, M. (Eds). *Child and Adolescent Mental Health Services: strategy, planning, delivery and evaluation.* Oxford: Oxford University Press.

Gillberg, C. (1999). Autism and its spectrum disorders. In: Bouras, N. (Ed.). *Psychiatric and Behavioural Disorders in Developmental Disabilities and Mental Retardation.* Cambridge: Cambridge University Press.

Gravestock, S. & Bouras, S. (1997). Emotional disorders. In: Holt, G. & Bouras, N. (Eds). *Mental Health in Learning Disabilities: a training pack for staff working with people who have a dual diagnosis of mental health needs and learning disabilities.* Brighton: Pavillion.

Hardy, S. & Bouras, N. (2002). The presentation and assessment of mental health problems in people with learning disabilities. *Learning Disability Practice*, **5** (3), 33–38.

Hardy, S., Essam, V. & Woodward, P. (2004). The Tuesday group: promoting mental health. *Learning Disability Practice*, (23), 20–23.

Healthcare Commission (2004). *Patient survey report 2004 – Mental Health.* London: Healthcare Commission.

Hollins, S. & Downer, J. (2000). *Keeping Healthy 'Down Below'.* London: Gaskell.

Jackson, S. & Stevenson, C. (2000). What do people need psychiatric and mental health nurses for? *Journal of Advanced Nursing*, **31** (2), 378–88.

Jaydeokar, S. & Piachaud, J. (2004). Out-of-borough placements for people with learning disabilities. *Advances in Psychiatric Treatment*, (10), 116–23.

Jenkins, R. & Davies, R. (2004). The abuse of adults with learning disabilities and the role of the learning disability nurse. *Learning Disability Practice*, **7** (2), 30–38.

Jones, J. (2004). *The Post-registration Education and Training Needs of Nurses Working with Children and Young People with Mental Health Problems in the UK: a research study conducted by the Mental Health Programme, Royal College of Nursing Institute, in collaboration with the RCN Children and Young People's Mental Health Forum.* London: RCN.

Le Couteur, A. & Baird, G. (2003). *National Autism Plan for Children.* London: National Autistic Society.

Levitas, A. (2001). The mental state examination in patients with mental retardation and developmental disabilities. *Mental Health Aspects of Developmental Disabilities*, **4** (2), 2–16.

Lindsey, M. (2001). Comprehensive healthcare services for people with learning disabilities. *Advances in Psychiatric Treatment*, (8), 138–48.

Loudon, M., Day, R. & Duke, E. (1985). Thyroid dysfunction in Down's Syndrome. *Archives of Disease in Childhood*, (80), 1149–51.

Lowe, K. & de Paiva, S. (1991). *NIMROD: an overview.* London: HMSO.

Lyon, C. (1995). *Legal Issues Arising from the Care, Control and Safety of Children with Learning Disabilities Who also Present Severe Challenging Behaviour.* London: Mental Health Foundation.

McDougall, T. (2000). Violent incidents in a forensic adolescent unit: a functional analysis. *NT Research*, **5** (5), 346–63.

McDougall, T. (2003). Every Child Matters: Green Paper on children at risk. *Learning Disability Practice*, **6** (9), 17.

McDougall, T. (2004). In the frame. *Learning Disability Practice*, **7** (9), 28–29.

McDougall, T. & Crocker, A. (2002). Referral pathways through a specialist child and adolescent mental health service: the role of the specialist practitioner. *Mental Health Practice*, **5** (1), 16–20.

McIntosh, B. & Whitaker, A. (1998). *Days of Change: a parental guide for developing better day opportunities with people with learning difficulties.* London: Kings Fund.

McKenzie, K., Paxton, D., Loads, D., Kwaitek, E., McGregor, L. & Sharp, K. (2004). The impact of nurse education on staff attributions in relation to challenging behaviour. *Learning Disability Practice*, **7** (5), 15–20.

Manthorpe, J., Alaszewski, A., Gates, B., Ayer, S. & Motherby, E. (2003). Learning disability nursing: user and carer perceptions. *Journal of Learning Disabilities*, **7** (2), 119–35.

Moore, D. (2000). Pathways to better health. *Learning Disability Practice*, **3** (4), 11–16.

Morris, J. (1999). *Hurtling into a Void.* Brighton: Pavillion.

National Assembly for Wales (2002). *The Review of Safeguards for Children and Young People Treated and Cared for by the NHS in Wales. Too Serious a Thing: the Carlisle Review.* Cardiff: National Assembly for Wales.

National Assembly for Wales (2005). *National Service Framework for Children, Young People and Maternity Services in Wales.* Cardiff: National Assembly for Wales.

Nursing & Midwifery Council (2004). *The NMC Code of Professional Conduct: standards for conduct, performance and ethics.* London: NMC.

Offler, E. (2000). Bullying: everybody's problem. *Paediatric Nursing*, **12** (9), 22–26.

Pearson, M. (1999). *Positive Health in Transition: a guide to effective and reflective transition planning for young people with learning disabilities.* Manchester: National Development Team.

Prior, M., Smart, D., Sanson, A. & Oberklaid, F. (1999). Relationships between learning difficulties and psychological problems in preadolescent children from a longitudinal sample. *Journal of the American Academy of Child and Adolescent Psychiatry*, (38), 429–36.

Quine, L. (1991). Sleep problems in children with mental handicap. *Journal of Mental Deficiency Research*, (35), 269–90.

Quine, L. (1992). Severity of sleep problems in children with severe learning disabilities: description and correlates. *Journal of Community and Applied Social Psychology*, (2), 247–68.

Quine, L. (1993). Teaching parents of children with severe handicaps to manage sleep disturbance by using behavioural methods. In: Harris, J. (Ed.). *Innovations in Training For Those Working With People Who Have Severe Learning Difficulties.* Kidderminster: BIMH.

Roeleveld, N., Zeilhuis, G. & Gabreels, F. (1997). The prevalence of mental retardation: a critical review of recent literature. *Developmental Medicine and Child Neurology*, (39), 125–32.

Royal College of Psychiatrists (2004). *Psychiatric Services for Children and Adolescents with a Learning Disability. Council Report CR70.* London: Royal College of Psychiatrists.

Scottish Executive (2000). *The Same as You?: a review of services for people with learning disabilities.* Edinburgh: Scottish Executive.

Scottish Executive (2002). *Promoting Health, Supporting Inclusion: the National review of the contribution of all nurses and midwives to the care and support of people with learning disabilities.* Edinburgh: Scottish Executive.

Simonoff, E. (2005). Children with psychiatric disorders and learning disabilities. *British Medical Journal*, **2** (5), 742–43.

Singh, P. (1997). *Prescription for change*. London: Mencap.

Slevin, E. & Sines, D. (1996). Attitudes of nurses in a general hospital towards people with learning disabilities: influences of contact and graduate non contact status: a comparative study. *Journal of Advanced Nursing*, **24** (12), 1116–26.

Stavrakaki, C. (1999). Depression, anxiety and adjustment disorders in people with developmental disabilities. In: Bouras, N. (Ed.). *Psychiatric and Behavioural Disorders in Developmental Disabilities and Mental Retardation*. Cambridge: Cambridge University Press.

Stores, R., Wiggs, L. & Stores, G. (2000). Management of sleep disorders in children with learning difficulties. In: Bage, R. & Jeffreys, K. (Eds). *Positive Initiatives For People With Learning Difficulties*. London: McMillan.

Strafford, B. & Gunn, P. (1996). *New Approaches to Down's Syndrome*. London: Cassell.

Thomson, R. & McKenzie, K. (2005). What people with a learning disability understand and feel about having a learning disability. *Learning Disability Practice*, **8** (6), 28–32.

Thorpe, B. (2005). Managing sleep disturbances in children with learning disabilities. *Nursing Times*, **101** (12), 42.

Ward, L., Mallett, R., Heslop, P. & Simons, K. (2003). Planning for health at transition. *Learning Disability Practice*, **6** (3), 24–27.

Wyman, R. (2000). *Making Sense Together*. London: Souvenir Press.

Williams, R. (2003). *Literature Review of Services for Children with Special Health Needs in Wales: Lot 3: mental health in childhood, children and young people who have mental health problems and mental disorders and mental health services for young people*. Cardiff: National Assembly for Wales.

Wilson, D. (1997). Psychiatric disorders and mild learning disability. In: Russell, O. (Ed.). *Seminars in the Psychiatry of Learning Disabilities*. London: Gaskell.

YoungMinds (2000). *Whose Crisis?: meeting the needs of children and young people with serious mental health problems*. London: YoungMinds.

Chapter 10

Child and Adolescent Forensic Mental Health Nursing

Paul Mitchell

Key points

- Young people in the youth justice system are up to three times more likely to have mental health problems than their peers in the general population.

- Mental health nurses are in key positions to play a prominent role in the development and delivery of forensic services for children and young people. This is due to both their specialist knowledge of mental health problems, and a broad-based understanding of the holistic needs of children and young people.

- For most young people in contact with the youth justice system, their mental health needs should be regarded as one element in their wider range of needs.

- The large majority of young people in contact with adolescent forensic mental health services meet the criteria for a diagnosis of conduct disorder, including subgroups such as mixed disorders of conduct and emotion, hyperkinetic disorder, depressive conduct disorder and ADHD (attention deficit hyperactivity disorder).

- Nurses undertaking forensic assessments should always seek to obtain information from as many sources as possible. Information provided by parents, or carers and professionals currently or previously involved with a young person, is crucially important.

- Adolescent forensic mental health provision is a rapidly developing field which provides nurses with a range of opportunities and challenges. The challenge is not only to implement change as services evolve, but also to innovate and influence how services for young people in contact with the youth justice system will be delivered.

Introduction

Young people in contact with the youth justice system are up to three times more likely to have mental health problems than their peers in the general population (Department of Health 2004). In recent years increasing attention has been paid to the mental health needs of children and young people within the criminal justice system by both clinicians and policymakers. This interest has been driven by a realisation that this population's mental health needs often go unrecognised and unmet (Teplin et al. 1992; Dolan et al. 1999); and also by the recognition of the long-term psychosocial implications which arise from the failure to recognise and address these needs (Kurtz et al. 1996).

Across the United Kingdom there are differences in legislation and the way in which services for young people are configured. In England the recently published National Service Framework (NSF) for Children, Young People and Maternity Services (DoH 2004) emphasises the need for equality of access to services, particularly for groups such as young offenders who often have complex health needs and find it difficult to access services. Standard 8 of the NSF specifically states that young people with complex needs should have access to services that promote social inclusion. Standard 9 states that all young people from birth to their eighteenth birthday should have access to timely, integrated services (DoH 2004). The range of mental health provision available to young people in contact with the criminal justice system remains inadequate but has developed significantly over the past few years. Services available include a range of options from mental health screening for young people in court, to long-term secure placements for young people with serious and enduring mental disorders. Between these two extremes a variety of new initiatives have also emerged. These include joint appointments between child and adolescent mental health services (CAMHS) and youth offending teams (YOTs); dedicated teams providing in-reach to secure units and young offender institutions (YOIs); and consultation and training by adolescent forensic nurse specialists or professionals in residential care, prison and community settings.

The following chapter does not address nursing care for the highly specialised needs of the relatively small population of young people with serious and enduring mental disorders who are cared for in conditions of medium security. This information can be accessed elsewhere (McDougall 1998; 1999). Nor will it look at the needs of the very small group of pre-adolescent children who come into contact with youth justice agencies. Rather, it will concentrate on the interface between CAMHS and the youth justice system. Mental health nurses are in key positions to play a prominent role in the development and delivery of these services. This is due to both their specialist knowledge of mental health problems affecting young people, and their broad-based understanding of the holistic needs of children and young people. By looking at the mental health needs of young people in contact with the youth justice system, it is possible to demonstrate that their needs are often the same as their peers. It can be argued therefore, that provided risk-management is addressed, mental health services for young people in general can be applied directly in the youth justice system. By addressing issues of risk assessment and management, mental health nurses can apply their knowledge and skills base to meeting the mental health needs of young offenders.

Mental health services for young people within the youth justice system

The youth justice system in the UK is overseen by the Youth Justice Board (YJB). The YJB is responsible for custodial provision for 'juveniles', under 18 years of age and 'young offenders', aged between 18 and 21. The majority of secure places for under-18s are in YOIs (*see Glossary*) but younger offenders, or those considered to be particularly vulnerable, are placed in local authority secure units which are smaller than YOIs and staffed by residential care workers. The YJB also oversees the work of local YOTs (*see Glossary*), which are responsible for working with young offenders in the community. YOTs have staff from multiple agencies (probation, social services, education, police and health) and are expected to form part of a 'joined-up' service to meet the wider needs of young offenders as well as supervising their non-custodial sentences.

It is often assumed that young people within the youth justice system have highly specialised mental health needs that are profoundly different to those of their peers. For a small number of young people this is undoubtedly true; young people who have committed serious acts of violence in response to command auditory hallucinations or paranoid delusions require highly specialised interventions. Particular differences relate to the legal process and include the young person's fitness to stand trial and their status as a remanded or sentenced offender. However, for most young people in contact with the youth justice system their mental health needs should be regarded as one element of their wider range of needs. For some of these young people particular concerns may exist in relation to risk. This often justifies referral to a specialised service for assessment and intervention. However, for many young people, there may not be a complex interrelationship between their high-risk or offending behaviour and mental health needs. Indeed, some young people in contact with the youth justice system have mental health needs not related to their offending behaviour. Here, mental health nurses can play a pivotal role. Skills to determine how specific mental health needs and problems relate to a wider range of personal and social needs are invaluable in determining an appropriate assessment and intervention strategy.

Which young people are likely to be referred for a mental health assessment?

Referrals of young people for mental health assessment come from a range of sources, including specialist CAMHS at Tiers 3 and 4. Many young people will be known by their local specialist CAMHS, and referral for a forensic assessment has usually been precipitated by a general increase in the severity of need, or an unanticipated change in behaviour or an increase in risk. As such, whilst such change may generate new needs for the young person, many other aspects of their overall needs will remain the same. Young people can also be referred for a forensic mental health assessment by their GP (general practitioner). This is often at the request of another professional working with a young person, such as a social worker or YOT worker. Other referrals are taken from adult psychiatrists, paediatricians and occasionally health service directors. In many cases, these young people will also be known to their local CAMHS. However, for some young people, a forensic assessment may be the first contact with mental health services and prior information may be limited.

Not surprisingly, the average age of young people referred for a forensic assessment is higher than those referred to mainstream CAMHS. Increasingly, CAMHS are required to provide services for young people aged between 16 and 18 (DoH 2004). Nurses working with this age-group must be aware that the mental health needs and other needs of older adolescents change as they near adulthood. Nurses must also establish links with adult mental health services (including forensic services) in order to ensure that transitional arrangements are in place before young people reach adulthood. More boys than girls are referred to community adolescent forensic services. This trend is to be expected since it is predominately boys and young men who come into contact with the youth justice system (National Association for the Care and Rehabilitation of Offenders 2001; Armstrong et al. 2005). There are undoubtedly some differences in the type of mental health problems which present in girls compared to boys. However, it is important to avoid stereotypes based on gender. For instance, there is increasing recognition of conduct disorder in girls (Storvoll & Wichstrom, 2002; Delligatti et al. 2003), and at the same time there are indications that the prevalence of self-harm amongst boys may be increasing (Hawton et al. 2003).

Historically, the principle task of the criminal justice system has been to manage adult male offenders. Young people, particularly young women and girls, constitute a minority group within the system. As such, nurses need to be aware about how the specific needs of certain young people can remain unmet. Many young people referred to adolescent forensic mental health services are in contact with the youth justice system, either in custody, on bail or subject to a community sentence. Many will be accommodated or the subject of a local authority care order (Hagell 2003; NACRO 2005). The high level of multiagency involvement with young people in contact with the youth justice system requires competent communication, liaison and consultation by nurses. These issues are explored later, with particular reference to the care programme approach (CPA).

What kind of mental health problems do they have?

Mental health problems are diagnosed using the World Health Organization's (WHO's) multiaxial classification of child and adolescent psychiatric disorders, ICD-10 (WHO 1992). This method of classification is valuable since it focuses specifically on child and adolescent disorders (Axis 1), but also broadens the context of diagnosis to account for other factors such as developmental disorders (Axis 2), intellectual functioning (Axis 3) and medical conditions (Axis 4). Axis 5 is also useful for classifying child and adolescent disorders as it addresses social factors (current and historical) which contribute to the generation, maintenance and exacerbation of a young person's mental health problems.

A large proportion of young people in contact with the youth justice system meet the criteria for a diagnosis of conduct disorder (Mental Health Foundation 2002), including subgroups such as mixed disorders of conduct and emotion, hyperkinetic disorder, depressive conduct disorder and ADHD (Fonagy & Kurtz 2002). High rates of conduct disorders are not surprising as persistent behavioural problems are likely to be the reason young people come into contact with the youth justice system in the first place. Increased prevalence of conduct disorder in this population has been consistently cited in the research literature (McManus et al. 1984; Nichol et al. 2000; Papageorgiou & Vostanis 2000; Carswell & Davenport 2000; Royal College of Psychiatrists 2004). In addition to conduct disorder, many young people in contact with the youth justice system meet the criteria for diagnosis of an emotional disorder (Lader et al. 2000; Mental Health Foundation 2002). As well as post-traumatic stress disorder (PTSD) which is common (Steiner et al. 1997), personality disorders (McManus et al. 1984; Lader et al. 2000) and drug and alcohol problems are also higher amongst this group (Watt et al. 1993; Dolan et al. 1999; Nichol et al. 2000). Young offenders have many of the same emotional, psychological and family problems as adolescents who are referred to mainstream CAMHS. However, the principle difference in young people referred for a forensic assessment is usually the coexistence of conduct disorders and associated high-risk behaviours.

Nurses should be aware that the presenting diagnosis may not be exhaustive. Furthermore, diagnostic categories are not mutually exclusive. For instance, a diagnosis of emotional disorder such as depression or anxiety does not preclude the possibility of conduct disorder and vice versa. Indeed, it is not unusual for young people referred to adolescent forensic services to have more than one disorder. Additionally, some young people may not meet the diagnostic threshold for some disorders but nevertheless display some of the signs and symptoms. This may be particularly true for young people with subtle neurological difficulties who present with partial symptoms of several disorders such as ADHD, Tourette's Syndrome or autistic spectrum disorders. A substantial number of young offenders have learning disabilities (Hall 1999; 2000) and a large proportion have speech and language problems (Bryan 2004). Again, multiple diagnoses, and the presence of complex needs which do not fit easily within any diagnostic framework, emphasise the importance of a comprehensive needs-based assessment. Although Axis 5 of the ICD-10 focuses on some of the psychosocial factors that may cause a young person's mental health problems to persist, the nurse should perform a more thorough needs assessment in order to determine the current levels of unmet need across multiple domains. This is illustrated next.

What are the social, personal and health needs of young people in contact with the youth justice system?

The value of needs-based assessment over traditional diagnostic assessment is that the nurse can assess and consider a wider range of factors. Also, the threshold for identifying an area of unmet need is lower than that required to make a formal psychiatric diagnosis. Needs can be considered to be unmet if they create difficulties for the young person in their day-to-day functioning, whereas the criteria for formal diagnosis are based on clinical benchmarks. A large majority of young people in contact with the youth justice system have unmet needs (Kroll et al. 1999). Without necessarily meeting the criteria for specific psychiatric disorders, many young people will be assessed to be in need of some type of psychological intervention (Mental Health Foundation 2002). A wide range of unmet needs can be generated from needs-based assessment. In relation to mental health, many young people in contact with the youth justice system have needs of a physical nature (Baker 1997; Home Office 1998). Young people with unstable lifestyles often fall through the net in terms of access to healthcare. Many miss routine health screening and inoculation opportunities and are often not registered with a GP. Here the CAMHS Tier 1 role of nurses can be seen to interface with their Tier 4 role and function.

Other areas of unmet need in this population of young offenders and those requiring similar services can arise in the context of behavioural difficulties. A significant proportion of young people in custody or in contact with YOTs have some degree of difficulty with substance or alcohol misuse (Rutter & Smith 1995; Hammersley et al. 2003). Nursing young people who misuse drugs and alcohol is explored elsewhere in this book. Nurses should also regard these young people vulnerable to acts of self-harm. Some young people in contact with the youth justice system will also have some degree of unmet need in relation to sexual functioning (YJB 2003). This may reflect a lack of psycho-sexual education in some cases; for the majority of young people however, their own sexualised behaviour, their vulnerability or a combination of both factors contribute to this. In terms of access to education, many young people in contact with the youth justice system are also experiencing difficulties, some will have special educational needs and a proportion will be excluded (Kendall et al. 2005). As well as the long-term future implications, these are significant day-to-day risk factors since a lack of structure, routine and purpose increases opportunities for antisocial behaviour. Helping create structure in the young person's life and facilitating purposeful activity are important strategies to help meet young people's needs and manage their risk behaviour. Many young people in contact with the youth justice system will be experiencing difficulties in terms of social functioning (Lader et al. 2000). This may be in the context of peer-group contact, bullying or general vulnerability. Many have unmet needs associated with family relationships (Lobley & Smith 1999). Family-based needs may be generated by lack of access or contact, negative past events and current family dysfunction.

Young people in contact with the youth justice system are often on a negative trajectory. In many cases the number of their unmet needs increases as the young person's emotional and behavioural problems increase or persist. Schools, other educational settings and care placements have limits in relation to the degree and range of behaviours they feel confident to manage safely. Multiple disrupted care and residential placements can lead to problems accessing healthcare and maintaining family contact. As family contact decreases, the psychological distress experienced by the young person may well increase and so the problems continue. Many of the unmet needs of young people described will be familiar to nurses in mainstream CAMHS and childcare settings. For the forensic population it is the number and complexity of unmet needs in this group that distinguishes them from their peers. Of course, many of these needs are beyond the scope and resources of nurses to address. However, a holistic view which considers how different areas of need may be interdependent is critical in developing a coordinated, comprehensive strategy for the young person's care and management.

Assessing needs

We have seen that in many respects, the needs of young people in contact with the youth justice system are the same as for young people in general. It therefore follows that the type of intervention which may benefit a young person is likely to be the same. Cognitive behavioural therapy (CBT), counselling, non-verbal therapy and family work have each been shown to be helpful for young people in contact with the youth justice system and for those in contact with mainstream care and treatment services (Kazdin 1993; Harrington et al. 1998; Harrington et al. 2005). All are likely to be helpful for this population. However, two key differences need to be highlighted. First, unlike some young people in mainstream services, those in contact with the youth justice system usually require multiagency intervention. Second, unlike their peers, young people in contact with the youth justice system are more likely to present significant risks to others that require systematic assessment and management. There are many reasons why nurses should base their assessment of young people on needs as well as problems. Although existing risk-assessment tools tend to concentrate on one area of risk (self-harm, aggression, sexualised behaviour), comprehensive risk-assessment should take account of a wide range of social and personal factors as part of the process. Therefore, the basis of good risk-assessment is likely to be found in a thorough assessment of all areas of social and personal functioning. In some situations, such as health screening interviews or assessment in custody, the nurse is likely to have little prior information on which to base their assessment. In other circumstances it may be possible to perform an assessment which is detailed, comprehensive and based on multiple sources of information. In either case, it is important that the nurse performs an assessment that is structured.

It is also important that nurses are able to justify the decisions they make, regardless of whether the decisions are about meeting a young person's needs or managing their risk. The use of structured assessment tools, particularly those that have been researched, developed and validated in clinical practice, should inform decisions about the most effective way to meet needs and manage risk. This is particularly important when such decision-making processes have resource implications for agencies involved in risk-assessment and management. There is at times a misperception that structured assessment tools limit the scope of judgement and decision-making by the individual practitioner. Indeed, it is true that all assessment tools have limitations to their scope and validity; they sometimes over-estimate (false positives) or under-estimate (false negatives) needs or risks. For any assessment tool to be used effectively, it is important that the nurse administering the tool has been trained to use it. They must also be aware of the specific strengths and weaknesses of that particular assessment tool. Good assessment tools do not disempower the nurse or stifle individual clinical judgement. Indeed, where an assessment tool produces an outcome that the nurse considers to be unrealistically high or low, it is important that clinical judgement and discussion with the multidisciplinary team is factored into the evaluation and outcome process of assessment. It is the combination of an experienced nurse using a structured, validated tool which is likely to produce the best outcomes whether it is needs or risks that are being assessed.

Many young people in contact with the youth justice system have been subjected to numerous assessments by professionals in the various agencies they have come into contact with. Assessment of their educational needs, social needs or mental health needs may well have been completed in the past. However, understanding about how such needs impact on the overall functioning of a young person is often lacking. Again, holistic assessment of need is important in order to understand how an unmet need in one domain of need (for instance housing) may affect need in another domain (such as mental health). Whereas previous assessments may be limited in their scope, they may contain important information that will inform decision-making in terms of meeting needs and managing risks. Therefore, nurses undertaking forensic assessments should always seek to obtain information from as many sources as possible. Information provided by parents or carers and professionals currently or previously involved with a young person is crucially important. Multiple sources of information also produce comparisons that may reveal contradictions or inaccuracies not previously recognised by other professionals. Sometimes such inaccuracies are propagated from one report to another until the original source material is verified. It is easy to see how myths about diagnosis, needs and risks are generated and perpetuated. Once in circulation, such myths can easily distort the assessment of needs, risks and the service a young person receives as a result.

Which assessment tools should nurses use?

There are a number of standardised tools for assessing the mental health of young people, including the Achenbach system of empirically based assessment (ASEBA) (Achenbach & Rescoria 2001). In many areas, clinicians including nurses have adapted these tools to meet local needs. Many tools are limited in their scope and concentrate more on diagnosis than assessment of need. Locally developed protocols are often wider in their scope but have not been developed and validated through clinical research. As a basis for the general assessment of needs, two tools are worthy of mention since they are both research-based, validated in clinical practice and can be used in a range of settings. The Salford needs assessment schedule for adolescents (S-NASA) (Kroll et al. 1999) has been developed as a generalised needs-assessment tool for young people, but has been used extensively for young people in contact with the youth justice system. It is comprehensive and addresses multiple domains of need. Outcomes are generated from both current and historical information provided by the young person and their parent, carer or other significant adult. A brief two-stage assessment tool known as SQUIFA (screening questionnaire interview for adolescents) and SIFA (mental health screening interview for adults) has been derived from S-NASA in conjunction with the YJB (Kroll et al. 2003). This is for use within the youth justice system and focuses on assessing acute mental health concerns such as low mood, PTSD and drug and alcohol misuse. The first stage of the tool is a brief questionnaire designed to be administered by YOT workers with minimal training. A high score at stage one triggers an in-depth interview lasting up to half-an-hour. Stage two is completed by a mental health practitioner who has undergone further training (Kroll et al. 2003).

Assessing and managing risk

The primary purpose of any risk assessment should be to inform a subsequent risk-management strategy. Risk assessment and risk management should be considered as two sides of the same coin. That is, it is pointless to undertake an assessment of risk unless consideration is given as to how that risk will be managed. Equally, it is difficult to evaluate the effectiveness of a risk-management strategy unless this has first been informed by a structured assessment of that risk. In general, risk-assessment tools are developed by looking at how specific factors affect the likelihood of future adverse events within a population. Trends within populations are helpful in identifying generalised areas of risk. For example, the link between substance misuse and offending behaviour is relatively well understood (Elliot et al. 1985; Fonagy et al. 2002).

On the other hand, a clinically useful risk-assessment tool should enable the nurse to make informed risk-management decisions about individual young people rather than just give a score to the risk being measured.

It is important that nurses recognise that risk assessment is a detailed and dynamic process rather than a one-off procedure. Risk changes over time, and even factors which appear to be consistent may not occur on either a regular or a purely random basis. For instance, a young person may have a two-year history of persistent aggression in their care placement. Though the frequency of aggressive incidents may have been generally uniform during the two-year period, closer scrutiny of the incidents is likely to reveal patterns within the young person's behaviour. Time of day, gender and personalities of adults they come into contact with, and presence of peers are just a few of the idiosyncratic factors that impact to influence the likelihood of acts of aggression occurring. Generally speaking, the more information that can be gathered about risks, the better the assessment is likely to be.

It is important to record specific details about specific aggressive incidents, particularly those which lead either to criminal charges or a change in the way the young person is perceived by those who know them. Simple statements such as 'he tried to stab him' should not be accepted at face value as an assessment of risk may reveal little about the act itself. It is critically important to contextualise the event. Did the young person use a carving knife or butter knife? Whereabouts on the body and how many times did the young person attempt to strike? Was there evidence of provocation or premeditation? What was the intention of the young person making the attack? Did they understand the potential consequences of their actions? These are just a few of the questions a nurse might ask before making any statements regarding the likelihood of future risk.

As well as exploring specific risk events in detail, it is important to consider these in the context of the young person's behaviour and social functioning. The wider context may highlight factors that appear to increase risk. By comparison, protective factors that may reduce the likelihood of future risk behaviour should also be identified. A risk-assessment measure designed specifically for use with young people in contact with the youth justice system is the Structured Assessment of Violence Risk in Youth (SAVRY) (Borum et al. 2003). This measures the risk of violence and is not designed for the assessment of risk for general offending or other high risk or antisocial behaviours such as sexual aggression or fire-setting. However, since managing the risk of interpersonal violence is a key part of the nurse's role, the value of such an assessment tool is clear. As with all structured assessment measures, nurses and other practitioners using SAVRY must undergo training and receive appropriate supervision.

Some risk-assessment tools are designed to enable the practitioner to consider a range of factors and give clear indications regarding which strategies are likely to be effective in managing risk (Steadman 1993). However, it is important for nurses to remember that all risk-assessment tools have their limitations.

For example, a measure used to evaluate the likelihood of violent behaviour is unlikely to assist the nurse in assessing the risk of sexually abusive behaviour. Within adult forensic mental health services, many risk-assessment tools have been developed for use in a wide variety of settings. However, these are not generally transferable for use with young people and nurses only have access to a limited number of risk-assessment tools specifically designed for adolescents (McDougall 2000). Whilst adult risk-assessment tools address historical variables, they do not usually take developmental factors into account. This is a central part of risk assessment with young people. Just as capacity for moral reasoning, empathy and understanding consequences all change over the course of life, so too do risk behaviours. Additionally, since adolescents are prone to sudden mood changes and tend to be sensitive to environmental changes, the factors that impact to produce risk can also change rapidly. It is therefore important that nurses working with young people in contact with the youth justice system reassess risk on a regular basis.

Case management and the care programme approach

As with the assessment of needs and risk, the most effective approach to case management is generated by a structured strategy which enables decision-making to be consistent and justifiable. The CPA was specifically developed to provide a framework for effective mental health care. This was initially in relation to case management where mental health needs were complex, risks required management and several agencies were involved in the careplan (DoH 1990). The four elements of the CPA are as follows:

- Systematic arrangements for assessing the health and social needs of people in specialist mental health services.
- Formation of a careplan which identifies the health and social care required from a range of agencies.
- Appointment of a Care Coordinator to monitor the careplan and keep in close touch with the service user.
- Regular review of the careplan.

As the CPA was essentially developed for meeting the mental health needs of adults, nurses will be required to adapt its use with young people. For example, involving parents and carers, teachers or education staff, and making the language accessible to young people, are all important. Any adaptations to the CPA should retain the principles of effective communication, effective risk-assessment and effective case-management, and must take account of policy and best practice guidelines. The careplan is essentially an agreement between the nurse or other mental health worker, the young person and their family or carers and other agencies who are involved. It is based on consultation and discussion with all those involved and results in agreement about who has responsibility for meeting each element of the young person's needs. The careplan should also identify areas of unmet need which the involved agencies feel unable to meet. Here, it is particularly important to identify unmet needs which are associated with risk. Early warning signs for potential relapse and resilience factors that might prevent this should also be highlighted. There should be a clear strategy for action in the event of a crisis and all parties should have a copy of the careplan. This should be reviewed on a regular basis or more frequently if there are significant changes to the young person's circumstances.

There are two levels of need identified within the CPA. Young people with multiple needs requiring a multiagency intervention are likely to fulfil the criteria for an enhanced CPA. Young people with mental health problems who are in contact with the youth justice system should usually be managed using an enhanced CPA (NHSE 1999; Care Programme Approach Association 2001). Crucial to the effective implementation of the CPA is the role of care co-ordinator. This person is not responsible for implementing all aspects of the careplan. Rather, the care coordinator oversees the careplan which specifies which individuals from which agencies are undertaking specific interventions. Professionals from any discipline may act as the care coordinator. However, NHSE guidelines state that the care coordinator should be competent in delivering mental health care, have knowledge of the service user, and of the other agencies involved. It is most often the case that nurses are the professionals who most easily meet these criteria. It is not possible to cover in detail all aspects of a CPA implementation. National policy (DoH 1999; NHSE 1999) and local guidance should be sought. The CPA Association (CPAA) handbook is also a valuable source of information and guidance for nurses (CPAA 2001). At the time of writing, a draft common assessment framework for helping children, young people and their families is out for consultation (Department for Education and Skills 2004). This is likely to result in a standardised format for assessment to facilitate coordinated interagency working to meet the needs of young people.

Conclusion

In conclusion, adolescent forensic mental health provision is a unique and rapidly developing field which provides nurses with a range of opportunities and challenges. The challenge is not only to implement change as services evolve, but also to innovate and influence how services for young people in contact with the youth justice system will be delivered. The untreated mental health needs of young people in contact with the youth justice system increases the demands placed on health and social services, education, youth justice and prison systems. In order to meet the needs of this particularly challenging group of young people, nurses must continue to develop a specialist knowledge base, develop and create benchmarks for evidence-based interventions, and disseminate best nursing practice.

John

John is a 14 year-old boy who has been in the care of the local authority since the age of 12. Since that time he has lost contact with his family, though it is known that he had contact with the local CAMHS team when he was younger because of concerns regarding his behaviour. Over the past six months he has had increasing contact with the youth justice system, mainly for driving stolen cars.

John recently received a supervision order and during health screening by the local YOT he received high scores for both depressed mood and for drug and alcohol use. He was referred to the mental health nurse who works between CAMHS and the YOT. She conducted a more detailed mental health assessment and there were clear signs and symptoms of depressed mood. There was no evidence of intent to self harm, but John was indifferent regarding his own safety and welfare. The mental health nurse wanted John to see the psychiatrist in the CAMHS team but he refused. However, he did agree to maintain contact with the mental health nurse either at his placement or at the YOT office.

John's social worker had organised a review meeting and John was agreeable to the mental health nurse liaising with his social worker and attending the meeting. At the meeting an agreement was reached between John, the mental health nurse, his social worker, his YOT worker and his key worker at the care home. The mental health nurse wrote up the agreement as a careplan under local CPA guidelines and the plan was circulated to all those present at the meeting. The plan contained the contact details of all those present and identified a review date in three months' time (or sooner if there was a significant change in John's circumstances). The mental health nurse agreed to act as the CPA coordinator in John's case. The careplan contained the following points:

- The care home staff agreed to monitor John for any significant changes in his mood and liaise with the mental health nurse regarding this. The residential staff already had a plan in place regarding John's frequent absconding which involved notifying his social worker and the local police.

- The YOT worker also agreed to monitor John's mood and notify the mental health nurse of any changes. He also agreed to inform John's social worker if John failed to attend any of the planned appointments.

- John's social worker agreed to monitor John's compliance with both his residential placement and appointments with the YOT worker so that if John disengaged from services working with him this would be spotted quickly.

- The mental health nurse arranged weekly appointments to monitor John's mood and report any changes to the care staff, his YOT worker and his social worker. She also agreed to inform John's social worker if he failed to attend any appointments. The mental health nurse also liaised with the CAMHS team to keep them updated.

- John agreed to attend appointments at the YOT office and also to see the mental health nurse but it was acknowledged that John's compliance with professionals was often erratic.

From her discussions with John the mental health nurse was able to identify the likely warning signs of a deterioration in John's mood (isolating himself, increasing alcohol use) and also the strategies that John thought had helped him in the past (diversional activities, talking to his key worker) and incorporated these into the careplan. Contact details for the CAMHS Team, the local Accident & Emergency department and John's GP were also included. Those at the meeting agreed that the two most likely scenarios for a crisis were that John either suffered a rapid deterioration in his mood or was arrested for further offences and placed in custody. The mental health nurse wrote a covering letter summarising her contact with John, her assessment of his mental state and concerns about the possible risk of self-harm if his mood deteriorated. The care home staff and John's social worker had copies of the letter in case they felt he needed an urgent assessment of his mental state via the A&E department. Both John's GP and his YOT worker also had a copy of the letter so that if John were to be arrested and placed in custody an urgent review of his mental state could be arranged. A copy of the letter was also placed in John's CAMHS file in case he was referred to them on an urgent basis.

References

Achenbach, T.M., Recorla, L.A. (2001). *Manual for the Achenbach System of Empirically-Based Assessment (ASEBA) School-Age Forms and Profiles*. Vermont: ASEBA.

Armstrong, D., Hine, J., Hacking, S., Armaos, R., Jones, R., Klessinger, N. & France, A. (2005). *Children, Risk and Crime: the on track youth lifestyles surveys*. London: Home Office Research, Development and Statistics Directorate.

Bailey, S. (2002). Violent children: a framework for understanding. *Advances in Psychiatric Treatment*, (8), 97–106.

Baker, G. (1997). *A Brief Introductory Survey of Health Care Needs*. Glen Parva Young Offenders Institution (YOI): Personal communication.

Borum, R., Bartel, P. & Forth, A. (2003). *Manual for the Structured Assessment of Risk in Youth (SAVRY)*. Tampa: University of South Florida.

Bryan, K. (2004). Preliminary study of the prevalence of speech and language difficulties in young offenders. *International Journal of Language and Communication Disorders*, (39), 391–400.

Care Programme Approach Association (2001). *The CPA Handbook*. Chesterfield: CPAA Walton Hospital.

Carswell, K. & Davenport, F. (2000). *The Psychosocial Problems of Young Offenders and Young People at Risk of Offending*. London: Lambeth, Southwark & Lewisham Health Commission.

Delligatti, N., Akin-Little, A. & Little, S. (2003). Conduct disorder in girls: diagnostic and intervention issues. *Psychology in the Schools*, **40** (2), 183–92.

Department for Education and Skills (2004). *Common Assessment Framework: consultation*. London: HMSO.

Department of Health (1990). *Joint Health and Social Services Circular: the care programme approach for people with a mental illness referred to specialist psychiatric services*. HC(90)23/LASSL(90)11. London: Department of Health.

Department of Health (2004). *National Service Framework for Children, Young People and Maternity Services*. London: HMSO.

Dolan, M., Holloway, J., Bailey, S. & Smith, C. (1999). Health status of juvenile offenders: a survey of young offenders appearing before the juvenile courts. *Journal of Adolescence*, (20), 137–44.

Dolan, M. & Smith, C. (2001). Juvenile homicide offenders: 10 years' experience of an adolescent forensic psychiatry service. *Journal of Forensic Psychiatry*, (12), 313–29.

Elliot, D., Huizingo, D. & Ageton, S. (1985). *Explaining Delinquency and Drug Use*. London: Sage.

Fonagy, P. & Kurtz, Z. (2002). What works for whom? In: Fonagy, P., Target, M., Cottrell, D., Phillips, J. & Kurtz, Z. (Eds) *A Critical Review of Treatments for Children and Adolescents*. London: Guilford Press.

Hagell, A. (2003). *Understanding and Challenging Youth Offending*. London: Quality Protects Research briefings.

Hall, I. (1999). *Young People with a Learning Disability in Secure Health and Social Services Care: a descriptive study*. St George's Medical School, London: Unpublished MPhil thesis.

Hall, I. (2000). Young offenders with a learning disability. *Advances in Psychiatric Treatment*, (6), 278–86.

Hammersley, R., Marsland, L. & Reid, M. (2003). *Substance Use by Young Offenders*. London: Home Office Research, Development and Statistics Directorate.

Harrington, R., Campbell, F., Shoebridge, P. & Whittaker, J. (1998). Meta-analysis of CBT for depression in adolescents. *Journal of the American Academy of Child and Adolescent Psychiatry*, (37), 1005–1006.

Hawton, K., Harris, L., Hall, S., Simkin, S., Bale, E. & Bond, A. (2003). Deliberate self-harm in Oxford, 1990–2000: a time of change in patient characteristics. *Psychological Medicine*, **33**, 987–995.

Home Office (1998). *Literature Review on the Health of Young People Aged 16–24 Detained in Young Offender Units or Prisons in England and Wales*. London: HMSO.

Kazdin, A. (1993). Treatment of conduct disorder: progress and directions in psychotherapy research. *Development Psychopathology*, (5), 76–85.

Kazdin, A. & Holland, L. (1997). Barriers to treatment participation scale: evaluation and validation in the context of child out-patient treatment. *Journal of Child Psychology and Psychiatry*, (38), 1051–62.

Kendall, S., Johnson, A. & Martin, K. (2005). *Vulnerable Children's Access to Examinations at Key Stage 4*. London: National Foundation for Educational Research.

Kroll, L., Woodham, A., Rothwell, J., Bailey, S., Tobias, C., Harrington, R. & Marshal, M. (1999). Reliability of the Salford needs assessment schedule for adolescents. *Psychological Medicine*, (29), 891–902.

Kroll, L., Bailey, S., Myatt, T., McCarthy, K., Shuttleworth, J., Rothwell, J. & Harrington, R. (2003). *The Mental Health Screening Interview for Adolescents*. London: Youth Justice Board.

Kurtz, Z., Thornes, R. & Bailey, S. (1996). *A Study of the Demands and Needs for Forensic Child and Adolescent Mental Health Services in England and Wales*. Manchester: Salford Mental Health Services.

Lader, D., Singleton, N. & Meltzer, H. (2000). *Psychiatric Morbidity Among Young Offenders in England and Wales*. London: Office for National Statistics.

Lobley, D. & Smith, D. (1999). *Working with Persistent Juvenile Offenders: an evaluation of the Apex Cue Ten project*. Edinburgh: Scottish Executive.

McDougall, T. (1998). Adolescent forensic mental health nursing. *Mental Health Practice*, **1** (4), 13–16.

McDougall, T. (1999). Adolescent forensic mental health nursing. In: Chaloner, C. & Coffey, M. (Eds). *Forensic Mental Health Nursing: from principles to practice*. Oxford: Blackwell.

McDougall, T. (2000). Violent incidents in a forensic adolescent unit: a functional analysis. *NT Research*, **5** (5), 346–63.

McManus, M., Alessi, N., Grapentine, W. & Brickman, A. (1984). Psychiatric disturbance in serious delinquents. *Journal of the American Academy of Child and Adolescent Psychiatry*, (23), 602–15.

Mental Health Foundation (2002). *The Mental Health Needs of Young Offenders: bright futures: working with vulnerable young people*. London: MHF.

National Association for the Care and Rehabilitation of Offenders (2001). *Youth Crime Briefing: girls in the youth justice system*. London: NACRO.

National Association for the Care and Rehabilitation of Offenders (2005). *A Handbook on Reducing Offending by Looked After Children*. London: NACRO.

Nichol, R., Stretch, D., Whitney, I., Jones, K., Garfield, P., Turner, K. & Stanion, B. (2000). Mental health needs and services for severely troubled and troubling young people including young offenders in an NHS region. *Journal of Adolescence*, (23), 243–61.

Papageorgiou, V. & Vostanis, P. (2000). Psychosocial characteristics of Greek young offenders. *Journal of Forensic Psychiatry*, (11), 390–400.

Royal College of Psychiatrists (2004). *About Us: treating conduct disorder in adolescents and young offenders: findings from research*. London: FOCUS.

Rutter, M. & Smith, D. (1995). *Psychosocial Disorders in Young People: time trends and their causes*. Chichester: John Wiley.

Steadman, H., Monaghan, J. & Robbins, P. (1993). From dangerousness to risk assessment: implications for appropriate research strategies. In: Hodgins, S. (Ed.). *Crime and Disorder*. London: Sage.

Stiener, H., Garcia, I. & Matthews, Z. (1997). Post-traumatic stress disorder in incarcerated juvenile delinquents. *Journal of the American Academy of Child and Adolescent Psychiatry*, (36), 357–65.

Storvoll, E. & Wichstrom, L. (2002). Do the risk factors associated with conduct problems in adolescents vary according to gender? *Journal of Adolescence*, (25), 183–202.

Teplin, L., Abram, K. & McLelland, G. (2002). Psychiatric disorders in youth in juvenile detention. *Archives of General Psychiatry*, (59), 1133–43.

Watt, F., Tomison, A. & Torpy, D. (1993). The prevalence of psychiatric disorder in a male remand population: a pilot study. *Journal of Forensic Psychiatry*, **4** (1), 75–83.

World Health Organization (1992). *The ICD-10 Classification of Mental and Behavioural Disorders: clinical descriptions and diagnostic guidelines*. Geneva: WHO.

Youth Justice Board (2003). *Screening for Mental Disorder in the Youth Justice System: supporting notes*. London: YJB.

Chapter 11

Substance Misuse, Young People and Nursing

Debra McKay, Tina Hatton and Tim McDougall

Key points

- Substance misuse is harmful to children and young people in a variety of ways. From conception to adulthood, it threatens their health and welfare and prevents them reaching their full potential across a number of different domains.

- All young people with increased vulnerability to developing substance misuse problems should have their needs identified as early as possible, and they should have access to appropriate services to prevent their substance misuse problems escalating.

- Substance misuse by young people is a sensitive area and is often associated with risk, vulnerability and harm. Nurses need to be clear about their duties regarding confidentiality and information-sharing in the best interests of the young person.

- Before any therapeutic work can take place with young people who misuse drugs or alcohol, a trusting therapeutic relationship will need to be established. If a young person does not want treatment or is unwilling to address their substance misuse problems, it will be very difficult for nurses to engage them in meaningful work.

- As young people who misuse drugs and alcohol are a heterogeneous group, no single treatment strategy will be effective for all. The main treatment modalities for young people who misuse drugs and alcohol include motivational interviewing and comprise individual therapy, family interventions, group work and multimodal treatment strategies such as multisystemic therapy. This is in addition to emergency medical treatments, detoxification and withdrawal programmes and relapse prevention.

- Substance misuse nursing is a rapidly developing area of practice. Specialist substance misuse nurses provide a range of direct and indirect interventions. These include assessment and treatment for individual young people with drug or alcohol problems and mental health problems, as well as support, training and supervision for colleagues who have concerns about drug or alcohol use by the young people they are working with.

Introduction

Nurses who work in a variety of health, education and youth justice settings encounter young people who have tried illegal drugs or alcohol. Substance misuse nurses are usually mental health nurses that have specialised in working with young people whose drug or alcohol use impacts negatively on their mental health. The role of the specialist CAMHS (child and adolescent mental health services) substance misuse nurse has developed over the last five years. The function of the role is to integrate knowledge of drug and alcohol use and misuse within the wider CAMHS; to work directly with young people who have substance misuse problems; and to liaise with colleagues in other services when anything from residential to medical or social support is needed for young people. Throughout the chapter, substance misuse refers to alcohol abuse, illicit use of prescribed medication, and the misuse of volatile substances and illegal drugs. The chapter provides an insight into the specialist work of the CAMHS substance misuse nurse, and provides useful information for nursing colleagues on the resources that are available to support young people who use drugs or alcohol in a problematic fashion.

In taking the reader from the strategic development of drug and alcohol services for young people through to therapeutic strategies used to foster engagement and change with young people who misuse drugs and alcohol, it is hoped that theory can be linked to nursing practice. Although the areas of prevention and drug education are beyond the scope of this chapter, further information can be found in the recommended reading list. The chapter begins with a history of the service framework and describes how substance misuse services are funded and organised. A continuum of services is described, from health promotion through to specialist residential services, that aim to help young people with serious drug or alcohol use. This links to a discussion about groups of young people that may be at particular risk of substance misuse, and how patterns of drug and alcohol use may bring increasing psychosocial problems to the lives of these young people. The aim is to enable the reader to consider which type of service will be suited to a particular level of difficulty for the young person and their family or carers. Consideration will be given to sensitive issues of confidentiality and consent and information-sharing, and these will be discussed before providing a brief overview of nursing assessment and treatment interventions.

Background

The government's white paper and 10-year anti drugs strategy, *Tackling Drugs to Build a Better Britain* was published by the Cabinet Office in 1998. This aimed to enable young people to resist drugs in order to reach their full potential. The strategy required services and information to be available to all young people, particularly those who are at increased risk of drug and alcohol misuse (Cabinet

Office 1998). The national delivery plan for young people and substance misuse is an interdepartmental government strategy, based on the cabinet office report. It aims to ensure that all young people with increased vulnerability to developing substance misuse problems have their needs identified as early as possible, and that they have access to appropriate services to prevent their substance misuse problems escalating (Department for Education and Skills 2005).

What are substance misuse services?

In order to understand how treatment is provided for young people who use drugs or alcohol in a harmful way, it is useful to have an insight into how the services are organised and delivered. The National Treatment Agency (NTA) is a special health authority, created by the English government in 2001. The NTA functions to improve the availability, capacity and effectiveness of treatment for drug misuse services. In other words, to ensure that there is more treatment, better treatment and fairer treatment available to all those who need it. Treatment for drug misuse in England is organised and commissioned through Drug Action Teams (DATs). These were set up in 1995, following publication of *Tackling Drugs Together*, the UK government consultation strategy for England (Lord Presidents Office 1995). Key organisations such as local authorities, primary care trusts, police and probation services are represented on each DAT, the majority of which also have a coordinator and commissioning manager. Most substance misuse services are funded through the DAT with guidelines provided by the NTA. Drug action teams plan and organise services to meet the needs of local populations, eliminate gaps in service provision and maintain a workforce with a range of skills and competencies in the area of substance misuse. In some areas, DATs are also involved in planning services for young people who abuse alcohol. Drug and alcohol teams are identified by the acronym DAAT. It is important that services for young people who misuse drugs and alcohol should be sensitive to their needs (Department of Health 2004a; DfES 2005). A report entitled *Young People and Drugs* produced policy guidance for drug interventions and set out a number of underpinning principles for the development of effective substance misuse services for young people (The Children's Legal Centre and Standing Committee on Drug Abuse 1999) (see Box 11.1).

These principles reflect the principles for the provision of effective services for young people in general which are enshrined in the NSF (National Service Framework) for Children, Young People and Maternity Services (DoH 2004a) and Change for Children Programme: Every Child Matters (DfES 2003). Best practice in substance misuse services for young people is also based on the Health Advisory Service (HAS) four-tiered framework of service delivery. In promoting for the development of a four-tier approach to the needs of children and young people with alcohol or substance misuse, the HAS report highlighted the potentially crucial role played by specialist CAMHS, which could include

Box 11.1 Principles of effective substance misuse services for young people: The Children's Legal Centre and Standing Committee on Drug Abuse 1999.

- A child or young person is not an adult.
- The overall welfare of the individual child or young person is of paramount importance.
- The views of the young person are of central importance, and should always be sought and considered.
- Services need to respect parental responsibility when working with a young person.
- Services should recognise the role of, and cooperate with, the local authority in carrying out its responsibilities towards children and young people.
- A holistic approach is vital at all levels, as young people's problems do not recognise professional boundaries.
- Services must be child centred.
- A comprehensive range of services needs to be provided.
- Services must be competent to respond to the needs of the young person.

working with primary services to add skills in working with addiction to the existing assessment and treatment capabilities within mainstream CAMHS. The way in which the tiered model is used to organise drug and alcohol services for young people is shown below in Figure 11.1 (HAS 1995).

How are young people affected by alcohol and substance misuse?

Drug and alcohol misuse by children and young people is widespread and preventable. The risk factors that place children and adolescents on trajectories towards substance misuse problems are well documented and well understood. Young people are reported to be trying drugs and alcohol at a younger age over time (Hibbell et al. 1999) and substance misuse is now very common (Hammersley et al. 2003). It is estimated that one in ten young people aged between 11 and 15 uses drugs (HAS 2001). Indeed, some argue that the use of drugs and alcohol by young people has now become normalised and incorporated into young people's daily lives (Parker et al. 1998). Substance misuse and associated psychosocial problems are harmful to young people in a variety of ways; it threatens their health and welfare and prevents them reaching their full potential across a number of different domains; ultimately it threatens their life. The deliberate inhalation of volatile substances such as lighter fuel, aerosols or glue, is responsible for more deaths in young people aged 10 to 16 in England and Wales than illegal drugs (HAS 2001). One-third of suicides by young people are thought to be intoxicated at the time of death (Williams & Morgan 1994) and substance misuse is a very strong predictor of completed suicide (Appelby et al. 1997).

Substance misuse rarely exists in isolation, but occurs in the context of other problems that affect young people in modern society (Melrose & Brodie 2000). At one end of a continuum it can be seen as part of growing up in modern

---

Tier 1 – generic and primary services
The frontline of service delivery to which children, young people and their families have direct access and which provide the first response to the needs of children and adolescents. These services are best placed to recognise and screen, and to provide some simple interventions with young people and their families. Here, professionals such as school nurses provide information and education about the harmful effects of drugs and alcohol as part of the education curriculum. Nurses at Tier 1 can also provide general medical services, routine health screening and vaccinations.

Tier 2 – firstline specialist services
First-contact young people's specialist services are critical to the early identification of vulnerable children. Professionals at this level should be concerned with the reduction of risks and vulnerabilities to substance misuse, and the reintegration and maintenance of young people in mainstream services. Nurses and other professionals working at Tier 2 may be providing substance misuse services as part of a YOT, and proving advice, guidance or counselling for young people.

Tier 3 – services provided by specialist teams
Tier 3 substance misuse services are multidisciplinary teams demonstrating a threshold of expertise and competence that is capable of comprehensive assessment and formulation of an overall plan for managing substance misuse and various other problems. The team will deal with the complex and often multiple needs of the young person, including substance misuse problems. The aim is to reintegrate and include the child or young person into his or her family, community, school, training or work. Nurses working at Tier 3 will also provide family assessment and support, and be involved in interagency planning and communication.

Tier 4 – highly specialised services
This refers to highly specialised young people's services used for intensive treatment interventions. This might consist of in-patient adolescent services; or forensic units complemented by specialist young people's addiction teams, paediatric beds; or intensive day centres for detoxification, crisis placements, specialist housing or fostering. The function of Tier 4 services is to provide specialist interventions after which may include in-patient treatment, as an adjunct to services provided by other tiers. Continuity of care before, during and, treatment by a Tier 4 service is important.

Figure 11.1   The tiered model of service delivery (based on Health Advisory Service report 1995).

society. It can be seen as a method of coping with negative emotions or bringing on a 'buzz'. At the other end of the continuum it is linked to a range of mental health problems and disorders including serious mental illness. Psychosis (Cantwell et al. 1999), major depression (King et al. 1996) and conduct disorder

(Young et al. 1995) have each been closely associated with substance misuse. However, the relationship between substance use and mental health problems is complex. Whether substance use triggers mental ill health in people who would not have experienced problems otherwise, or whether a predisposition to mental disorder existed all along is an area of debate (Bukstein et al. 1989; Wilens 1999; Crome 2004). A number of factors seem to play a part in problematic drug and alcohol use. Research suggests that alcohol and substance misuse has a negative impact on relationships (McGilvarry & Crome 2004); prevents educational fulfilment and achievement (DfES 2005); and leads to a number of general health problems (Crome et al. 2004).

Which groups of young people are at risk?

An evidence base for the effectiveness of young people's drug and alcohol services is currently lacking. It is difficult to measure accurately drug use amongst young people, and therefore difficult to attribute trends of cause and effect. However, due to new government priorities, and increased funding for services and research activity, the next few years are likely to see the evidence base for young people's substance misuse services develop significantly. But given that the evidence-based practice is currently lacking, the links drawn about the causes of young people's drug and alcohol use are still tentative. Despite this, it is known that some groups of young people are at higher risk than others. The HAS report, *The Substance of Young Needs* (HAS 2001) identified several groups of young people whom research has shown to be at higher risk of substance misuse. These include those who are:

- In contact with specialist mental health services.
- Looked after by the local authority or in contact with social services.
- Homeless.
- Runaways.
- Involved in prostitution.
- Young offenders and those involved in the criminal justice system.
- Young people with educational problems, and those who are absent or excluded from school.
- Young people with recurrent and substantial disruptive behavioural problems.
- Children whose parents misuse drugs or alcohol.

The costs of substance misuse to young people are extensive and span all domains of functioning. However, problematic or dependent drug use is often diagnosed by specialist practitioners and surveys of this client group are targeted in specialist drug services. This inevitably means that a proportion of young people at risk will not be identified as having a substance misuse problem, and many will not receive professional help or treatment. Young people with significant needs may not have engaged with specialist services or may be wary about having information about them shared with others. The way in which drug and alcohol statistics are recorded may also fail to reflect a true picture of prevalence rates. Availability of particular substances in different local areas can create idiosyncratic patterns that tend to be discounted by national studies. Similarly, surveys of Class A drugs will not necessarily quantify the negative effects of daily cannabis use or alcohol binges.

Despite difficulties in measuring young people's drug and alcohol use, a review of the research reveals a number of trends. It is important to understand that these do not point to clear causal factors for dependency. That is, not all vulnerable young people will take drugs and those that do will not always develop problems. Numerous research studies show that children who are looked after by the state and those leaving care have higher rates of mental health problems than those in family homes (Phillips 1997; Saunders & Broad 1997; Richardson & Joughin 2000; DoH 2002; Meltzer et al. 2004). They are also much more likely to misuse drugs and alcohol (Craig et al. 1996). The higher prevalence of drug misuse by children and young people who are homeless or runaways has been previously reported (Fitzpatrick & Klinker 2000; Wincup & Bayliss 2001). It has also been suggested that homeless people are particularly difficult to engage and retain in treatment (Kazdin 1997). Nurses should also be aware that many young people who are homeless are multiple drug users and approximately one-quarter of these injects drugs, as well as having very high levels of tobacco and alcohol use (Wincup et al. 2003). Such a lifestyle presents numerous health concerns. The physical health implications of intravenous drug-use, intoxication and overdose are well understood but poorly acknowledged by young people, particularly those who are homeless. The Health Protection Agency (HPA) reports that cases of Hepatitis C have doubled in the last three years among adults who have recently started injecting, and that Methicillin-resistant Staphylococcus Aureus (MRSA) and severe Group A Streptococcus (GAS) linked to intravenous drug use is on the increase (Gilbert et al. 2004).

There are indisputable links between offending, antisocial behaviour and substance misuse (Elliot et al. 1985; Rutter & Smith 1995). Young people in contact with the criminal justice system are also at higher risk of substance misuse than their non-offending peers (Hammersley et al. 2003). In a large study of young people in contact with YOTs (Youth Offending Teams), 85% had used cannabis and alcohol, substances that are more strongly associated with offending than other drugs. This is in addition to almost a fifth who had used Class A drugs such as crack cocaine or heroin (Hammersley et al. 2003). The backgrounds of this population reveal high rates of family disruption, poor social skills, school-based difficulties and low self-esteem. Surveys of school-age children and substance misuse focus on those who are in school rather than targeting young people who are truanting or being educated in special services. It is these groups that are more likely to be involved in drug use than their peers in mainstream education. Young people's education can deteriorate over time due to intoxication or truanting, or end completely because of school exclusion.

It is widely acknowledged that parental drug use can and does cause serious harm to children at every stage, from conception to adulthood (Home Office 2003a; DfES 2005). However, substance misuse is sometimes described by young people as having an element of family culture and heritage. Some young people have become socialised into accepting that substance use appears to be a regular part of life and their own substance use is condoned; but others may find the experience of their parents' addiction puts them off using drugs themselves. Young people who have been abused and those who are involved in prostitution are also at greater risk of substance misuse (Social Services Inspectorate 1997). Nursing interventions with these groups is discussed later in the chapter.

Why do young people misuse drugs and alcohol?

There are many reasons why young people misuse drugs and alcohol. Nowinski (1990) has defined various patterns of use in Box 11.2.

Central to this debate of why young people misuse drugs is the use of so-called 'gateway drugs'. This is a term used to describe a drug whose use is likely to lead on to other types of drug use. Cannabis, described as such a gateway drug, is the most frequently used illicit drug among 11–24 year-olds in the UK (Ramsey & Partridge 1999; Royal College of Psychiatrists 2004).

Box 11.2 Nowinski's patterns of substance use.

(1) Exploratory or experimental
Here, the primary reason for using drugs or alcohol is curiosity. The mood-altering effects are secondary to the adventure of use.

(2) Social use
Here, the context in which young people take drugs is social. Substance use takes place at social events such as parties, friends' houses or parks. The primary motive for social substance use is acceptance and peer pressure.

(3) Emotional or instrumental
Here, the young person learns to use substances purposely to manipulate feelings and behaviour. This may be to seek pleasure and fun or cope with stress and negative emotions.

(4) Habitual
Here, patterns of substance use start to show compulsiveness and preoccupation and levels of tolerance may increase. Lifestyle converges around psychoactive substances. Behavioural problems may increase and school performance becomes seriously affected.

(5) Dependent or addictive
Here, physical and/or psychological addiction becomes the main feature. Tolerance, craving, withdrawal and compulsion become prominent.

Some research suggests that the use of cannabis will make a person more vulnerable and addicted to other drugs by way of the reaction in the brain to the active ingredients in cannabis. Others believe that it is more likely that young people who use cannabis will be more vulnerable to other drug use due to the circles they socialise in and their exposure to drug dealers (Home Office 2002; Home Office 2003b). It has been estimated that as many as half of all young people between 11 and 15 who use cannabis more than once per week develop mental health problems (Meltzer et al. 2000). It is important to remember that not all substance misuse will result in problematic behaviour and that young people may pass through the different levels described in the above table. Substance misuse nurses should perform a thorough assessment of drug and alcohol misuse to determine levels of risk and associated problems.

Consent and confidentiality

Substance misuse by young people is a sensitive area and is often associated with risk, vulnerability and harm. During work with a young person who has become involved in problematic drug use, the potential to hear about serious crime and child protection issues increases. When working with young people who use drugs or alcohol, it is important that nurses are clear about their duties of confidentiality from the outset. Supervision and consultation should also be used to address these issues and protect the young person and nurse. All nurses and other professionals have a duty to protect the best interests of young people and inform others if they are at risk of harm. General issues of consent and confidentiality have been covered elsewhere in the book. However, when nursing young people who misuse drugs and alcohol, the nurse should also explore the potential for involvement in crime, issues of child protection and, in particular, sexual exploitation. The young person may be associating with adult drug users, involved in acquisitive crime or violence. Young people may consider high-risk activities along a continuum, culminating in selling sex to finance drug use. Children and adolescents involved in high-risk activities such as prostitution should be treated primarily as victims of sexual abuse. The young person may have disclosed sensitive information that leads the professional to suspect grooming or confirm that abuse is occurring, or has occurred. It is important for the nurse not to work alone on such issues. They should always seek advice, support and guidance from colleagues with statutory responsibilities for the welfare and protection of children. Guidance is available for professionals concerned with children at risk of prostitution or other areas of harm (DoH 2000a).

Whilst consent will be required in order to share information across agencies and refer the young person to other professionals, there are occasions when consent will not necessarily be needed. These include instances such as disclosure from a young person that they may be at significant risk from or towards others. Here, the nurse should fulfil their duty to safeguard children, by alerting social services or the police, even if the young person does not give their consent for this. It is vital that nurse's record-keeping is always clear, concise and contemporaneous. This is because clinical notes may be used in any investigations conducted by social services and the police in the interests of child protection and public welfare. Each NHS (National Health Service) trust will have policies and procedures in relation to consent, confidentiality and child protection. Each organisation is also required to have a designated nurse for child protection who is able to provide advice and guidance to nurses and other professionals on child protection matters (DoH 2000b). Some aspects of working with young people who use drugs and alcohol require further consideration in terms of consent and confidentiality. These include school-based interventions such as clothing and bag searches, drug-screening and the use of police drug sniffer dogs. School nurses may have a role to play in helping develop policies and procedures that appropriately address issues of consent and confidentiality, whilst ensuring that the problem of drug and alcohol misuse is tackled.

Sarah

Sarah, aged 15, was referred to the substance misuse nurse in the Tier 3 CAMHS by her social worker. Sarah has recently been injecting heroin and living in a squat. Sarah and her parents were given an appointment on the day of referral due to concerns about vulnerability and risk.

Sarah and her parents looked devastated on arrival. The parents were initially seen alone, as Sarah refused to enter the assessment room. The mother explained that the problems had started because Sarah had been sexually abused by an uncle when she was 10, and described how the family had tried to get through the trauma together. It seemed that Sarah felt loyal to her abuser and as she entered adolescence brought up conversation that others in the family found difficult to cope with. It became apparent that anger and shame had contributed to relationship breakdowns, culminating with Sarah entering local authority care 12 months earlier. The parents stated that she spent evenings on the streets and tended towards relationships with adult men, rather than boys and girls her own age. Having not seen Sarah for almost three months prior to the assessment, the parents were shocked to notice her weight-loss, pallor and withdrawal symptoms. A friend had recently alerted Sarah's parents to say that she had been visiting for loans and had disclosed that she was living with a man called Rob, who was in his 30s and living in a squat. The friend noticed that Sarah had marks on her arms which she believed were heroin injection sites.

Sarah eventually agreed to see the nurse alone. She described feeling ashamed, felt increasingly cut off and believed her parents didn't want to know her. During the assessment Sarah complained of chills, nausea, irritability and bouts of rage. She talked about her relationship with Rob and knew early on that he used heroin and visited a clinic to collect equipment. She felt a bond with him in that they both felt like outsiders because of the legacy of abuse. She described that when sad and disconnected she let Rob inject her and found refuge in the sensations. She learnt to inject, and seemed knowledgeable about safety. This may have helped her health as testing revealed that she did not have any of the long-term infections or physical health difficulties associated with injecting. Sarah was keen to be understood, helped and supported through her struggles. Following the initial assessment the child protection concerns in relation to Rob were reported to the social services. Sarah was also referred to an adolescent in-patient service for detoxification and rehabilitation. A waiting list at the adolescent unit meant that interim measures were required. The nurse arranged a professionals' meeting and a safety plan was agreed between health, social services and the family. Sarah was admitted to the adolescent unit after 10 days.

After a programme of detoxification, Sarah began a programme of individual therapy focused on relapse prevention and understanding the sexual abuse she had experienced as a child. Prior to discharge, a multiagency follow-up plan was agreed. This involved a day programme including support from a Connexions worker, social services and the substance misuse nurse who continued the work on relapse prevention and sexual abuse. Several months on, Sarah has avoided all drugs except tobacco. She attributes this to reinventing her appearance, avoiding people and places from her 'old life', and understands that she took heroin to dissociate herself from the abuse she had experienced. However, she continues to require support from the substance misuse nurse and Connexions worker as she is struggling to make new friends, relate to her family and maintain an interest in education.

Engagement

Before any therapeutic work can take place with young people who misuse drugs or alcohol, a trusting therapeutic relationship will need to be established. In order to enable the young person to feel safe to discuss their drug or alcohol misuse, the nurse should attempt to create a climate of trust and acceptance. The nurse should try to be neutral, believe what they are told, and allow the young person to lead the discussion. It is common for young people to underestimate the severity of their substance misuse and the consequences of their actions. Young people may be ill-informed of the associated problems, which may include mental health problems, family and social breakdown, school exclusion and the risk of overdose or death. It is not uncommon for young people with substance misuse problems to resist professional help. However, if a young person does not want treatment or is unwilling to address their substance misuse problems it will be very difficult to engage them in meaningful work. In this case it may be wise to offer a brief advice or drug education session followed by the offer that they can return for an assessment if they want help and support with their substance misuse. This brief intervention may lead to engagement for assessment or treatment at a later date.

The process of engagement starts before the nurse even meets the young person. If an appointment letter is to be sent, the information and language used needs to be in a form that is appropriate to their age and developmental status. This may be the first point at which the nurse may need to consider issues of consent, parental responsibility and information-sharing. It is not unusual to send separate letters to the young person and to their parents. This can help achieve a balance between ensuring that the parents are kept informed about their child and that the young person's right to privacy is maintained. If a young person has asked for help it is imperative that they are given an appointment as quickly as possible. This is because waiting extended periods of times for meetings may decrease the opportunities for engagement and reduce the willingness of the young person to address the adversities they face. Collaboration is the key to successful treatment with young people who misuse drugs and alcohol. The nurse should approach the assessment with the aim of 'getting alongside' the young person to discover their priorities and view of the situation. At this stage the nurse should avoid giving advice and acting as an expert. Instead they should be aware of the personal aspirations of the young person and attempt to embark on the process of assessment and treatment in partnership with the young person. Evocation is also important during the treatment process. Here, the therapeutic aim is for the nurse to identify motivation from the young person with the basic assumption that this is essential for treatment. The nurse may have a good idea about what may be shaping and maintaining a young person's substance misusing behaviour, but it is the young person themself that holds the key to positively changing such behaviour.

Assessment

The venue for the assessment meeting requires consideration, in terms of accessibility, privacy and safety. Nurses must be flexible about where the assessment takes place since young people may be concerned about confidentiality. As well as specialist CAMHS bases, substance misuse nurses work in a range of settings including YOT offices, children's homes, GP surgeries, youth centres, schools and hospital wards. In addition, neutral venues such as cafes or libraries can often be used. Accessibility needs to be balanced with safety and the need for privacy. Information being discussed may be of a sensitive nature and the nurse should consider whether the environment where the assessment is taking place is fit for purpose. Nurses who are working away from their base should always be aware of safety, and risk-management will need consideration.

Comprehensive history-taking is fundamental to therapeutic intervention with young people who misuse drugs or alcohol (DoH 1999). The role of the nurse during the process of assessment includes gathering general information about personal and social functioning, as well as specific information about drug or alcohol misuse. Consideration should be given to the hierarchy of needs in relation to safety, accommodation, good care, education and therapeutic intervention (Crome et al. 2004). Information should be recorded in relation to which drugs or alcohol the young person is using, as well as details about duration of use, age of first use, first intoxication, first regular use, and events coinciding with regular drug or alcohol misuse. The nurse should also seek to understand how use is financed and how much money the young person spends on their drug or alcohol dependency. Perceptions of drug or alcohol use that the young person believes to be both positive and negative should be explored. Sometimes a young person will use terms about their drug use similar to those used when talking about relationships; 'it's like a friend that's always there for me'; or 'it kicks me when I'm down'. The nurse should also explore how family and friends may be involved in substance misuse. Young people who do not view themselves as having problems or mental health needs in relation to parental addiction may still value talking through issues and concerns with a substance misuse nurse or other professional. The impact of parental drug or alcohol addiction on a child or young person's development is an area of growing interest in substance misuse services.

During the assessment process, it is also important for the nurse to explore whether the young person is engaging in risky or harmful behaviour. This might include self-harm, harm to others or antisocial behaviour such as damage to property. For example young people may participate in risky sexual behaviour, fights or criminal activities which they might have avoided when not under the influence of drugs or alcohol. However, it is important to recognise that young people will be unlikely to answer questions about their behaviour honestly if a therapeutic relationship has not been established. It may take several hours or appointments before any of these questions are answered. Some young people will be uncomfortable with a formal interview and the nurse may gather more information by just chatting with them. However, the nurse's duty of confidentiality applies during both formal and informal discussions. A balancing and engaging style of communication, which nevertheless manages to convey professional boundaries, requires care and consideration on the part of the nurse. It is not unusual for children and young people involved in substance misuse to be suspicious of mental health and social care professionals, citing previous experiences as negative. The Chief Nursing Officer's review of the nursing contribution to vulnerable children and young people demonstrated that looked-after children often experience a lack of privacy, and highlighted a tendency among professionals to respond to them as a collection of problems outlined in case notes rather than real people (DoH 2004b).

Jake

Jake, aged 14, was referred to the substance misuse nurse by his GP. This followed his mother's concerns that Jake was using drugs. Initially both Jake and his mother were seen together. The mother explained that she had discovered Jake was using cannabis when he had returned from the park and appeared intoxicated. Jake had later admitted that he was using cannabis with his friends, but denied it was a problem. The mother was concerned that Jake's behaviour had recently deteriorated and that this was as a result of his cannabis use.

Jake was reportedly doing well at school. His parents had divorced two years ago and Jake has limited contact with his father who had a new family. Jake has two sisters and one brother, Hannah aged 16, Leanne, aged 10 and Ryan, aged 3. His relationship with his sisters appeared to be mixed. He described feeling close to Leanne, but said that he did not get on with Hannah. Jake described his brother, Ryan, as a nuisance.

His mother explained that there were often physical fights between Jake and Hannah. The mother had a new partner, Steve, who had grown-up children of his own. The family lived in their own home and the mother did not work. Steve was self-employed and was out of the house for long hours. Recently there had been some money worries and the mother was looking for part-time work. Jake had recently been having arguments with his mother about pocket money, and had been very irritable and restless when he was not allowed out with his friends. The school was not aware of Jake's drug use, and there had been no reports of bad behaviour at school. He denied any other drug use and said he had only been drunk once which his mother was aware of. Jake reported that he now disliked alcohol and did not drink. He smoked 5–10 cigarettes per day.

After being seen with his mother, the nurse assessed Jake on his own. He continued to deny any other drug use but admitted to regular cannabis use. This was smoked with his peer group in the park on Friday, Saturday and Sunday evenings. He spends £5–10 per week on cannabis which his friend gets from a dealer. Jake had been smoking cannabis regularly for about 18 months but stated that he never smoked alone. Jake said that he used cannabis to help him relax and deal with his feelings. During the assessment, Jake became very tearful and said that since his parents had divorced he felt his mother and stepfather had very little time for him. He felt his mother spent more time with his siblings, and his father with his new family and felt that his stepfather was always at work. Jake felt he no longer had anyone to discuss his problems with, and felt that he was just expected to just get on with things. Jake wanted his mother to know how he felt, but had not been able to find the words to tell her. He also wanted time on his own with his mother but had not been able to ask her. Jake told the nurse that he found that cannabis made him forget about being lonely and he enjoyed the relaxed feeling the drugs gave him. He believed that he would be able to stop using cannabis if things got better at home. The nurse advised Jake that cannabis could be making his mood more depressed. He acknowledged that the next day after taking cannabis, his mood would be down and he would often feel irritable. Jake recognised that this was making his relationship with his mother more difficult. The nurse also informed Jake that if he was caught with a large amount of cannabis, he might be charged with possession with intent to supply. He was unaware that smoking cannabis was illegal.

After the individual assessment, the mother was invited back into the room. With support from the nurse, Jake was able to tell her how he had been feeling. She was also very tearful and had not been aware of the full impact of her divorce on Jake. She promised him that they could have some individual time together as long as he gave up smoking cannabis. Jake agreed and another appointment was made for review in three months' time. At follow-up, Jake and his mother were seen together. Both said things at home were much better. Jake had stopped smoking cannabis and was having 'special time' with his mother once a week. Jake reported that he had also made contact with his uncle who he had been close to in the past. Jake said that since stopping cannabis, his mood was much better and that he was far less irritable. His mother agreed and said that Jake was more like his old self and less argumentative. Neither felt the need for another appointment. After discharging Jake, the nurse advised his GP of the intervention and brief outcome.

Treatment

The aim of treatment is to increase intrinsic motivation so that change arises from within the young person. The responsibility to change behaviour rests with the young person rather than the nurse, other professional, parent or carer. The role of the nurse is the help the young person describe their hopes and aspirations and the goals and values that are theirs. Treatment interventions with young people who misuse drugs or alcohol are largely based on work documented with adults. Motivational interviewing, cognitive behavioural therapy, harm-reduction and abstinence models are drawn upon. Using a family therapy approach, multigenerational influences can be considered and each family member is given an opportunity to share their concerns about substance misuse, mental health and behaviour. Theory and therapy related to young people allows developmental aspects of language, understanding and power differentials to be factored into the work. Creative approaches using music, drama and art therapy that rely less on spoken communication can also be utilised. Since not all teams will have access to such therapeutic approaches, it is important that nurses investigate the provision of services in their local area in order to enable young people to make the best use of them. Some specialist teams may have the full range of treatment services including individual work through to in-patient assessment and detoxification services. In another area there may just be an individual clinician attached to a community mental health team.

It is important to remember that young people who misuse drugs and alcohol are not a homogenous group. This means that no single treatment strategy will be effective for all young people. The main treatment modalities for young people who misuse drugs and alcohol include motivational interviewing (Aubrey 1998) and comprise individual therapy, family interventions, group work and multimodal treatment strategies such as multisystemic therapy. This is in addition to emergency medical treatments, detoxification and withdrawal programmes and relapse prevention. Motivational interviewing as an ethos and therapeutic technique is used widely with people who are ambivalent about change (Miller & Rollnick 1991). Individual approaches for both drug and alcohol misuse may include brief intervention work (Longabaugh et al. 2001) and solution-focused therapy (Hanton 2003). Since the involvement of parents or carers of young people who misuse drugs or alcohol is often central to successful treatment, family interventions are crucially important and are associated with positive outcomes (Deas & Thomas 2001).

One of the most advanced models of intervention with young people who misuse drugs or alcohol is multidimensional family therapy (Liddle 2001). However, as well as formal family therapy, work with families or carers can also be exploratory, supportive or psycho-educational. Sometimes the family does not have to be present to be considered during therapeutic sessions, thus becoming part of the family work. It can sometimes be useful for the nurse to ask the young person to bring anyone with an important view of the situation to sessions. This can result in friends, associates, other family members or community support workers contributing to the therapeutic process. Group work with young people who misuse drugs and alcohol is an undeveloped area of practice. Whilst self-help groups are often an important part of treatment programmes, bringing together young people with drug or alcohol problems may propagate misuse (Crome et al. 2004). However, nurses often run groups for young people based on social skills-building, anger management, assertiveness or conflict resolution, and these may be a positive part of the overall treatment strategy.

Conclusion

Substance misuse is a major psychosocial problem facing young people in modern society. The prevention and treatment of drug and alcohol problems requires a multiagency effort, and nurses in a range of settings share responsibility for improving services for young people with substance misuse problems. Nurses play a number of key roles in terms of health promotion, the prevention of substance misuse and early identification of drug or alcohol problems. Through their work in schools, hospitals and prison settings, nurses are well-placed to help children and young people develop an understanding of the potential risks and harmful effects of drugs and alcohol. They also have a role to play in identifying young people with substance misuse problems and help ensure they can access specialist services for assessment and treatment for their addiction. To ensure that nurses are able to help improve substance misuse services for young people, they must develop basic competencies in the areas of drug and alcohol awareness, recognition of vulnerabilities and child protection.

Substance misuse nursing is a rapidly developing area of practice. Specialist substance misuse nurses provide a range of direct and indirect interventions. These include assessment and treatment for individual young people with drug or alcohol problems and mental health problems, as well as support, training and supervision for colleagues who have concerns about drug or alcohol use by young people. Through their work in YOTs, they can also identify and signpost young people with complex, severe or persistent mental disorders to specialist CAMHS. Specialist substance misuse nurses should also help ensure that drug and alcohol services for young people are planned, commissioned and delivered as part of the wider children's services agenda.

Sources of further information

'Talk to Frank' is a free confidential drugs information and advice line www.talktofrank.com www.wrecked.co.uk

References

Appelby, L., Shaw, J. & Amos, T. (1997). *Safer Services: report of the national confidential inquiry into suicide and homicide by people with mental illness.* London: HMSO.

Aubrey, L. (1998). *Motivational Interviewing with Adolescents Presenting for Out-patient Substance Abuse Treatment. Doctoral dissertation.* University of New Mexico: dissertation abstracts DAI-B 59-03 1357.

Bukstein, O., Brent, D. & Kaminer, Y. (1989). Comorbidity of substance abuse and other psychiatric disorders in adolescents. *American Journal of Psychiatry*, (146), 1131–41.

Cabinet Office (1998). *Tackling Drugs to Build a Better Britain: the government's 10-year strategy for tackling drugs misuse.* London: HMSO.

Cantwell, R., Berwin, J., Glazebrook, C., Dalkin, T., Fox, R., Medley, I., & Harrison, G. (1999). Substance misuse: prevalence of substance misuse in first episode psychosis. *British Journal of Psychiatry*, (174), 150–53.

Children's Legal Centre and Standing Conference on Drug Abuse (1999). *Young People and Drugs: policy guidance for drug interventions.* London: SCODA.

Craig, T., Hodson, S., Woodward, S. & Richardson, S. (1996). *Off to a Bad Start: a longitudinal study of homeless young people in London*. London: Mental Health Foundation.

Crome, I. (2004). Psychiatric comorbidity. In: Crome, I., Ghodse, H., Gilvarry, E., & McArdle, P. (Eds). *Young People and Substance Misuse*. London: Gaskell.

Crome, I., Ghodse, H., Gilvarry, E., & McArdle, P. (2004). *Young People and Substance Misuse*. London: Gaskell.

Crome, I., McArdle, P., Gilvarry, E. & Bailey, S. (2004). Treatment. In: Crome, I., Ghodse, H., Gilvarry, E., & McArdle, P. (Eds). *Young People and Substance Misuse*. London: Gaskell.

Crome, I., Rumball, D. & London, M. (2004). Health issues. In: Crome, I., Ghodse, H., Gilvarry, E., & McArdle, P. (Eds). *Young People and Substance Misuse*. London: Gaskell.

Deas, D. & Thomas, S. (2001). An overview of controlled studies of adolescent substance abuse treatment. *American Journal of Addictions*, (10), 178–89.

Department for Education and Skills (2003). *Every Child Matters*. London: HMSO.

Department for Educational and Skills (2005). *Government Response to Hidden Harm: the report of an inquiry by the advisory council on the misuse of drugs*. London: HMSO.

Department of Health (1996). *Children and Young People Substance Misuse Services*. London: HMSO.

Department of Health (1999). *Drug Misuse and Dependence: guidelines on clinical management*. London: HMSO.

Department of Health (2000a). *Safeguarding Children Involved in Prostitution: supplementary guidance to Working Together to Safeguard Children*. London: HMSO.

Department of Health (2000b). *Working Together to Safeguard Children*. London: HMSO.

Department of Health (2002). *Promoting the Health of Looked After Children*. London: HMSO.

Department of Health (2004a). *National Service Framework for Children, Young People and Maternity Services*. London: HMSO.

Department of Health (2004b). *The Chief Nursing Officer's Review of the Nursing, Midwifery and Health Visiting Contribution to Vulnerable Children and Young People*. London: HMSO.

Elliot, D., Huizingo, D. & Ageton, S. (1985). *Explaining Delinquency and Drug Use*. London: Sage.

Fitzpatrick, S. & Klinker, C. (2000). *Research on Single Homelessness in Britain*. London: Joseph Rowntree Foundation.

Gilbert, T., O'Connor, S., Mathew, S., Allen, K., Piper, M. & Gill, O. (2004). Hepatitis A vaccine: a prison-based solution for a community based outbreak? *Communicable Disease and Public Health*, **7** (4), 289–93.

Hammersley, R., Marsland, L. & Reid, M. (2003). *Substance Use by Young Offenders*. London: Home Office Research, Development and Statistics Directorate.

Hanton, P. (2003). Solution focused therapy and substance misuse. In: O'Connell, B. & Palmer, S. (Eds). *Handbook of Solution Focused Therapy*. London: Sage.

Health Advisory Service (2001). *The Substance of Young Needs*. London: The Home Office Drugs Prevention Service.

Hibbell, B., Anderson, B. & Bjamason, T. (1999). *Alcohol and Other Drug Use Among Students in 30 European Countries – the 1999 ESPAD report*. Stockholm: Council for Information on Alcohol and Other Drugs, Council of Europe, Pompidou Group.

Home Office (2003a). *Hidden Harm: responding to the needs of children of problem drug users: the report of an inquiry by the advisory council on the misuse of drugs*. London: HMSO.

Home Office (2003b). *Substance Misuse by Young Offenders: the impact of the normalisation of drug use in the early years of the 21st century*. London: Home Office Research, Development and Statistics Directorate.

Kazdin, A. (1997). Practitioner review: psychosocial treatments for conduct disorder in children. *Journal of Child Psychiatry and Psychology*, (38), 161–78.

King, C., Guaziuddin, N. & McGovern, L. (1996). Predictors of comorbid alcohol and substance misuse in depressed adolescents. *Journal of the American Academy of Child and Adolescent Psychiatry*, (35), 743–51.

Liddle, H., Dakof, G., Parker, K., Diamond, G., Barrett, K. & Tejeda, M. (2001). Multidimensional family therapy for adolescent drug abuse: results of a randomised clinical trial. *American Journal of Drug and Alcohol Abuse*, **27** (4), 651–88.

Lloyd, C. (1998). Risk factors for problem drug use: identifying problem groups. *Drugs: Education, Prevention and Policy*, (3), 217–32.

Longabaugh, R., Woolard, R. & Nirenberg, T. (2001). Evaluating the effects of a brief motivational intervention for injured drinkers in the emergency department. *Journal of Studies on Alcohol*, (63), 806–16.

Lord President's Office (1995). *Tackling Drugs Together: a consultation document on a strategy for England 1995–1998*. London: Lord President's Office.

McGilvarry, E. & Crome, I. (2004). Implications of parental substance misuse. In: Crome, I., Ghodse, H., Gilvarry, E., & McArdle, P. (Eds). *Young People and Substance Misuse*. London: Gaskell.

Melrose, M. & Brodie, I. (2000). *Vulnerable Young People and their Vulnerability to Drug Misuse*. London: Drugscope.

Meltzer, H., Gatward, R., Goodman, R. & Ford, T. (2000). *The Mental Health of Children and Adolescents in Great Britain*. London: HMSO.

Meltzer, H., Lader, D., Corbin, T., Goodman, R., & Ford, T. (2004). *The Mental Health of Young People Looked After by Local Authorities in Wales: the report of a survey carried out in 2002/2003 by the Office for National Statistics on behalf of the Welsh Assembly Government*. London: HMSO.

Miller, W. & Rollnick, S. (1991). *Motivational Interviewing: preparing people to change addictive behaviour*. New York: Guilford Press.

Nowinski, J. (1990). *Substance Abuse in Adolescents and Young Adults: a guide to treatment*. New York: Norton.

Parker, H., Aldridge, J. & Measham, F. (1998). *Illegal Leisure: the normalisation of adolescent recreational drug use*. London: Routledge.

Phillips, J. (1997). Meeting the psychiatric needs of children in foster care: social workers views. *Psychiatric Bulletin*, (21), 609–11.

Ramsey, M. & Partridge, S. (1999). *Drug Misuse Declared in 1998: results from the British Crime Survey*. London: Home Office.

Richardson, J. & Joughin, C. (2000). *The Mental Health Needs of Looked After Children*. London: Gaskell Royal College of Psychiatrists.

Royal College of Psychiatrists (2004). *Mental Health and Growing Up Factsheets: alcohol and drugs (30a)*. London: Royal College of Psychiatrists.

Rutter, M. & Smith, D. (1995). *Psychosocial Disorders in Young People: time trends and their causes*. Chichester: John Wiley.

Saunders, L. & Broad, B. (1997). *The Health Needs of Young People Leaving Care*. Leicester: De Montfort University.

Social Services Inspectorate (1997). *Young People and Substance Misuse: the local authority response*. London: Department of Health.

Wilens, T., Biederman, J., & Millstein, R. (1999). Risk of substance use disorders in youths with child and adolescent onset bipolar disorder. *Journal of American Academy of Child and Adolescent Psychiatry*, (38), 680–85.

Williams, R. & Morgan, H. (1994). *Suicide Prevention: the challenge confronted.* London: HMSO.

Wincup, E. & Bayliss, R. (2001). Problematic substance use and the young homeless: implications for wellbeing. *Youth and Policy*, (71), 44–58.

Wincup, E., Buckland, G. & Bayliss, R. (2003). *Youth Homelessness and Substance Misuse: report to the drugs and alcohol research unit.* London: Home Office Research, Development and Statistics Directorate.

Young, S., Mikulich, S., & Goodwin, M. (1995). Treated delinquent boys: substance misuse onset pattern relationship to conduct and mood disorders. *Drug and Alcohol Dependence*, (37), 149–62.

Chapter 12

Nursing and School-Based Mental Health Services

Sharon Leighton

Key points

- Schools have been identified as an ideal place to begin to address the crisis in child and adolescent mental health.

- Research evidence for school-based mental health services (SBMHS) in the UK is sparse. The majority of the research relating to SBMHS originates in the US.

- Although there are no definitive approaches to providing mental health services within schools, there are several factors associated with the success of a service.

- Models for SBMHS include consultation with teachers and other professionals in schools, and training for educational staff and school nurses.

- Nurses at different CAMHS (child and adolescent mental health services) tiers can be seen to have a role to play in the development of SBMHS.

- School nurses are ideally placed to assist in the provision of mental health services within schools as they work across education, health and social care boundaries.

Introduction

This chapter is based on a review of the research and practice literature currently available on SBMHS and reference is made to pertinent key policies. Studies were obtained through electronic and manual searches. Although SBMHS represent an area of growing interest, the research literature and evidence base is limited. The majority of the references relating to SBMHS originate from the US and therefore caution is needed in applying findings to the UK. This chapter provides an overview of child and adolescent mental health services and the provision of SBMHS and focuses on the implications for nurses, particularly school nurses. A reflective exercise is provided after the conclusions.

Readers may wish to peruse this beforehand and hold the questions in mind as they read the chapter. Key texts for further reading, and internet resources, are listed at the end of the chapter.

Child and adolescent mental health

Mental health is a socially created and described concept. Professionals from different backgrounds – e.g. health, education, social care – may react differently to the term, possibly preferring to substitute the word 'emotional' for 'mental'. In a chapter on SBMHS, it is important to recognise that different terminologies are often used by professionals in schools and health services in the UK. In schools, professionals may use the term educational and behavioural difficulties (EBDs) when the problems encountered by children are severe, persistent and associated with other problems. Another term which is commonly used by educational staff is special educational needs (SENs). This may apply to developmental or learning disabilities, as well as to emotional, behavioural and mental health problems. It is usually the case that educational and behavioural difficulties, special educational needs and mental health problems and disorders overlap to a great extent. In health services, problems encountered by children and young people are usually understood within a broad biopsychosocial model. Nurses in both schools and in health services such as specialist CAMHS are in key positions to help ensure that differences in language and understanding do not compromise the mental health services provided for individual children and young people.

For the purpose of this chapter the World Health Organization (WHO) definition is used. This describes mental health as a fundamental component of health, through which a person realises their intellectual, emotional and social abilities. Positive mental health helps a person to cope effectively with life's stressors, work productively and profitably, and make a contribution to the community (WHO 2000). For children and adolescents this means achieving at school, establishing and maintaining supportive relationships and progressing successfully into adult and working life (Department for Education and Skills 2001). Mental health and mental illness can be viewed as existing on a continuum, with mental illness being diagnosed from a clinically recognisable set of symptoms, associated in most cases with distress and with interference with daily life (WHO 1992).

In the UK, the prevalence of mental health problems amongst children and adolescents is high. One in twenty young people is reported to be experiencing mental health problems at any given time (Mental Health Foundation 1999; Meltzer et al. 2000; Green et al. 2005). These problems include emotional and behavioural problems such as stress, self-harm and drug or alcohol misuse. Furthermore, one in ten young people suffers from a diagnosable mental illness such as depression or an eating disorder (Mental Health Foundation 1999; Meltzer et al. 2000; Green et al. 2005). Such problems have a negative impact on a child's physical, emotional, social and cognitive development, reducing their quality of life (Mental Health Foundation 1999; Meltzer et al. 2000; Department of Health 2004; Green et al. 2005). The burden of childhood mental health problems and illness represents a vast financial cost to individuals, families and society. This includes poor academic achievement, loss of earnings for parents, as well as costs to the NHS (National Health Service) and government departments (Appleton & Hammond-Rowley 2000). Despite the extent of the problem, mental health services in general, and CAMHS in particular have been under-funded and under-resourced (Health Advisory Service 1995; Mental Health Foundation 1999). Fewer than half of young people experiencing mental health problems ever reach specialist services (Laurence 2003; DoH 2004). It is families, local communities, primary care agencies and schools who attempt to compensate for this discrepancy, providing what assistance they can (HAS 1995; Mental Health Foundation 1999; Mitchell et al. 2004). According to the four-tier model of CAMHS (HAS 1995), Tier 1 comprises non-mental health professionals such as school nurses and teachers – i.e. those professionals who are trying to cope with the burgeoning mental health problems of young people, which can present as challenging, disruptive, antisocial and self-harming behaviour. This is despite often feeling neither confident nor competent in this area (HAS 1995; YoungMinds 2001).

However, CAMHS are evolving. Policy and practice changes across health, education, social services and youth justice agencies emphasise multiagency working and the need to configure local services to reflect the needs of local populations. The DoH and DfES (Department for Education and Skills) in the UK have documented the need for coordinated and integrated partnerships working across health, education, social care, youth justice and the voluntary sector agencies in relation to meeting the mental health needs of children and adolescents (DoH 2004; DfES 2005). Clear pathways which specify how the range of mental health needs of children and adolescents are to be addressed, whether from within mental health services or from other services where mental health is not the primary focus, have been recommended (DoH 2004; DfES 2005). This generates opportunities for working differently and for interagency cooperation across seamless services. Partnership working across agencies working with children and young people with mental health problems and learning disabilities can be a challenging task. The lack of understanding of the respective roles, duties, responsibilities and organisation of the different agencies and professionals involved, and their different language, may lead to poor communication, misunderstandings and frustration. Effective partnership working can improve children and young people's experience of services and lead to improved outcomes (DfES 2003).

A similar picture can be seen in the US with regard to child and adolescent mental health problems. Research has identified that between 12% and 20% of children and adolescents experience mental health problems, with very few obtaining appropriate services (Adelman et al. 1997). Epidemiological studies indicate that fewer than 20% of young people who need mental health care actually receive a service. Earlier studies showed that of those who did receive services, fewer than half received services appropriate to their need (Atkins et al. 2003). Barriers to accessing specialist mental health services include poor knowledge of services; stigma associated with mental illness; transport difficulties; limited resources; and long waiting lists (Weist & Albus 2004). This resulted in two important developments in CAMHS in the US – the advocation of evidence-based practice; and calls for alternative models of working (Atkins et al. 2003). The need to provide services in natural community settings such as schools was also highlighted (Weist & Albus 2004).

School-based mental health services (SBMHS)

Schools have been identified as ideal places to begin to address the crisis in child and adolescent mental health, since a large percentage of childhood and adolescence is spent within this environment. The Healthy Schools Initiative, as part of the wider public health agenda, *Our Healthier Nation* set improvement in mental health as a target (DoH 1999). Schools can therefore be considered to have a key role to play in influencing the mental health of the children of today and the adults of tomorrow (Adelman et al. 1997; WHO 1998; Mental Health Foundation 1999; DfES 2001; Hales et al. 2003; Richardson & Partridge 2003). Though there are distinct differences between the US and the UK in terms of health care, social policy and culture there are also similarities in that increasing numbers of children and adolescents are presenting with mental health problems. Additionally, there are comparable issues and challenges involved in working across agency and professional boundaries. For these reasons the ideas and experiences reported in the US merit consideration and reflection within a UK context. The evolution of school mental health services in the US spans several decades. It reflects changes in dominant philosophies and approaches to public education, and development in professional fields that relate to school mental health (Flaherty & Osher 2003). The biggest period of growth in SBMHS has occurred within the last decade and has been influenced by such factors as the following (McMahon et al. 2000; Weist et al. 2003; Weist & Albus 2004):

- An increased awareness of the enormous gap between, demand for, and supply of CAMHS.
- The beginnings of an evidence base in child and adolescent mental health.
- Reforms in health, social care and education services.
- Systematic efforts to influence policy, expand and improve funding, technical assistance and training at federal, state and local levels.
- Emerging research evidence that SBMHS are reaching those most in need and/or at risk and having a positive effect.

SBMHS in the US are deemed to be very much in their infancy, with considerable variation at local and state levels (Weist et al. 2003). Nevertheless, early findings suggest that the provision of access and early intervention is cost-effective in the long term, with SBMHS considered as effective as out-patient CAMHS (Armbruster & Lichtman 1999), and as associated with improved learning and behavioural outcomes for children and adolescents (Weist & Albus 2004).

Research evidence for SBMHS in the UK is sparse. The Mental Health Foundation (MHF) conducted a research project for the DfES, which focused on the links between CAMHS and schools and on four funded pilot projects (Pettitt 2003). CAMHS structures were found to vary greatly across the UK and, whilst 89% of CAMHS professionals who responded to their survey did work with schools, the majority of these provided consultation and liaison in an *ad hoc* manner, rather than on a regular basis. Work in schools represented a tiny proportion of CAMHS resources. The professionals most involved with schools were clinical psychologists, specialist CAMHS nurses and social workers (Pettitt 2003). The MHF project (Pettitt 2003) reported on four different projects in the UK involving joint work between CAMHS and schools. Two projects involved the secondment of CAMHS staff to schools where they were involved in providing a range of services. Another consisted of specialist school teams located within Tier 2 CAMHS, providing a variety of school-based interventions. The fourth consisted of local teams staffed jointly by education and health and supplying an assortment of interventions. Specialist CAMHS nurses were actively involved in three of the projects (Pettitt 2003). The research identified several advantages of joint working between CAMHS and education services. These included a positive impact on children and education staff; relationships between parents and school; accessing children in need of mental health services who would not normally be reached; and an earlier identification of children's mental health problems (Pettitt 2003). Unfortunately information provided concerning evaluation measures and outcomes was limited.

Government initiatives in England in relation to SBMHS include behaviour and education support teams (BESTs). These are multiagency teams which support schools in identified deprived areas of England. The aim is to promote emotional wellbeing, positive behaviour and improve school attendance. The Department for Education and Skills commissioned the National Foundation for Education Research to undertake an independent evaluation of BESTs (www.dfes.gov.uk). The results of the evaluation were not in the public domain at the time of writing. The CAMHS Innovation Projects (Kurtz & James 2002) included school-based initiatives. These included the Child Behaviour Intervention Initiative in Leicester, the Excluded Children's Project in Rochdale and the York and North Yorkshire Schools Project. The executive summary of the evaluation of all the projects was positive (Kurtz & James 2002). Independent evaluation of individual projects was completed by local universities but reports relating to school-based projects are not yet available.

Summarising the research evidence from both the US and the UK, it has been suggested that the provision of SBMHS can be seen as making a positive contribution to meeting the mental health needs of children and adolescents. They provide access to services for disadvantaged and disenfranchised young people. There is also system-wide collaboration; outreach and community-based care is provided with systematic evaluation in naturalistic settings; they act as gatekeepers for more acute or specialised care; professionals are trained to work within a range of systems and cultures; and there is a positive impact on children, staff and relationships between parents and school (Armbruster 2002; Pettitt 2003; Weist & Albus 2004).

Different models of school-based mental health services

In their review of the literature on SBMHS in the US between 1985 and 1999, Rones & Hoagwood (2000) concluded that though there was no definitive approach to providing mental health services within schools, there were several factors associated with the success of a service. These included consistent programme implementation; the use of multiple modalities; involvement of parents, teachers and peers; the integration of programme content into the general curriculum; and approaches that were developmentally appropriate (Rones & Hoagwood 2000). Recent research conducted by the MHF outlines some key issues for consideration to improve joint working between CAMHS and schools (MHF 2004). In addition, there have been several good practice recommendations from the reviewed literature for establishing an SBMHS project in schools. These include the need to ensure that all school staff be made aware of the function of the project; the need to be clear about the role of project workers; and the need to identify clear referral routes. It is also suggested that expectations should be realistic and a written agreement about how the project will operate should be negotiated between the school and CAMHS. The importance of strong links with CAMHS is stressed, ideally with professionals remaining part of the CAMHS team and receiving clinical supervision (McMahon et al. 2000; Armbruster 2002; Leighton 2003; Pettitt 2003; Massey et al. 2005). Various models of SBMHS are discussed below. The available published literature is extremely sparse. This is with the exception of school-based health centres and professionals, which is the main model used in the US. This model of intervention has more of an evidence base in comparison to the others. Consultation with teachers and other professionals in schools and training for educational staff and school nurses are often provided jointly, but have been separated here for clarity of discussion.

School-based health centres and professionals

Despite the relatively large evidence base that has been generated in the US, school-based health centres and professionals have not been widely reported in literature on SBMHS in the UK, and it is difficult to draw comparisons. Although there are several models of SBMHS, two prominent models exist in the US: the mental health component of a school-based health clinic (SBHC); and an independent school-based mental health programme (Armbruster 2002). These are models that could be considered within the context of UK initiatives and anecdotal evidence exists for embryonic projects of this nature. Both models have common developmental and administrative issues that require ongoing attention. These include funding, needs assessment and resources, local politics, legal and ethical considerations, programme structure, staffing and training, partnerships and collaboration, unrealistic expectations, quality assurance and evaluation (McMahon et al. 2000; Armbruster 2002; Massey et al. 2005). It can be contended that these issues are pertinent for any SBMHS initiative, irrespective of locality or model used. Although an article by Hales et al. (2003) provides limited information, it is of interest as it focuses on the role of a mental health clinical nurse specialist working in conjunction with a school nurse in an SBHC. This pilot study involved much ongoing collaboration between the stakeholders and was perceived as a way of accessing vulnerable young people in a non-stigmatising environment (Hales et al. 2003). Information regarding evaluation was limited, with reference made to the use of validated rating scales to evaluate treatment efficacy over time. Nonetheless, the idea of a working partnership between mental health and school nurses in school-based clinics can be viewed as a powerful alliance, acting in the interests of children and adolescents (Hootman et al. 2003). This is an alliance that could be fostered between CAMHS and school nurses within the UK context.

Consultation with teachers and other professionals in schools

There is a dearth of published literature evaluating the process and outcomes associated with the provision of consultation to teachers and other professionals in schools. Interestingly, Cvejic & Smith, as far back as 1979, described a Canadian programme whereby a school nurse with training in mental health acted as a consultant to school staff. The school nurse was in turn supervised by a psychiatrist (Cvejic & Smith 1979). Regrettably, the information provided about the programme was limited, and further reports on the initiative were not found. Teachers can be regarded as being under increasing pressure, with larger classes, the integration of children with special needs into classes, and an emphasis on academic ability and examination results (DfES 2001). Teachers who feel overwhelmed by such stressors may find it difficult to attend to the emotional wellbeing of their pupils. Therefore appropriate and accessible support from specialist CAMHS can be viewed as essential (Richardson & Partridge 2003). The provision of such support can be seen to offer teachers, and other professionals in schools, an opportunity to contain their anxieties, learn new skills and gain confidence (Jackson 2002; Richardson & Partridge 2003). An ongoing project in the UK was reported whereby a child psychotherapist had provided regular work discussion groups and individual consultation with teachers in a mainstream secondary school over a three-year period (Jackson 2002). Evaluation involved regular reviewing on a formal and informal basis with teachers, the head teacher and the SEN coordinator (SENCO). The most valuable outcome reported in the evaluation was that the project enabled teachers to step back and create a space to reflect on the emotional factors that could be affecting behaviour, learning and teaching. In another small-scale UK project the provision of regular CAMHS consultation to school nurses led to a reported increase in confidence amongst school nurses working with adolescents presenting with mental health problems (Richardson & Partridge 2000).

A further article summarised US research related to mental health collaboration between school social workers and teachers. School social workers were perceived as being key players in the development of SBMHS, through the process of collaborating with teachers and other school staff (Lynn et al. 2003). Collaboration involved regular consultation about mental health issues and classroom interventions plus direct work with children and their families. Whilst social workers in the US have a different remit from social workers in the UK, the same principles of collaboration and consultation can be applied to other CAMHS professionals in the UK. From the limited evidence available it can be suggested that opportunities for collaboration between teachers and other professionals in schools and specialist CAMHS professionals, such as nurses, are positive. Such collaboration allows relationships to be developed, and confidence and skills in dealing with mental health issues to be increased. Concerns and anxieties held by teachers and other professionals in schools can be contained, and more appropriate referrals made to specialist CAMHS (Jackson 2002; Richardson & Partridge 2003).

Training for educational staff and school nurses

This model of intervention will be reviewed briefly here and explored in more detail later in the chapter. Whilst the importance of CAMHS training has been widely recognised (DoH 2004; 2005; DfES 2005), there are few published studies on training initiatives available to date. The information presented focuses on local initiatives involving school nurses although one makes a recommendation to include future training for teachers (Clarke et al. 2003). One school nurse-led project in the UK focused on screening and providing initial support for Year 9 students. The school nurses involved received monthly supervision from specialist CAMHS professionals (DfES 2001). Unfortunately no information about outcomes was available for this project. Another school nurse-led clinic for children and adolescents with emotional and mental health difficulties was set up after school nurses had received training in mental health issues. Monthly supervision and consultation was provided by specialist CAMHS. Initial feedback from children, adolescents and their families and from teachers and other professionals was reported to be positive (Chipman & Gooch 2003). Unfortunately, other than reference to a satisfaction survey, little information was provided about how the service was evaluated. Another small-scale local pilot study involving partnership between various stakeholders, e.g. CAMHS, school nurses, school personnel and adolescents was reported. Training and supervision were provided to three school nurses in order to enhance their skills in addressing mental health issues presented by pupils from Years 10 and 11 at drop-in clinics (Clarke et al. 2003). Again, information on the evaluation of the project was limited, with the authors acknowledging the evaluative process as a project limitation. Nevertheless, feedback from the school nurses was reported to be positive and funding was secured to provide core mental health training for school nurses in the area (Clarke et al. 2003).

Outreach clinics from specialist CAMHS

Another potential model of SBMHS is the provision of outreach clinics or services from specialist CAMHS. Two project examples were found in the literature (Turpin & Titheridge 2001; Pettitt 2003). In the first project, two specialist CAMHS professionals, one of whom was a CAMHS clinical nurse specialist, piloted a group project in a primary school (Turpin & Titheridge 2001). The group was for children with behavioural and social difficulties, and included five 7–9 year-olds, and ran weekly for two terms. Evaluation was obtained by feedback from parents and carers, class teachers and the SENCO. The authors concluded that supervision was essential when working with difficult and challenging behaviour in a group context and that two terms were necessary for the children to consolidate the behaviour they had learnt (Turpin & Titheridge 2001). The second project was one of the MHF's pilot projects and involved a specialist schools team working within Tier 2 CAMHS (Pettitt 2003). The team comprised various professionals including CAMHS nurses, was managed by the local specialist CAMHS and operated across primary and secondary schools in a disadvantaged area. The overall aim was to improve emotional wellbeing and learning by providing a range of services, including outreach clinics for children and adolescents; consultation; and training for staff and health promotion (Pettitt 2003). Several different approaches to evaluation were used, including service evaluation packs consisting of standardised measures and questionnaires. Minimal information was provided about outcomes other than reference to generally positive results.

School nurses and SBMHS

In this section the issue of providing mental health training and supervision to school nurses in order to support such endeavours is explored. It can be argued that school nurses are ideally placed to assist in the provision of mental health services within schools as they work across education, health and social care boundaries (DoH 2005, in press). The September 2004 NHS workforce census identified that there were nearly 2500 qualified school nurses working in the NHS, with most working part-time or term-time only. A significant number of school nurses also work in the independent sector. School nurses have always played a vital role in promoting health and helping students. In the UK their roles are widening to incorporate early identification of, and intervention for, students experiencing mental health problems (Hootman et al. 2003; Mitchell et al. 2004; DfES 2005). The *Choosing Health* White Paper (DoH 2004b) has called for new roles for school nurses which are relevant to today's society. The new roles include a focus on tackling mental ill-health in children and adolescents at both Tiers 1 and 2 CAMHS (DoH 2004b).

In order for school nurses to be successful in their extended roles, continuing education and training are deemed necessary (Adelman et al. 1997; United Kingdom Central Council 2000; DfES 2001). A UK survey identified that 80% of Tier 1 staff, such as teachers, social workers and school nurses had not received appropriate training in child and adolescent mental health issues (YoungMinds 2001). The United Kingdom Central Council (UKCC), now known as the NMC (Nursing & Midwifery Council), identified that non-mental health nurses, that is, those working in areas other than mental health, did not have the confidence and skills necessary to deal with the increasing number of mental health problems they were encountering, nor did they consider themselves sufficiently well-trained to provide mental health services (UKCC 2000). Despite the perceived lack of confidence and skills it could be argued first that, school nurses already deal with a large quantity of mental health issues in their work with children and adolescents; and second, with appropriate additional training and supervision they would be in a position to take on work that might otherwise be referred to specialist CAMHS (Richardson & Partridge 2003). Specialist CAMHS are seen as having a pivotal role in providing clinical training, supervision and consultation for school nurses. This is in order to develop their knowledge and skills, clarify the role of CAMHS and increase their confidence in dealing with students presenting with mental health problems (Richardson & Partridge 2000; 2003; Clarke et al. 2003; Hootman et al. 2003; Leighton et al. 2003). All specialist CAMHS professionals including nurses have a role to play in helping to develop mental health knowledge, skills and competencies in the non-specialist CAMHS workforce. There have been several CAMHS training initiatives in recent years to develop school nurses' knowledge and skills in mental health, but there are few published articles available.

Two small-scale local UK studies, where training based on needs identified by local school nurses and supervision were provided, demonstrated positive results at initial evaluation (Richardson & Partridge 2000; Leighton et al. 2003). A further local study involved CAMHS consultation with school nurses in order to ascertain their mental health training needs (Mitchell et al. 2004). A range of training needs were identified which included the need for knowledge and skills in relation to emotional and behavioural problems, family relation-ships, self-harm and psychosis (Mitchell et al. 2004).

In the US, an internet-based mental health education programme exists for school nurses, which aims to enable them to provide direct services to students, to coordinate and develop resources and to enhance access to community resources (Adelman et al. 1997). Though the resources are still available online at http://smhp.psych.ucla.edu, it is regrettable that published reports on the evaluation of this programme were not found in the literature searches under-taken, as lessons could be learnt from this initiative in terms of providing training in the UK.

Whilst school nurses have an advantage in that they are already work-ing within the school environment, it is important to consider that there are challenges involved in focusing on school nurses in relation to the provision of mental health services in schools. These include the following: they are a limited resource and thus there are negative implications for time out for training and supervision; there are competing demands on their time; mental health might not be considered to be a priority at primary care trust or even at individual team level; and providing ongoing consultation and supervision may not be possible within existing specialist CAMHS resources. Never-theless, from the limited evidence available, it would appear that training school nurses in mental health interventions could help to strengthen the critical mass of those who can provide mental health care to children and adolescents.

Conclusion

The need to proceed with caution when generalising to the UK findings which originate largely from the US was highlighted in the introduction to this chapter. It is essential to establish an evidence base of SBMHS that have originated within the UK. We know that projects are being undertaken, but there is a dearth of published evidence to date. The research data and anecdotal evidence indicate that there are a range of options to choose from when considering a model for a school-based mental health service. The evid-ence points to the need for individual projects to be grounded in an analysis of local demographic information, the unique aspects of an individual com-munity and available specialist CAMHS resources. Robust and transparent evaluation of projects is also essential. Nurses at different tiers can be seen to have a role to play in the development of SBMHS. School nurses in par-ticular have been identified as a potential vital resource in the provision of SBMHS. However, caution is necessary, given that school nurses are limited in number and have many competing demands on their time. Nevertheless, the provision of SBMHS can be perceived as an approach with the potential to offer a positive contribution to meeting the increasing mental health needs of children and adolescents.

Reflective exercise

Consider how you might develop school-based mental health services in the school(s) you work in or with. Reflect on the following questions:

- Which model might work best within the local context?
- What could be the advantages of using this model?
- What challenges could you be faced with?
- How might you work with these challenges?
- What resources are available locally that could prove helpful?
- What might be the role(s) of a nurse in such a project?

References

Adelman, H.S., Taylor, L., Bradley, B. & Lewis, K. (1997). Mental health in schools: expanded opportunities for school nurses. *Journal of School Nursing*, **13** (3), 6–12.

Appleton, P. & Hammond-Rowley, S. (2000). Addressing the population burden of child and adolescent mental health problems: a primary care model. *Child Psychology and Psychiatry Review*, **5** (1), 9–16.

Armbruster, P. (2002). The administration of school-based mental health services. *Administrative Psychiatry*, **11** (1), 23–41.

Armbruster, P. & Lichtman, J. (1999). Are school-based mental health services effective? evidence from 36 inner city schools. *Community Mental Health Journal*, (35), 493–504.

Atkins, M., Frazier, S., Adil, J. & Talbot, E. (2003). School-based mental health services in urban communities. In: Weist, M., Evans, S. & Lever, N. (Eds). *Handbook of School Mental Health: advancing practice and research*. New York: Kluwer Academic & Plenum Publishers.

Chipman, M. & Gooch, J. (2003). Community school nurses and mental health support: a service evaluation. *Paediatric Nursing*, **15** (3), 33–35.

Clarke, M., Coombs, C. & Walton, L. (2003). School-based early identification and intervention service for adolescents: a psychology and school nurse partnership model. *Child and Adolescent Mental Health*, **8** (1), 34–39.

Cvejic, H. & Smith, A. (1979). *The Journal of School Health*, January 1979, 36–39.

Department for Education and Skills (2001). *Promoting Children's Mental Health Within Early Years and School Settings*. London: DfES.

Department for Education and Skills (2005). *Common Core of Skills and Knowledge for the Children's Workforce*. London: DfES.

Department of Health (1999). *Saving Lives: our healthier nation*. London: HMSO.

Department of Health (2004). *National Service Framework for Children, Young People and Maternity Services*. London: HMSO.

Department of Health (2004b). *Choosing Health: making healthier choices easier*. London: HMSO.

Flaherty, L. & Osher, D. (2003). History of school based mental health services in the United States. In: Weist, M., Evans, S. & Lever, N. (Eds). *Handbook of School Mental Health: advancing practice and research*. New York: Kluwer Academic & Plenum Publishers.

Green, H., McGinnity, A., Meltzer, H., Ford, T. & Goodman, R. (2005). *Mental Health of Children and Young People in Great Britain*. London: ONS.

Hales, A., Karshmer, J., Montes-Sandoval, L., Glasscock, F., Summers, L., Williams, J. & Robbins, L. (2003). Psychiatric – mental health clinical nurse specialist in a public school setting. *Clinical Nurse Specialist*, **17** (2), 95–100.

Hootman, J., Houck, G. & King, M. (2003). Increased mental health needs and new roles in school communities. *Journal of Child and Adolescent Psychiatric Nursing*, **16** (3), 93–101.

Jackson, E. (2002). Mental health in schools: what about the staff? *Journal of Child Psychotherapy*, **28** (2), 129–46.

Kurtz, Z. & James, C. (2002). *What's New: learning from the CAMHS innovation projects summary*. London: HMSO.

Laurence, J. (2003). *Pure Madness*. London: Routledge.

Leighton, S. (2003). *School-Based Mental Health Services: a way forward?*: Observational Visits to SBMHS in Baltimore, Washington DC, Denver and New Haven. Report produced for the Florence Nightingale Foundation (unpublished report).

Leighton, S., Worraker, A., Scattergood, S. & Nolan, P. (2003). School nurses and mental health: part 2. *Mental Health Practice*, **7** (4), 17–20.

Lynn, C., McKay, M. & Atkins, M. (2003). School social work: meeting the mental health needs of students through collaboration with teachers. *Children and Schools*, **25** (4), 197–209.

McMahon, T., Ward, N., Pruett, M., Davidson, L. & Griffith, E. (2000). Building full-service schools: lessons learned in the development of interagency collaboratives. *Journal of Educational and Psychological Consultation*, **11** (1), 65–92.

Massey, O., Armstrong, K., Boroughs, M., Henson, K. & McCash, L. (2005). Mental health services in schools: a qualitative analysis of challenges to implementation, operation and sustainability. *Psychology in Schools*, **42** (4), 361–72.

Meltzer, H., Gatward, R., Goodman, R. & Ford, T. (2000). *The Mental Health of Children and Adolescents in Great Britain*. London: The Stationary Office.

Mental Health Foundation (1999). *Bright Futures: promoting children and young people's mental health*. London: Mental Health Foundation.

Mental Health Foundation (2004). *Effective Joint Working Between CAMHS and Schools: research report 412*. London: MHF.

Mitchell, G., Baptiste, L. & Potel, D. (2004). Developing links between school nursing and CAMHS. *Nursing Times*, **100** (5), 36–39.

NHS Health Advisory Service (1995). *Together We Stand: the commissioning, role and management of child and adolescent mental health services*. London: HMSO.

Pettitt, B. & Mental Health Foundation (2003). *Effective Joint Working Between Child and Adolescent Mental Health Services (CAMHS) and Schools*. London: HMSO.

Richardson, G. & Partridge, I. (2000). Child and adolescent mental health service liaison with tier 1 services: a consultation exercise with school nurses. *Psychiatric Bulletin*, **24** (12), 462–63.

Richardson, G. & Partridge, I. (2003). Liaison and consultation with tier I professionals. In: Richardson, G. & Partridge, I. (Eds). *Child and Adolescent Mental Health Services: an operational handbook*. London: Gaskell.

Rones, M. & Hoagwood, K. (2000). School-based mental health services: a research review. *Clinical Child & Family Psychology Review*, **3** (4), 223–41.

Turpin, A. & Titheridge, A. (2001). Groupwork in schools: supporting children with behavioural difficulties. *Young Minds Magazine*, (50), 21–24.

United Kingdom Central Council (2000). *The Nursing, Midwifery and Health Visiting Contribution to the Continuing Care of People with Mental Health Problems: a review and UKCC action plan*. London: UKCC.

Weist, M., Evans, S. & Lever, N. (2003). Advancing mental health practice and research in schools. In: Weist, M., Evans, S. & Lever, N. (Eds) *Handbook of School Mental Health: advancing practice and research*. New York: Kluwer Academic & Plenum Publishers.

Weist, M. & Albus, K. (2004). Expanded school mental health: exploring program details and developing the research base. *Behavior Modification*, **28** (4), 463–71.

World Health Organization (1992). *The ICD-10 Classification of Mental and Behavioural Disorders: clinical descriptions and diagnostic guidelines*. Geneva: WHO.

World Health Organization (1998). *WHO's Global School Health Initiative: health promoting schools*. Geneva: WHO.

World Health Organization (2000). *World Mental Health Day: mental health: stop exclusion – dare to care*. www.who.int/world-health-day

YoungMinds (2001). Training analysis. *YoungMinds Magazine*, (March), 21–22.

http://smhp.psych.ucla.edu last visited 26/07/05

http://www.dfes.gov.uk last visited 26/07/05

Recommended Reading

Department for Education and Skills (2001). *Promoting Children's Mental Health Within Early Years and School Settings*. London: HMSO.

Department for Education and Skills (2004). *Draft Common Assessment Framework*. London: HMSO.

Department for Education and Skills (2004). *Five-Year Strategy for Children and Learners*. London: HMSO.

Department of Health (2004). *National Service Framework for Children, Young People and Maternity Services*. London: HMSO.

Department of Health (2004b). *Choosing Health: making healthier choices easier*. London: HMSO.

Mental Health Foundation (1999). *Bright Futures: promoting children and young people's mental health*. London: Mental Health Foundation.

Mental Health Foundation (2003). *Effective Joint Working Between Child and Adolescent Mental Health Services (CAMHS) and Schools*. London: MHF.

Richardson, G. & Partridge, I. (2003). *Child and Adolescent Mental Health Services: an operational handbook*. London: Gaskell.

Weare, K. (1999). *Promoting Mental, Emotional and Social Health: a whole school approach*. London: Routledge.

Weist, M., Evans, S. & Lever, N. (2003). *Handbook of School Mental Health: advancing practice and research*. New York: Kluwer Academic & Plenum Publishers.

World Health Organization (1998). *WHO's Global School Health Initiative: health promoting schools*. Geneva: WHO.

Website Resources

www.dfes.gov.uk Department for Education and Skills website – includes policy information.

www.dh.gov.uk Department of Health website – includes policy documents.

www.everychildmatters.gov.uk/multiagencyworking A resource to support managers and practitioners delivering school-based, multiagency services.

www.kidscape.org.uk A resource for children, parents and professionals addressing issues such as bullying, making friends and online safety.

www.mentalhealth.org.uk Mental Health Foundation – mental health resource for professionals, parents, children and young people.

www.ncb.org.uk National Children's Bureau (NCB) – includes information on policy, research and best practice relating to children and adolescents.

www.smallwood.co.uk Smallwood Publishing – supplies books on mental health issues for children, adolescents, parents and professionals.

www.teachernet.gov Includes sections dedicated to child and adolescent mental health and whole school issues.

www.tsa.uk.com Trust for Study of Adolescents (TSA) – includes resources for professionals and parents.

www.wiredforhealth.gov.uk Part of Our Healthier Nation Strategy, linked to the Healthy Schools initiative.

www.youngminds.org.uk YoungMinds – the children's mental health charity. Includes a series of information booklets aimed at young people that can be downloaded as well as resources for parents and professionals.

Chapter 13

Nursing Children and Young People in a Multicultural Society: an acculturation model

Ray McMorrow

Key points

- Concepts of mental health, mental illness and the factors that produce mental health or illness vary dramatically across cultures. CAMHS (child and adolescent mental health services) need to be sensitive to such differences and nurses must have the knowledge and understanding of the different groups represented within the communities they serve.

- Although ethnicity *per se* does not affect mental health, the experience of racism, poverty and disadvantage, often associated with minority status within the UK, is closely linked with adversity and poor mental health.

- Exploration of culturally competent CAMHS provision is not only about minority ethnic communities, but also must focus on the needs of other groups who may be unable to access child and adolescent mental health services. These include hearing-impaired communities, sight-impaired communities and travelling communities.

- Cultural competence should be seen as a central element in nursing children and young people with mental health problems. All nurses working in child and adolescent mental health services should have a personal development plan that includes training in this area.

- Though the challenge of providing culturally competent CAMHS is significant, this should not be regarded as an optional extra. The model of acculturation needs to be developed at a number of strategic and organisational levels, from policymakers through to the activity of each nurse who works with a particular child or their family or carers.

- Those commissioning and planning CAMHS should engage with voluntary organisations, religious groups, ethnic minority community leaders and advocacy services where this may help to foster understanding of the particular needs of the various groups of children and young people in our community.

Introduction

The presence of a chapter in such a book on the subject of culturally competent care and treatment reflects rapid changes in our society. In an era of increasing opportunity for world travel and global communication, nursing care takes places in an international and multicultural context. Until recently the cultural needs of people with mental health problems received very little attention in mental health settings in the UK, and this despite the enormous cultural complexity found in our society. For example, over 300 languages are spoken by London schoolchildren (Baker & Eversley 2000) and at least three million people living in the UK were born in countries where English is not the national language (Department for Education and Employment 2001). Concepts of mental health, mental illness and the factors that produce mental health or illness vary dramatically across cultures. Nurses and other professionals in CAMHS need to be sensitive to such differences and have knowledge and understanding of the different groups represented within the communities they serve. The challenge for nurses to provide culturally competent CAMHS is significant and it is not possible to cover all the issues surrounding culture in one chapter. However, there are a number of fundamental principles that can be applied in order to work towards achieving culturally competent nursing and child and adolescent mental health services.

Background

Although the terms ethnicity, race and culture are often used interchangeably these words have different meanings. Ethnicity refers to a broad range of factors and cannot easily be defined. This is because it is a fluid concept, influenced by social, political, historical and economic factors (Smaje 1995). It has been suggested that memories of colonialism, imperialism and slavery, and refugee and immigration status as well as skin colour are all important factors that determine mental health treatments and outcomes (Sue & Sue 1999). The concept of ethnicity is complex, incorporating religious and cultural background, shared history and common descent (O'Hara 2003). Although ethnicity *per se* does not affect mental health, the experience of racism, poverty and disadvantage, often associated with minority status within the UK, is closely linked with adversity and poor mental health. Migration to the UK, whether forced or voluntary, has a long and rich history. Despite this, minority groups have a history of poor mental health outcomes in the UK. For example, Afro-Caribbean men have been over-represented in mental hospitals (National Institute for Mental Health in England 2003), referral pathways for Irish immigrants have been shown to be different (Mental Health Act Commission 2004; Greensdale 1992), and the uptake of mental health services by black and south Asian young people remains low (Neale et al. 2005). This is partly due to prejudiced, stereotyped and racist perceptions that have permeated through mental health service planning and delivery. These are important issues to consider when working with immigrant groups that have more recently arrived in the UK from eastern Europe.

The impact of moving house is recognised as one of the highest stress factors we experience. It is therefore hard to appreciate the impact of changing continents, with new languages, customs and possible hostilities on arrival in the UK. In some cases the journey has not been a planned life choice but is the result of war and atrocities. It is not surprising that this may affect parenting and the ability to provide a secure base in which children can grow and flourish. Children and young people sometimes arrive in the UK as unaccompanied minors, having lost their family, friends and possessions. They may have witnessed trauma and violence and their mental health is likely to be suffering (Wood 1995; Izycki 2001; Save the Children et al. 2002). Refugees and asylum seekers are predominately young, with as many as 40% below the age of 18 years (Hodes 2002). Compared with immigrant or indigenous children, most refugee children are at increased risk of psychological distress and mental disorders. However, despite experiencing terrible trauma, some children and young people appear to cope well, do not suffer significantly from mental health problems and achieve good social adjustment upon arrival in the UK (Hodes 2000). The rights and welfare of refugee and asylum-seeking children are covered by the provisions of the Children Act 1989 which includes a requirement for local authorities to consider the psychological and cultural development of such children.

The legal and policy context

The Race Relations Act (1976) stated that, amongst other things, public service providers have a duty not to discriminate on the grounds of race. The Race Relations (Amendment) Act (2000) made this duty enforceable, and public service providers can now be held accountable in a court of law if they fail to promote equality of opportunity and provision of culturally competent services. Ensuring equal access to healthcare is a core component of the NHS (National Health Service) Plan (2000), and these commitments are reflected in *Your Guide to the NHS* (DoH 2001). This report states that the NHS will be required to shape its service around the needs and preferences of individual patients, their families and carers, and will have to respond to different needs of different populations. A number of important reports have raised awareness about the particular issues facing minority ethnic groups in accessing mental health services. *Breaking the Circles of Fear*, published by the Sainsbury Centre for Mental Health (SCMH), demonstrated that the care pathways for black people are problematic and influence the nature and outcome of treatment and the willingness of these communities to engage with mainstream mental health services (SCMH 2002). This was followed by *Delivering Race Equality*, published by the Department of Health (DoH) in 2003. This included an action plan to achieve equality and tackle discrimination in mental health services for all people of black and minority ethnic status, including those of Irish or Mediterranean origin and east European migrants. *Delivering Race Equality* set out two core standards: for mental health organisations to challenge discrimination, promote equality and respect human rights; and for organisations to enable all members of the population to access mental health services equally.

Concern about racial attitudes in public services has been highlighted by high-profile reports such as the Stephen Lawrence Inquiry (Home Office 1999) and the Independent Inquiry into the death of David Bennett (DoH 2005). Both reports highlighted the need to tackle institutional racism across all public services. The NHS has been the focus of the DoH's spotlight on institutional racism in a report called *The Vital Connection* (DoH 2000). This document focuses on the strategic aims of developing and retaining a varied workforce in which diversity is celebrated and valued. In addition to legislation, the provision of services to our population should be of concern to all professionals who work with children, their families and carers. Issues of discrimination, migration and ethnicity are central to our ability to provide effective mental health service outcomes. Cultural competence should be seen as a crucial element of nursing children and young people with mental health problems.

Improving access to specialist CAMHS

In their report, *Inside Outside*, the National Institute for Mental Health in England found evidence that people from non-white backgrounds under-utilise mental health services in general (NIMHE 2003). This is also reflected within specialist CAMHS where the uptake of mental health services is poor (Neale et al. 2005), and the needs of minority ethnic communities are not specifically met (DoH 2004). There are many reasons for this. The needs of specific minority ethnic groups are not being assessed or included in CAMHS needs assessments, and people from minority ethnic groups are not routinely invited to contribute to the planning and evaluation of CAMHS services (Malek & Joughin 2004). This means that the cultural needs of children and young people from minority ethnic backgrounds are often overlooked in service design, delivery and evaluation (Saxena et al. 2002; National Assembly for Wales 2004; Webb 2004). As a result, children and young people as well as their families and carers may feel marginalised and fail to access CAMHS (Clarke 2003). It is essential that CAMHS engage with local minority ethnic communities to improve access to CAMHS. This is to ensure that needs assessments are representative of the local communities, that mental health needs can be identified and addressed in a non-stigmatising manner and that the voluntary sector can be properly involved in the strategic planning and delivery of CAMHS.

A lack of awareness of what CAMHS can offer is another reason why children and young people from minority ethnic backgrounds do not access services. There is a wider priority in public services to ensure that mental health promotion is improved through the use of a range of media; but nurses in all settings need to ensure that children and young people from minority ethnic groups have access to information about mental healthcare and treatment services. This needs to be in appropriate languages and formats, and be sensitive to their cultural background. To engage service users effectively, nurses may have to demystify concepts of psychiatry and mental health, legitimise critical and alternative perspectives about health and illness and identify and create safe spaces in local communities for children, young people and their families and carers to access CAMHS (Kurtz et al. 2005).

Care and treatment pathways

Information about referral pathways of children and young people to community-based CAMHS is poorly understood. This is because commissioners and local organisations frequently do not record information about level of need, unmet need, demand and supply and there is only very limited data from contact with specialist CAMHS (Hodes 2002). The Mental Health Act Commission (MHAC) (2004) found that where ethnicity is stated, admissions for people from black and minority ethnic backgrounds represented 11.9% of formal admissions of children to adult mental health wards. This is despite very few staff on adult wards having either the training, skills or experience to work with adolescents and a lack of advocacy services for young people in adult settings. Those of an Afro-Caribbean black-British background represented 13.1% of MHAC notifications of detention on adult wards (MHAC 2004). These figures represent just 2.7% of the general population detained on adult mental health wards in England and Wales and show a significant over-representation in this group. This is in stark contrast to the figure of 3% of admissions identified for black and minority ethnic groups to in-patient child and adolescent mental health units and the apparent under-representation of children and young people from minority ethnic groups accessing informal treatment within CAMHS in-patient units. For those young people who do gain access to specialist CAMHS, this is often at a late stage in the development of their problems, or in crisis (YoungMinds 2005). It is a current priority in England and Wales for all CAMHS to improve access to both community and in-patient mental health services for children and young people from minority ethnic backgrounds (DoH 2004; National Assembly for Wales 2005).

Shazeen

Shazeen, aged 14, was admitted to an in-patient adolescent psychiatric unit with a history of eating problems and low body weight. She had not attended mainstream school for 12 months and presented as introverted and depressed. The records note that Shazeen's family were of Pakistani origin and that her parents spoke very little English. The family did not visit the unit to discuss Shazeen's care and treatment with the nursing staff.

In the above vignette the nurses on the unit might interpret the actions of Shazeen's parents as uncaring and perceive that they want to dump Shazeen's problems onto the staff. However, this may be a defence against feeling hampered by their own lack of understanding about cultural differences. Before attempting any assessment or treatment intervention it is important for the nurse to identify language and communication needs. Many families from ethnic minority backgrounds do not possess a vocabulary equivalent to standard English and may at first appear 'flat', 'non-verbal', 'uncommunicative' or 'lacking in insight' (O'Hara 2003). It is important that communication needs are not misunderstood as symptoms of mental health problems and disorders. Young people with eating disorders, such as anorexia nervosa, are often un-communicative and difficult for the staff to reach. Nursing staff who have not received adequate training may feel persecuted by the presentation of such hostile non-conformity. This can lead them to develop basic assumptions about the behaviour which are based on the cultural experiences of the staff group. These assumptions might include the following:

(1)   Shazeen is displaying somatised distress because of an intercultural iden-
      tity crisis.
(2)   Shazeen's parents are ashamed of their daughter's mental health problems.
(3)   Family work is impossible because of the language barriers.

However, after cultural competence skills and awareness training, and after engaging in supported family work, the picture of this family can be quite different. As with many families who have a child with an eating disorder, the family may indeed reach a state of hopelessness and fatigue, as well as experience a sense of parental shame. In the above scenario it is also possible that, like the nurses, Shazeen's parents had preconceived ideas. They may have believed that:

(1)   They had no authority over their daughter after she was admitted to an
      in-patient setting.
(2)   They must await the results of the treatment.
(3)   The adolescent unit is the authoritative domain of staff and the parents
      had no clear right to be there.

Some members of the family actually spoke English well but the engagement of an interpreter, professionally employed, allowed for a greater dialogue between staff and family members. In some cases interpreters are used only in therapeutic work such as family therapy. But by using an interpreter in the assessment, planning and evaluation of care the family, the young person and staff group were able to develop a shared programme of care and treatment in which the values of the staff and the family were explored and shared. The family advised the staff on dietary norms, which included providing food and recipes. They also explained which staff behaviours were acceptable and unacceptable within the family's culture and religious heritage. The nurses were in turn able to share the goals and philosophy behind the treatment model of the CAMHS service. This resulted in a closer partnership between the staff and the family, better family engagement in the treatment programme and alleviation of the persecutory relationship that had been developing.

An acculturation care model and issues of bridging

Inherent in attempting to achieve an acculturated care model in nursing, is engagement with notions of cultural practices of healing. Migrant communities bring with them their own understanding of health and mental health, and understanding of helpful interventions and healing. The term 'acculturation' has been used to explore how migrant individuals and communities relate their cultural heritage or history with that of the indigenous culture, focusing on the domains of integration, assimilation, separation and marginalisation (Berry 1992; 1997). This model can be adopted to develop culturally competent care pathways in CAMHS. The key domains for this model are family culture and institutional culture. The family culture contains the individual and the family experience. As well as religious and ethnic identities, it embraces local communities, relationships and friendships. Service providers and organisations that commission and deliver CAMHS also have complex ethnic and cultural identities (Neale et al. 2005). The institutional culture will be multilayered, including the individual nurse's culture and beliefs, along with the service and organisational culture. One of the central aims of a service striving towards cultural competency is always to work with young people and their families towards integration. However, integration has been a recent buzz-word in political circles but should not be a cover for assimilation. To achieve integration, marginalisation, assimilation and separation must also be addressed.

The multidisciplinary team working in CAMHS also needs to focus on their own experiences of culture. Included in this should be an exploration of being marginalized by the institutional system, areas where they feel assimilated and areas where they feel separation or separateness is an important part of their integration. The aim of nursing interventions should not be to educate the child and family in a linear manner in order for them to participate in treatment plans led solely by the staff group. This would constitute a drive towards assimilation that would continue to marginalise the family's understanding of healing. To achieve true integration would mean 'bridging' the institutional culture of nursing with that of the child's personal and family culture. Barker & Buchanan-Barker (2004) describe bridging as an appropriate term to describe nursing activities in the twenty-first century. It involves constructing a means of crossing the gap, in this case the gap in cultural understanding. Separateness or difference in understanding has to be accepted, and the bridge provides the means of experiencing the other. Here the role of interpreters and bilingual CAMHS workers can be critical in bridging differences.

Interpreters not only assist with understanding spoken language, but can also assist in sign language and sometimes same language advocates for groups such as migrant travelling communities. Similarly, the role of bilingual workers is not only limited to interpreting and liaison but involves helping to develop transcultural frameworks, different theoretical perspectives and intelligence about local resources. Tribe (1999) focuses on the need for interpreters to work as bicultural workers, bridging the gap of cultural understanding and language. To achieve this they need to be trained in understanding the cultural model that we bring to the bridge as nurses or other professionals, as well as that of the child and family culture.

Nathan

Nathan, aged 14, is an Afro-Caribbean boy who has been referred to a community CAMHS team. He recently arrived in the country from Trinidad and was living with his mother. She worked long hours to support them financially but this has meant that Nathan has spent long periods of time at home alone. There were grave concerns about his behaviour as he had been fighting at school and failing to complete his homework. Nathan had also made unwelcome sexual advances to girls at school. When Nathan was assessed by the community psychiatric nurse he was initially assessed as aloof and uncommunicative.

When first meeting Nathan, the CAMHS team were concerned that his sexual behaviour and aggression might require a forensic intervention. However, further assessment revealed the picture of a marginalised and lonely young man with a poor attachment to his mother. Nathan had no history of disruptive behaviour in school in the Caribbean, where he had been a model student and high academic achiever. He had also attended church on a regular basis. However, Nathan had previously lived in a large multigenerational family and had been brought up by his grandparents whilst his mother worked towards their financial security in England. During the course of individual sessions with the community nurse, it became clear that Nathan had little understanding of 'how to be' in England, and he had very little experience of living with his own mother. In school, Nathan's black Caribbean culture was interpreted by other young people as negative and associated with gangsters and 'rap', and he experienced hostility and bullying. Nathan's behaviours were not only a response to the hostility, but also a systemic response to how others engaged with the stereotype of how a black Caribbean boy should be. In his marginalized position Nathan's responses were both defensive and a search for identity. His mother had limited understanding of parenting expectations within Britain and was anxious not to overwhelm her son. Her socioeconomic need to work was substantial. The community psychiatric nurse involved himself at a systemic level, engaging Nathan in seeking to understand the relationship between his home Caribbean experience and life in England, exploring with both Nathan and his mother their shared experience of migration and separation.

This case study represents the activity of bridging at a systemic level. The migration of parents for economic reasons and multigenerational parenting is long established as a 'norm' within the Caribbean community (Arnold 1997). While this may be due to economic necessity, it is not always in the best interests of family mental health. The community psychiatric nurse went on to engage a wide network of agencies and community services to support Nathan and his mother. These included education services, Connexions and the family church. The use of positive role models in social care, health services or an appropriate community group, can help integration, protect cultural identity, and enable service users to achieve an acculturated understanding of a place in their new surroundings. Some CAMHS services, in seeking to engage service users that may feel excluded have been effective in using befriending schemes, faith-based support and community volunteers to help improve access and engagement (Street et al. 2005). In Nathan's case we see how the Caribbean 'Diaspora' may be difficult for a young man coming into the country due to its connections with gangster culture. This young man arrived in the country with a positive cultural engagement, but during his accultura-tion in Britain, became engaged in negative and destructive behaviour. The use of the 'big brother' model ideally engages someone of a similar cultural background and again provides for bridging of culture between the young person's own experience and that of the host culture.

Workforce development

Child and adolescent mental health services in the UK should be provided by professionals and teams with the skills, competencies and capabilities to respect the values, beliefs, customs and cultures of an increasingly diverse population. Recruitment and training are important issues, as users need to see evidence that CAMHS are focused on and engaged with their community and culture (Malik & Joughin 2004). This is no easy task and we have a long way to go to achieving culturally competent CAMHS for children and young people from ethnic minority backgrounds. One of the major challenges facing child and adolescent mental health services is to achieve an integrated and culturally sensitive workforce. There are particular problems in recruiting nurses from ethnic minorities, particularly those from Asian backgrounds (Qureshi et al. 2000). In addition, education and training opportunities which enable CAMHS staff to provide services that are sensitive to racial and cultural differ-ences are not widely available. However, it is not just a matter of achieving a culturally representative CAMHS team and providing adequate education and training. Some young people may want support from a nurse or professional from their own culture, whereas others may not for fear that their confiden-tiality may be breached (YoungMinds 2005), or the perception of others that they are 'going outside the family' (Kurtz et al. 2005). Much more than provid-ing individual staff with cultural awareness training, the organisation needs to promote an inclusive, non-Eurocentric and faith-sensitive vision of services on offer (Shafi 1998; Neale et al. 2005). Indeed, over-investing in minority ethnic CAMHS staff as 'specialists' in relation to minority ethnic issues runs the risk of leaving other staff uninformed and unskilled to work with minority ethnic groups. Though the challenge of providing culturally competent CAMHS is significant, this should not be regarded as an optional extra. The model of acculturation needs to be developed at a number of strategic and organisational levels, from policymakers through to the activity of each nurse who works with a particular child or their family or carers.

Conclusion

It is only in recent years that we have seen an increased sensitivity to the role of ethnic and cultural factors as moderators of treatment effects and outcomes in CAMHS. It is not possible to address all the issues in relation to providing culturally competent CAMHS in one chapter. Exploration of culturally competent CAMHS provision not only is about minority ethnic communities, but also must focus on the needs of other groups who may be unable to access child and adolescent mental health services. This includes hearing-impaired communities, sight-impaired communities and travelling communities. There is no simple solution to providing culturally competent care. Cultural presentations are too complex to be addressed by standardised protocols or careplans. A systemic understanding of each family culture is required and nurses will need to explore the unique needs of each child and their family in detail. Here, the systemic concept of maintaining curiosity and using enquiry as a portion of cultural neutrality is a valuable tool. It is essential that cultural competence is woven into the thread of the CAMHS system. This is in relation to commissioning, care pathways and multidisciplinary or multiagency development programmes. Those commissioning and planning CAMHS should engage with voluntary organisations, religious groups, ethnic minority community leaders and advocacy services, where this may help to understand the particular needs of the various groups of children and young people in our community. Organisations commissioning and providing CAMHS must also engage with individuals and their communities to identify the best way to deliver effective services. This will mean working flexibly, creatively and in new ways in order to improve cultural competence in CAMHS.

References

Arnold, E. (1997). Issues of re-unification of migrant west Indian children in the United Kingdom. In: Roopnarine, J. & Brown, J. (Eds). *Caribbean Families: Diversity Among Ethnic Groups*. London: Greenwood.

Baker, P. & Eversley, J. (2000). *Multilingual Capital*. London: Battlebridge.

Barker, P. & Buchanan-Barker, P. (2004). Bridging: talking meaningfully about the care of people at risk. *Mental Health Practice*, **8** (3), 29–30.

Berry, J. (1997). *Cultural and Ethnic Factors in Health*. Cambridge: Cambridge University Press.

Berry, J. (1992). Acculturation and adaptation in a new society. International migration, special issue: *Migration and Health*, (30), 19–22.

Clarke, J. (2003). Developing separate mental health services for minority ethnic groups: what changes are needed? *Mental Health Practice*, **6** (5), 22–25.

Department of Health (2000). *NHS Plan*. London: HMSO.

Department of Health (2000). *The Vital Connection*. London: HMSO.

Department of Health (2001). *Your Guide to the NHS*. London: HMSO.

Department of Health (2003). *Delivering Race Equality: a framework for action*. Mental Health Services Consultation Document. London: HMSO.

Department of Health (2004). *National Service Framework for Children, Young People and Maternity Services*. London: HMSO.

Department of Health (2005). *Delivering Race Equality in Mental Health Care: an action plan for reform inside and outside services and the government's response to the independent inquiry into the death of David Bennett*. London: HMSO.

Greenslade, L. (1992). White skins, white masks: psychological distress among the Irish in Britain. In: O'Sullivan, P. (Ed.). *The Irish World Wide, Vol. 2: The Irish in the new communities*, Leicester: Leicester University Press.

Hodes, M. (2000). Psychologically distressed refugee children in the United Kingdom. *Child Psychology and Psychiatry Review*, (5), 57–68.

Hodes, M. (2002). Implications for psychiatric services of chronic civilian strife: young refugees in the UK. *Advances in Psychiatric Treatment*, (8), 366–76.

Home Office (1999). *The Stephen Lawrence Inquiry. Report of an inquiry by Sir William Macpherson*. London: HMSO.

Izycki, K. (2001). A safe haven for asylum seekers. *Mental Health Practice*, **4** (6), 12–15.

Kurtz, Z., Stapelkamp, C., Taylor, E., Malek, M. & Street, C. (2005). *Minority Voices: a guide to good practice in planning and providing services for the mental health of black and minority ethnic young people*. London: YoungMinds.

Malek, M. & Joughin, C. (2004). *Mental Health Services for Minority Ethnic Children and Adolescents*. London: Jessica Kingsley.

Mental Health Act Commission (2004). *Safeguarding Children and Adolescents Detained Under the Mental Health Act 1983 on Adult Psychiatric Wards*. Nottingham: MHAC.

National Assembly for Wales (2005). *National Service Framework for Children, Young People and Maternity Services in Wales*. Cardiff: National Assembly for Wales.

National Institute for Mental Health England (2003). *Inside Outside: improving mental health services for black and minority ethnic communities in England*. London: NIMHE.

Neale, J., Worrell, M. & Randhawa, G. (2005). Reaching out: support for ethnic minorities. *Mental Health Practice*, **9** (2), 12–16.

O'Hara, J. (2003). Learning disabilities and ethnicity: achieving cultural competence. *Advances in Psychiatric Treatment*, (9), 166–176.

Qureshi, T., Berridge, D. & Wenman, H. (2000). *Where to Turn? Family support for south Asian communities*. London: National Children's Bureau.

Save the Children, the Children's Society & the Refugee Council (2002). *A Case for Change: how refugee children in England are missing out*. London: The Refugee Council.

Saxena, S., Eliahoo, J. & Majeed, A. (2002). Socioeconomic and ethnic group differences in self reported health status and use of health services by children and young people in England: cross sectional study. *British Medical Journal*, (325), 520–23.

Shafi, S. (1998). A study of Muslim Asian women's experiences of counselling and the necessity for a radically similar counsellor. *Counselling Psychology Quarterly*, **11** (3), 301–14.

Smaje, C. (1995). *Health, Race and Ethnicity: making sense of the evidence*. London: King's Fund.

Street, C., Stapelkamp, C., Taylor, E., Malek, M. & Kurtz, Z. (2005). *Minority Voices: research into the access and acceptability of services for the mental health of young people from black and minority ethnic groups*. London: YoungMinds.

Sue, D. & Sue, D. (1999). *Counselling the Culturally Different: theory and practice*. (3rd edn). New York: John Wiley.

Tribe, R. (1999). Bridging the gaps or damming the flow? some observations on using interpreters/bi-cultural workers when working with refugee clients, many who have been tortured. *British Journal of Medical Psychiatry*, (72), 567–76.

Webb, E. (2004). Discrimination against children. *Archives of Disease in Childhood*, (89), 804–808.

Wood, C. (1995). *The Settlement of Refugees in Britain – Home Office Research Study (141)*. London: HMSO.

YoungMinds (2005). *Minority Voices: research into what young people from black and minority ethnic backgrounds – and the staff who work with them – say about mental health services*. London: YoungMinds.

Chapter 14

Treatment Interventions for Children and Young People with Mental Health Problems

Eileen Woolley

Key points

- There are many different forms of therapy and treatment. Deciding which approach to use depends on the developmental status of the child, the evidence base for use and the specific wishes of the child, their family or carers.

- The importance of a structured assessment prior to treatment cannot be overstated. The process of assessment provides a rich source of information and awareness of family functioning. As well as the young person themselves, parents and carers and other family members should be involved wherever appropriate.

- Individual child psychotherapy refers to a number of different therapeutic approaches. It may be used to help the child explain emotions and relationships, learn how to change things or form a supportive therapeutic alliance.

- Group therapy can be facilitated by nurses to help children and young people discuss problems, identify with others and share strategies to resolve conflict and distress. Nurses should be aware that whilst groups can be useful for children who require the approval of their peers, they can provoke anxiety for children who are shy or lacking in confidence.

- Generic therapies and treatment orientations that focus exclusively on the child are declining. In their place, specialist strategies or multimodal treatment manuals represent a move towards systemic and contextual explanations of childhood mental disorders.

- Together with a range of psychological and social interventions, psychopharmacological treatments are one of the major therapeutic options available to help children and young people with mental health problems and disorders.

- Most nurses in specialist CAMHS (child and adolescent mental health services) work within a humanistic framework and apply an eclectic and holistic approach to the assessment and treatment of children and young people, their families and carers.

Introduction

The following chapter discusses a range of individual and group therapies carried out by nurses as part of a multidisciplinary team. Evaluating effective treatments for children and adolescents is problematic. A lack of well-conducted randomised controlled trials has resulted in a poorly developed evidence base for treating child and adolescent mental disorders. However, the last ten years has seen significant growth and development in treatment strategies and modalities. We have seen the increasing decline of generic therapies and treatment orientations that focus exclusively on the child. In their place have emerged systemic and contextual explanations for childhood mental disorder with the emphasis on highly specialist, multimodal or manualised approaches to treatment. A range of key treatment issues and trends are emerging. These demonstrate that children and their families or carers are increasingly involved in treatment decisions and the roles of family, school and peers are factored in as essential treatment mediators. As well as a range of individual and group treatments, the physical treatment of children with mental disorders is also discussed.

The importance of thorough assessment

The importance of a structured assessment cannot be overstated. The process of assessment provides a rich source of information and awareness of family functioning. As well as the young person themselves, parents and carers and other family members should be involved wherever appropriate. It is clear that the cause of the mental health problem has a significant bearing on the treatment strategy. For example, a comprehensive family history can reveal genetic trends that enable nurses to identify early onset disorders and many specific learning disorders. Alternatively, identifying dysfunctional family dynamics can exclude mental disorders and prevent a child being wrongly diagnosed, for example with ADHD (attention deficit hyperactivity disorder). Taking a full developmental history also helps nurses identify any birth trauma which may have little implication until the child reaches school age. For instance, children who have had hearing problems in their early years may experience difficulties with social functioning, and may be mistaken for children with problems on the autistic spectrum. There are a range of childhood neurodevelopmental disorders such as Tourette's Syndrome, ADHD and Asperger's Syndrome, which may at first appear to be disruptive behaviour. This is particularly evident where such children have learnt to mask their difficulties by making their peers laugh or by bullying them.

There are also clear links between speech and language development, learning difficulties and behaviour problems (Law & Garnett 2004). Intergenerational transmission of risks for mental health problems have been studied over many generations (Brook et al. 2002). Findings indicate that parental personality and behavioural difficulties are passed on through the parent–child relationship. Mental health treatment for children and young people rarely involves a single intervention or treatment approach with the child. Wherever possible and appropriate, as well as young people themselves, nurses should involve parents or carers and siblings in treatment decisions. Children and young people do not exist in isolation; they are part of a wider system which involves the extended family, the school and society as a whole. Treatment therefore must involve the wider system when this is appropriate.

What are the different psychotherapies?

There are many different forms of individual psychotherapy. Deciding which approach to use depends on the developmental status of the child, the evidence base for its use and the specific wishes of the child, their family or carers. For example, expressive therapies such as play or music therapy may be appropriate for younger children, whereas older children may benefit from talking therapies such as CBT (cognitive behavioural therapy) or family therapy. Children with a low IQ (intelligence quotient) or marked receptive speech difficulties and social impairment are less likely to benefit from talking therapies. Non-verbal therapies such as art, music and dance therapy are often used in CAMHS. Creative therapies often have a psychodynamic basis and may be used on an individual or group basis. Some children may benefit more from using expressive or creative media such as art, music or dance therapy (Nation 2003). Although music therapy is not widely available in CAMHS, the production of music, with the help of a therapist, can be a powerful experience containing elements of creativity, expression and socialising with others (Weaver 2001). Each such therapy is aimed at increasing self-awareness and all depend crucially on a positive relationship between the child and therapist.

Cognitive behaviour therapy

Cognitive interventions are designed to change negative beliefs by gaining insight into how one's thoughts, feelings and behaviour are connected. Young people are helped to first elucidate, and then challenge, aspects of their core beliefs and negative thoughts. Behavioural interventions apply learning theory to achieve specific behavioural changes. Key strategies include exposure and response prevention. CBT combines both strategies and is used for children and young people alone, in groups or with families or carers. We have heard that single interventions are most effective when used as part of a broader treatment strategy, and CBT is no exception. CBT works best when used as part of a multimodal treatment approach or alongside family work (Shortt et al. 2001) or medication. Due to the growing interest in the use of CBT in CAMHS, it is important to take account of developmental considerations in the design, implementation and evaluation of interventions.

Charlene

Charlene, aged 15, has a fear of balloons. She has lived with this fear since the age of six when a balloon burst in her face at a birthday party. Charlene now either avoids going to parties, or her mother asks for balloons to be removed beforehand. Charlene sees balloons everywhere she goes; in shops and in shopping centres and at places she would like to visit. The avoidance techniques taught to her by the school nurse are no longer working. She recently had a severe panic attack when faced with a large number of balloons decorating a clothes shop. She is now out of school and anxious about leaving home. Charlene was referred to the CAMHS nurse for CBT.

Behaviour, effect and cognition are part of the human condition. Being aware of our thinking allows us to understand feelings and behaviour and how they interact. CBT has a number of components, which can be useful for treating a range of problems across a variety of settings. CBT is based on the premise that cognition is a primary determinant of behaviour and mood. (Fonagy 2003). CBT therapists work on the principle that if a child can learn maladaptive, inaccurate or irrational beliefs and behaviours, they can 'unlearn' them. Therapy involves transforming passive suffering into active change. Negative generalisations about the world and future are dismantled and positive generalisations are unified. Treatment within a CBT framework is based on the assumption that inaccurate or maladaptive thoughts cause pathological effect and behaviour (Fonagy 2003). CBT interventions are aimed at targeting and changing faulty cognitions to produce a change in effect and behaviour. Therefore the removal of negatively distorted beliefs improves coping mechanisms.

For younger children, verbal instruction training can be used to reduce fears as part of phobic conditions (Mercherbaum & Goodman 1971). The therapist first models appropriate interactions with the phobic stimulus by using verbal self-instruction. After the child has listened to the therapist complete the same task with verbal instruction, they then complete this themselves using self-instruction. Verbal instructions are gradually replaced by whispering until this fades away and is internalised. The technique may be combined with relaxation training. Other practical CBT techniques are used to help children face their fears. This may be achieved by working through a hierarchy of situations that cause anxiety and fear. Using techniques such as roleplay and modelling, children can be helped to identify cognitions that generate anxiety and learn to challenge thoughts that are not based on fact. CBT has been shown to be effective for children and young people with depression (Harrington et al. 1998), anxiety disorders such as obsessive compulsive disorder (OCD) (March 1995) and specific phobias (Ollendick & King 1998). A combination of family intervention and CBT is also of some benefit for ADHD, post traumatic stress disorder (PTSD) and conduct disorder (Shortt et al. 2001).

Dialectical behaviour therapy (DBT)

Dialectical behaviour therapy (DBT) is a cognitive behavioural psychotherapy developed by Marsha Linehan to treat the chronically parasuicidal behaviours of women diagnosed with borderline personality disorder, as defined in DSM-IV (American Psychiatric Association, 1994). (Linehan 1993a; 1993b). Parasuicide can be defined as acute, deliberate nonfatal self-injury or harm that includes suicide attempts, and non-suicidal self-injurious behaviours (Linehan 1993a). This client group is particularly difficult to treat, as clients fail to stay in therapy; often fail to respond to therapeutic efforts; and place considerable demands on the emotional resources of the therapist (Linehan 1993a). DBT has been adapted for use with adolescents, and the principles can be used individually, in a group and in a family setting.

DBT involves building therapeutic alliances and teaching life skills which include problem-solving; self-soothing; removing negative images of the self; remaining in the present; keeping respect for oneself; maintaining and sustaining relationships; and asserting oneself. As well as being used individually, DBT can be used in groups and in the context of a family intervention. As stated earlier, DBT as part of a multimodal intervention aims to facilitate acceptance and validation of present behaviours. Emphasis is placed on addressing resistance to therapy, building therapeutic alliances, and developing life skills. These include assertiveness and problem-solving, removing negative self-images and making and sustaining positive relationships. DBT applied to children and adolescents has not been subject to systematic outcome evaluation, and has only been proved to be effective with adults (Williams 2002). Despite this, the model is receiving increasing attention in specialist CAMHS settings. An unpublished trial in Cambridge (2001) indicates that although young people understand the DBT skills they have acquired, they experience difficulty in applying them.

DBT for young people is based on a biosocial theory of borderline personality disorder described by Linehan (1993a; 1993b). She hypothesises that problems encountered by young people with borderline personality traits occur as a consequence of an emotionally vulnerable individual growing up within an 'invalidating environment'. Linehan suggests that an emotionally vulnerable person is one whose autonomic nervous system reacts excessively to relatively low levels of stress, and has a slow return to baseline. An invalidating environment is a situation where a child's emotional responses are ignored or invalidated by significant others. Typically, such young people are emotionally vulnerable, and may blame others for having unrealistic expectations of them. They internalise the characteristics of the invalidating environment, and tend to show 'self-invalidation'. Such young people invalidate their own responses, and have unrealistic goals and expectations, feeling ashamed and angry with themselves when they struggle to achieve their goals (Kiehn & Swales 1995).

It is not unusual for young people with borderline personality traits to engage in dysfunctional and high-risk behaviours, including suicidal, self-harming

(1) *Individual therapy*

In DBT the relationship between the young person and nurse is thought to be highly influential in the success of therapy. Linehan (1993a) suggests that at times the relationship with their therapist is the only thing that keeps the client alive. DBT is a collaborative therapy, and requires a level of motivation on the part of the young person who is coached in applying the strategies taught in skills-training and is assisted with problem-solving.

(2) *Telephone contact*

Between sessions the young person should be offered telephone support from the individual nurse, including out-of-hours contact. This provides help and support in the application of adaptive skills.

(3) *Skills training (group)*

Skills are taught which are relevant to the particular problems experienced by this client group. There are four modules, comprising: core mindfulness skills; interpersonal effectiveness skills; emotion modulation skills; and distress tolerance skills.

(4) *Therapist consultation*

Due to the emotionally demanding nature of DBT with young people who have borderline personality traits, nurses using DBT receive supervision in a regular therapists' consultation group. This is to enhance therapeutic ability and avoid 'burnout'.

Figure 14.1   Primary treatment modes (DBT).

and impulsive behaviours, to cope with the intense and painful feelings they experience. Suicide attempts may be seen as an expression of the fact that at times life does not seem worth living. As the name suggests, in DBT there is an emphasis on 'dialectics'. This refers to the reconciliation of opposites in a continual process of synthesis. The most fundamental dialectic is the need to accept the young person just as they are in the context of trying to teach them to change (Linehan 1993a). Dialectic strategies used in DBT provide the nurse with an opportunity to balance change and acceptance, and prevent the young person and nurse from becoming stuck with rigid thoughts and behaviours. The four primary treatment modes are shown in Figure 14.1.

Individual child psychotherapy

Individual child psychotherapy refers to a number of different therapeutic approaches. It may be used to help the child explain emotions and relationships; to learn how to change things; or to form a supportive therapeutic alliance.

Psychodynamic psychotherapies focus on unconscious processes and use the concepts of defence, resistance and transference analysis to understand and explain mental health problems and psychological distress. Transference is the projection onto the therapist of relationships with figures from the past, which the therapist can use to understand the child. Counter-transference is the projection of these feelings or emotions from the therapist to the child (Lask et al. 2003). With younger children, play is often used to help symbolise conflict and anxiety, whereas with older children and adolescents therapists use free association of ideas and focus on unconscious processes and the transference relationship (Fitzgerald 1998).

Joe

Joe, aged 7, was adopted as a toddler and had no contact with his birth parents. He was always described as a 'difficult' child by his adoptive parents, harmed himself and was frequently aggressive towards not only himself but also his adopted sister. Joe was diagnosed as having an attachment disorder and was referred for individual psychotherapy by a nurse therapist. During therapy, it became evident that Joe found it very difficult to make and sustain relationships with females. This caused problems at home and at school. Due to insecurity, Joe would characteristically 'destroy' such relationships before he could be rejected. After two years of psychotherapy, Joe found it easier to make and sustain relationships but his self-destructive behaviour continued.

Psychodynamic psychotherapy, derived from psychoanalysis, is based on the premise that the capacity for motivation to change and resistance to change exists in all people (Lask et al. 2003). An event that occurs during one stage of a child's life can affect them later on in life. By understanding the connections between life events, feelings, behaviour and relationships, children can gain a greater sense of control and reduce the potential for inner conflict. The therapeutic relationship between the child and therapist is of paramount importance. The concepts of transference and counter-transference are used to bring about therapeutic change. Nurses who have been trained to use individual psychodynamic psychotherapy usually see children once or twice per week, for between 50 and 60 minutes over a period of approximately two years. The aims are to work through a range of feelings such as anger, control, dependence and loss. Since loss is an essential part of living, loss of the nurse-therapist needs to be anticipated and prepared for with the young person. This is both in terms of therapy closure, and if the nurse leaves the service before therapy has finished.

Brief solution-focused therapy

Brief solution focused therapy (BSFT) was developed in the US during the mid 1980s, and is an approach to treatment or therapy which is based on solution-building rather than problem-solving (Iverson 2002). A small number of studies have demonstrated the efficacy of BSFT with children and young people (Zimmerman et al. 1996), in UK settings, including schools (Lethem 1994; Rhodes & Ajmal 1995). The technique is simple, interactive and of course, brief. Nurses using BSFT do not seek to explain the cause of a problem. Rather, children and their families or carers are helped to find solutions to their difficulties. Very small changes can often produce a solution to the presenting problem and the role of the nurse using BSFT is to build on strengths and resources to facilitate effective communication and cooperation between the child and their family or carers (Terry 2003).

BSFT is structured according to a series of questions aimed at obtaining information about interactions and relationships. Children and their families or carers often know what has caused their difficulties. However, they may be struggling to find ways to change or cope with these. Alternatively, children and young people may not imagine their life being different and struggle to identify anything positive or of value in their current circumstances (Iverson 2002). BSFT aims to produce change and to enable the child and their family or carers to understand why change has occurred. Using a rating scale of between one and ten, improvement can be tracked and explanations for what has caused the improvement can be identified (Iverson 2002). Comparing different ratings by family members may reveal useful information about relationships, perceptions of difficulties and parental coping styles. Since younger children often struggle to understand the language of adults, nurses using BSFT should talk in concrete language and avoid asking 'why' questions, which children often struggle to answer.

Psycho-educational interventions

School-based interventions are becoming increasingly common, as children with hyperactivity and concentration problems are a cause of great disruption in the educational setting. This has been discussed in greater detail in Chapter 12 on school-based mental health services, and is also explored in the context of nursing interventions with children who have ADHD in Chapter 3.

Oliver

Oliver, aged 8, was referred to the local Tier 3 CAMHS by his teacher. This followed oppositional behaviour, outbursts of anger and refusal to cooperate at school. His parents had two older children and were extremely concerned about Oliver's lack of education and increasingly disturbed behaviour. When he was globally tested by a clinical psychologist, Oliver was found to have a very large discrepancy between his verbal and performance IQ, which was only 70. Working in close liaison with the school, the family and a nurse specialist in the CAMHS team, Oliver was able to overcome his performance deficits with extra tuition on practical skills rather than verbal skills. Subsequently his self-esteem increased, he began to make progress and his behaviour improved with the help of behaviour management techniques involving his parents.

Close cooperation between nurses in the multidisciplinary team in the Tier 3 services, parents and schools can help children to avoid social exclusion. Global testing can show other specific learning difficulties as well as a low IQ. The phenomena of non-verbal learning difficulties (NVLD) are not fully understood, but it is accepted that some children have higher scores on verbal than performance IQ scales and deficiencies in visual spatial organisation and non-verbal integration (Snowling 2003). Dyslexia affects between 7% and 54% of children depending upon their age (Shaywitz et al. 1992). Dyslexia is a specific reading difficulty, which includes poor letter knowledge, idiosyncratic spelling and problems with copying. Dyscalculia, which involves specific difficulties with numeracy skills, is characterised by a problem in learning number facts. Arithmetic is therefore very weak compared with literacy. Dyspraxia is a term used to describe problems of motor coordination. This affects children's gross motor coordination (running, jumping, balancing, catching a ball) and fine motor coordination, which affects manual dexterity (holding a pencil, tying up laces, eating with a knife and fork). Recognition of these specific difficulties and educational support, together with behaviour management, family involvement and support helps to alleviate behaviour problems by increasing the child's ability to achieve, thus improving self-esteem.

The impact of bullying on children's mental health and general development cannot be over-emphasised. Bullying is the systematic abuse of power. It involves aggressive behaviour perpetrated against a victim who cannot defend him or herself (Rigby 2002). Bullying takes many forms and ranges from name-calling to direct physical attacks and includes spreading rumours, social exclusion, social isolation, threats of violence and destruction of the victim's property. It is not unusual for children being bullied to become anxious, depressed and refuse to attend school. School nurses and nurses in CAMHS are often involved in anti-bullying initiatives (Offler 2000). School programmes have been initiated which include awareness-raising, assertiveness-training, peer support and mentoring. Children who have developed mental health problems due to bullying need careful support to remain in the school setting, and close collaboration between the school, home and CAMHS nurse is essential if the child is to return to full-time education.

Family therapy

Since children grow up in families or alternative families, many solutions to problems can be found in the family context. Family therapy is based on the principles of a systemic or contextual approach. There are numerous models of systemic family therapy that are used by nurses either in their day-to-day work or in their role as family therapists. Though the two most common are structural family therapy and strategic family therapy, Milan family therapy, narrative, psychoeducational and behavioural therapy are also used (Asen 2002). Structural family therapy was pioneered by Minuchin (1974) and assumes that families require clear hierarchical structures and lines of communication and accountability. Various subsystems including the parents, siblings and the marital relationship need to have clear boundaries. Children's psychological distress is viewed as a result of these boundaries being blurred or breached. Techniques used in strategic family therapy include challenging rigid or absent boundaries, unbalancing the family equilibrium by temporarily joining with one family member against others, and setting 'homework' tasks designed to restore hierarchies (Asen 2002). Strategic family therapy was pioneered by Hayley (1963) and, like solution-focused therapy, concentrates on solving problems rather than searching for causes. It is based on the belief that psychological distress is maintained by behaviours that seek to suppress it. When children are highly anxious and need to control their behaviour, enabling the parents to take control may produce the change that is required.

Joanna

Joanna, aged 11 years, had behaviour problems and hysterical outbursts characterised by screaming. She was referred to the nurse specialist at the Tier 3 CAMHS. During the initial assessment it became clear that Joanna had obsessive preoccupations with her parents touching one another. If the parents held hands or kissed, Joanna would scream at her mum and hit her and become hysterical. This was not only very upsetting for the parents, but their marriage was becoming strained. The parents avoided each other because they were afraid of making Joanna upset. They were referred to CAMHS for family therapy.

A range of interpersonal and social stressors can impact negatively on family life and exacerbate a child's mental health problems. This can result in parental conflict and psychosocial adversity. Nurses working as family therapists encourage direct interactions between family members and ensure that parental authority is maintained. The contribution of each family member is valued and each person is encouraged to describe the difficulties from their own point of view. It is not unusual for parents to feel impotent in terms of their child's mental health problems. This is particularly common for parents of children with OCD. Such parents often seek permission to take control of situations and set boundaries in relation to their child's obsessive and ritualistic behaviour.

There is evidence to support the use of family therapy to treat a number of mental disorders (Senior 2003). Family therapy appears to be most effective as part of multimodal integrated programmes. For depression and self-harm, randomised controlled trials have not shown family therapy to be as effective as CBT, drugs or a combination of both (Senior 2003) However, since family dysfunction and poor relationships are predictors of persistence (Senior 2003), the commonly held view amongst CAMHS nurses is that family intervention alongside other treatments is likely to be helpful. Problems of conduct and behaviour have not been shown to improve with family therapy unless they are treated as part of a multisystemic treatment programme (McMahon &

Kotler 2004). Family therapy in both in-patient and out-patient settings is effective with eating disorders of short duration (NICE 2004). Family work with children and young people is beneficial in anorexia nervosa, and family work with CBT is most effective in bulimia nervosa, and is more effective than individual therapy alone (NICE 2004). There are no controlled outcome studies in relation to family therapy and specific phobias. However, as outlined previously, facilitating parental control and effective boundary-setting is part of the family therapy process. When treating phobias, nurses using a family therapy approach can support parents by training them in strategies for phobic exposure and response prevention. Despite widespread use in CAMHS settings, family therapy approaches in general have not been evaluated using well-designed studies. In order to assist with systematic evaluation of family therapy, it has been suggested that the different approaches should be set out in manuals to guide clinicians and aid evaluation (Fonagy 2003).

Parent training

Parent training strategies, such as the Webster-Stratton programmes (Webster-Stratton 1998) have grown out of treatment interventions with families of children with oppositional defiant disorder. Whilst their use may be limited in terms of preventing mental disorders (Scott et al. 2001), parent training programmes are used widely, particularly in Tier 3 specialist CAMHS, and appear to be effective when used as part of a multimodal treatment strategy for ADHD (Anastopoulos et al. 1993), autism (Rutter 1985) and behaviour problems in younger children (Fonagy & Kurtz 2002).

Group therapy

Group therapy is based on the premise that children's difficulties develop within a network of relationships and in the social context. Relationships are explored as part of a dynamic and changing process. Children and young people are able to discuss problems, identify with others and share strategies to resolve conflict and distress. Nurses should be aware that whilst groups can be useful for children who require the approval of their peers, they can provoke anxiety for children who are shy or lacking in confidence.

Chloe

Chloe, aged 16, had been harming herself for two years and had cut her arms and face on numerous occasions. Chloe was sexually abused by her paternal uncle between the ages of 7 and 10. When she disclosed the abuse, her parents separated and her father had had no contact with her since. Chloe had recently started to binge drink and to engage in unsafe sexual behaviour. Chloe was referred for family therapy and to a life-skills group run by a community mental health nurse trained in DBT.

Though it has been suggested that group therapy has been given a low profile in the UK (Fitzherbert 2005), there are several models of group therapy designed to facilitate social and life-skills training for children and adolescents. It is important that nurses who facilitate group therapy have completed training in relation to group dynamics and process. In order to facilitate therapeutic change, all groups require clear objectives, limits and boundaries. This is regardless of whether the groups are verbal or non-verbal, structured or unstructured, or open or closed to new members who wish to join. Cognitive behavioural group treatment (CBGT) has been used to develop social skills, problem-solving and assertiveness for young people. This is a modified version of CBGT for adults, and involves a 16-week programme of skills training and psychoeducation (Swales et al. 2000).

Multisystemic therapy

The move away from treatment orientations that focus exclusively on the child has brought with it systemic and contextual explanations for childhood psychosocial disorders (Fonagy 2003). The development of multisystemic therapy (MST) as a multimodal treatment strategy has its roots in the US, where it has been successfully used with young people with conduct disorder and antisocial behaviour (Henggeler et al. 1998). Whilst MST is relatively expensive to provide, governments in North America and Europe have been concerned with reducing the long-term costs of antisocial behaviour and crime, and have recognised the important 'invest-to-save' principles associated with these programmes. MST in the UK is in its infancy, but Belfast's Extern Project has shown positive results (Jefford & Squire 2004). Here, the potential benefits have been recognised by the Home Office and Youth Justice Board (YJB), where intensive supervision and surveillance programmes (ISSP) based on MST have been funded. Programmes based on MST are proving to be effective, reducing out-of-home placements; improving family functioning; and reducing reoffending rates (Ogden & Halliday-Boykins 2004; Jefford & Squire 2004).

In the US and other countries, MST has demonstrated positive outcomes for young people with antisocial behaviour. It is based on the premise that rather than provide individual treatment or family therapy, behavioural change is achieved through reorganisation of the young person's social environment (Bronfenbrennes 1979). Individual programmes are tailored to the needs of the young person. The family, peer group and school are involved in order to reduce barriers and promote generalisation of the interventions. Each problem area is individually targeted and action plans are generated. The young person and family are expected to achieve targets on a weekly or more frequent basis. Staff trained in MST are available to the family on a 24-hour basis. Therapeutic interventions used as part of MST programmes include strategic and structural family therapy, parenting programmes, anger management and CBT. A small amount of research into the use of MST with young offenders has been carried out in the UK. However, further research is required in order to focus on exploring which components of multicomponent packages are effective and which young people benefit from which interventions.

James

James, aged 13, had problems with anger and aggression. He had been known to his local Tier 3 CAMHS since the age of three when he witnessed his mother being murdered by his father. He had not seen his father since as he was raised by his maternal grandparents. They doted on him, but as James grew older, both grandparents found it increasingly difficult to control him. By the time James was 12 he was hitting his grandmother and mixing with older boys who were involved in petty crime. He had already seriously assaulted a younger boy in the community who was irritating him. James was assessed by the nurse specialist and referred to the MST programme.

Physical treatments

Physical treatments for childhood mental disorders are generally psychopharmacological. It is now widely accepted that pharmacological treatments have a central role to play in the treatment and management of some psychiatric disorders. On rare occasions electroconvulsive therapy is used with children and adolescents. Physical interventions such as restraint or seclusion are generally considered to be containment rather than treatment strategies and are not addressed in this chapter. Together with a range of psychological and social interventions, drug treatments are one of the major therapeutic options available to help people with mental health problems and disorders (Brimblecombe et al. 2005). Drug treatment plays an important role in the management of childhood mental disorders, particularly severe and persistent disorders such as schizophrenia and bipolar disorder. Pharmacological treatments are usually prescribed on a trial basis and as part of a multimodal treatment strategy implemented by the multidisciplinary team. However, most drugs that are commonly prescribed for mental disorder are not licensed for use with children (Johnson & Clark 2001). This is of concern for doctors, nurses and other professionals, as well as for children and young people, their families and carers (Sutcliffe 1999; Choonara 2000). However, the evidence base for psychopharmacological treatments is growing quickly (Coghill 2003).

Antipsychotics

Antipsychotic medication is used for the treatment of psychosis and bipolar disorder. Neuroleptic drugs can be categorised into two groups. First are traditional antipsychotics (e.g. chlorpromazine, haloperidol and thioridazine). These drugs are limited in their use with children and young people, due to significant and potentially serious side-effects such as extrapyramidal symptoms and tardive dyskinesia. Second, are so-called atypical antipsychotics (e.g. olanzapine, risperidone and clozapine). Due to their decreased side-effect profile, atypical antipsychotic drugs tend to be used instead of traditional neuropletics with children and adolescents. However, they are not free from side-effects. Weight gain, in particular, can be distressing for adolescents, many of whom may already have issues about body image. The choice of antipsychotic medication is generally based on the nature of the disorder; other medication that may be being taken; side-effect profile and the wishes of the young person, their family and carers.

Antidepressants

The treatment of choice for mild to moderate depression during childhood and adolescence is CBT (National Institute for Clinical Excellence 2005). However, for severe or persistent depression, a limited range of antidepressants can be beneficial; these are selective serotonin reuptake inhibitors (SSRIs). At the time of writing this chapter there are no antidepressant drugs with a current UK marketing authorisation for depression in children and young people under 18 years old. However, it is generally recognised that some children and young people will benefit from an antidepressant, and guidance on the prescription of unlicensed medicines has been published to assist doctors in making competent treatment decisions (Royal College of Paediatrics & Child Health 2000). This states that the use of unlicensed medicines is necessary in paediatric practice and that doctors are legally allowed to prescribe unlicensed medicines where there are no suitable alternatives, and where their use is justified by a responsible body of professional opinion. The SSRI of choice for children and adolescents is usually fluoxetine. However, a range of other SSRIs can be used (e.g. citalopram, sertraline, paroxetine) in exceptional circumstances; for instance, where the child or young person is moderately or severely depressed and is intolerant of fluoxetine.

Working with families, carers, teachers and social workers, as well as health professionals in primary and secondary care may be familiar for CAMHS nurses. However, they also need to understand the potential role that medication can play, particularly when psychological, psychosocial or psycho-educational approaches have not been successful. Medication is an integral part of the treatment for ADHD, and for children and young people with serious mental disorders. Which drugs are likely to work best for which children and adolescent depends on good assessment and knowledge about the young person. The process of selection and evaluation is a multidisciplinary activity in which nurses play an important role. Nurses who work with children or young people who have been prescribed medication for mental disorders have a duty to provide them with straightforward information about their treatment. When this involves taking medication, nurses must be able to describe why the drug has been prescribed, and what are the potential side-effects and anticipated treatment gains. This is particularly relevant for nurses who, in the future, may be in a position to prescribe medication within their sphere of competence, expertise and experience. A good understanding of the role of pharmacology is also necessary if nurses are to practice as supplementary or independent prescribers in the future.

Conclusion

Whilst the child and adolescent have been the focus of interventions for a number of years, it is clear that many childhood disorders present in a number of settings. Therefore it is necessary to use multicomponent therapeutic interventions to address their needs. Generic therapies and treatment orientations that focus exclusively on the child are declining. In their place, specialist strategies or multimodal treatment manuals represent a move towards systemic and contextual explanations of childhood mental disorder. Most nurses in specialist CAMHS work within a humanistic framework and apply an eclectic and holistic approach to assessment and treatment with children and young people, their families and carers. Many of these interventions are psychosocial or psychoeducational and are used as firstline interventions for some disorders such as anxiety and autism. Psychiatric disorders such as severe clinical depression, early onset psychosis and OCD, often require combination treatments or multimodal treatment strategies. Here nurses often work in partnership with their psychiatrist colleagues.

References

Anastopolous, A., Shelton, T., DuPaul, G. & Guevremont, D. (1993). Parent training for attention deficit hyperactivity disorder: its impact on parent functioning. *Journal of Abnormal Child Psychology*, (21), 581–96.

Asen, E. (2002). Outcome research in family therapy. *Advances in Psychiatric Treatment*, (8), 230–38.

Brimblecombe, N., Parr, A. & Gray, R. (2005). Medication and mental health nurses: developing new ways of working. *Mental Health Practice*, 8 (5), 12–14.

Brook, J., Whiteman, M. & Zheng, L. (2002). Intergenerational transmission of risks for problem behaviour. *Journal of Abnormal Child Psychology*, 30 (1), 65–76.

Bronfenbrennes, U. (1979). *The Ecology of Human Development*. Cambridge MA: Harvard University Press.

Choonara, I. (2000). Clinical trials of medicine in children. *British Medical Journal*, (321), 1093–94.

Coghill, D. (2003). Current issues in child and adolescent psychopharmacology. Part 1: anxiety and obsessive-compulsive disorders, autism, Tourette's and schizophrenia. *Advances in Psychiatric Treatment*, (9), 289–99.

Fitzgerald, M. (1998). Child psychoanalytic psychotherapy. *Advances in Psychiatric Treatment*, (4), 18–24.

Fitzherbert, K. (2005). The power of group work. *YoungMinds Magazine*, (74), 28–29.

Fonagy, P. & Kurtz, Z. (2002). Disturbance of conduct. In: Fonagy, P., Target, M., Cottrell, D., Phillips, J. & Kurtz, Z. (Eds). *What Works for Whom?: a critical review of treatments for children and adolescents*. London: Guilford Press.

Fonagy, P. (2003). *A Review of the Outcomes of all Treatments of Psychiatric Disorder in Childhood: (MCH 17–33)*. London: HMSO.

Fonagy, P. (2004). Psychosocial therapies for young people. In: Skuse, D. (Ed). *Child Psychology and Psychiatry: an introduction*. London: Martin Duntz.

Harrington, R., Whittaker, J., Shoebridge, P. & Campbell, F. (1998). Systematic review of efficacy of cognitive behaviour therapies in childhood and adolescent depressive disorder. *British Medical Journal*, (316), 1559–63.

Haley, J. (1963). *Strategies of Psychotherapy*. New York: Grune & Stratton.

Henggeleer, S., Schoenwald, S., Borduin, C., Rowland, M. & Cunningham, P. (1998). *Multisystemic Treatment of Antisocial Behaviour in Children and Adolescents*. New York: Guilford Press.

Iverson, C. (2000). Solution focused brief therapy. *Advances in Psychiatric Treatment*, (8), 149–57.

Jefford, T. & Squire, B. (2004). Model practice. *YoungMinds Magazine*, (71), 11.

Johnson, J. & Clark, A. (2001). Prescribing of unlicensed medicines or licensed medicines for unlicensed applications in child and adolescent psychiatry. *Psychiatric Bulletin*, (25), 465–66.

Kiehn, B. & Swales, M. (1995). An overview of dialectical behaviour therapy in the treatment of borderline personality disorder. *Behavior Therapy*, (32), 371–90.

Lask B., Taylor S. & Nunn, K. (2003). *Practical Child Psychiatry: the clinicians guide*. London: BMJ publishing group.

Law, J. & Garnett, Z. (2004). Speech and language therapy: its potential role in CAMHS. *Child and Adolescent Mental Health*, **9** (2), 50–55.

Letham, J. (1994). *Moved to Tears: Moved to Action: brief therapy with women and children*. London: BT Press.

Linehan, M. (1993a). *Cognitive Behavioural Therapy of Borderline Personality Disorder*. New York: Guilford Press.

Linehan, M. (1993b). *Skills Training Manual for Treating Borderline Personality Disorder*. New York: Guilford Press.

MacMahone, R. & Kotler, J. (2004). Treatment of conduct problems in children and adolescents. In Barrett & Olendick (Eds). *Handbook of Interventions that Work with Children and Adolescents Prevention and Treatment*. England: John Wiley.

March, J. (1995). Cognitive behavioural psychotherapy for children and adolescents with OCD: a review and recommendations for treatment. *Journal of the American Academy Child and Adolescent Psychiatry*, **34**, 7–18.

Meichembaum, D. & Goodman, J. (1971). Training impulsive children to talk to themselves, a means of developing self control. *Journal of Abnormal Psychology*, **70**, 117–26.

Minuchin, S. (1974). *Families and Family Therapy*. London: Tavistock.

Nation, K. (2003). Developmental language disorders. In: Skuse, D. (Ed). *Child Psychology and Psychiatry: an introduction*. 71–74.

National Institute for Clinical Excellence (2004). *Core Interventions in the Treatment and Management of Anorexia Nervosa, Bulimia Nervosa and Related Eating Disorders*. London: NICE.

National Institute for Health and Clinical Excellence (2005). *Depression in Children and Young People: identification and management in primary, community and secondary care*. London: NICE.

Offler, E. (2000). Bullying: everybody's problem. *Paediatric Nursing*, **12** (9), 22–26.

Ogden, T. & Halliday-Boykins, C. (2004). Multisystemic treatment of antisocial adolescents in Norway: replication of clinical outcomes outside of the US. *Child and Adolescent Mental Health*, **9**, (2), 77–83.

Ollendick, T. & King, N. (1998). Empirically supported treatments for children with phobic and anxiety disorders. *Journal of Clinical Child Psychology*, (27), 156–67.

Rhodes, J. & Ajmal, Y. (1995). *Solution Focused Thinking in Schools*. London: BT Press.

Rigby, K. (2002). *New Perspectives on Bullying*. London: Jessica Kingsley.

Robertson, M. (2003). Tourette's syndrome. In: Skuse (Ed). *Child Psychology and Psychiatry: an introduction*. 86–88.

Royal College of Paediatrics and Child Health (2000). *The Use of Unlicensed Medicines or Licensed Medicines for Unlicensed Applications in Paediatric Practice: policy statement*. London: Royal College of Paediatrics and Child Health.

Rutter, M. (1985). The treatment of autistic children. *Journal of Child Psychology and Psychiatry*, (26), 193–214.

Scott, S., Knapp, M., Henderson, J. & Maughan, B. (2001). Financial cost of social exclusion: follow-up study of anti-social children into adulthood. *British Medical Journal*, (323), 1–5.

Senior, R. (2003). Family and group therapies. In: Skuse (Ed). *Child Psychology and Psychiatry: an introduction*. London: The Medicine Publishing Company.

Shaywitz, S., Escobar, M., Shaywitz, B., Fletcher, J. & Makugh, R. (1992). Evidence that dyslexia may represent the lower tail of a normal distribution of reading ability. *New England Journal of Medicine*, **326**, 145–50.

Shortt, A., Barrett, P. & Fox, T. (2001). Evaluating the FRIENDS programme: a cognitive behavioural group treatment for anxious children and their parents. *Journal of Clinical Child Psychology*, **30**, 525–35.

Snowling, M. (2003). Specific learning difficulties. In: Skuse (Ed). *Child Psychology and Psychiatry: an Introduction*. London: The Medicine Publishing Company.

Sutcliffe, A. (1999). Prescribing medicines for children. *British Medical Journal*, (319), 70–71.

Terry, J. (2003). Brief intervention: a pilot initiative in a child and adolescent mental health service. *Mental Health Practice*, **6** (5), 18–19.

Weaver, A. (2001). Individual and group therapy. In: Gowers, S. (Ed). *Adolescent Psychiatry in Clinical Practice*. London: Arnold.

Webster-Stratton, C. (1998). Preventing conduct problems in Head Start children: strengthening parental competencies. *Journal of Consulting and Clinical Psychology*, (66), 715–30.

Williams, C. (2002). A sense of self and identity. *Mental Health Practice*, **5** (6), 24–27.

Yanof, J. (1996). Child analysis: language, communication, transference. *Journal of the American Psychoanalytic Association*, (44), 79–116.

Zimmerman, T., Jacobson, R., MacIntyre, Y. & Watson, C. (1996). Solution focused parenting groups: an empirical study. *Journal of Family Therapy*, **19**, 159–72.

Chapter 15

Clinical Governance for Specialist Child and Adolescent Mental Health Nurses

Ian Roberts and Tim McDougall

Key points

- Clinical governance is about striving towards a culture of excellence in CAMHS (child and adolescent mental health services) service provision. Nurses in specialist CAMHS must help contribute to service planning, design and evaluation through a continuous process of lifelong learning, quality improvement and standard-setting.

- Whilst listening to what children and young people want has previously been a challenge to CAMHS providers, there is good evidence that the rhetoric of user-involvement is being translated into reality. The growing voice of service users is bringing welcome pressure to bear on CAMHS who have a responsibility to ensure that current and future services meet the needs of local children and families.

- Policymakers, commissioners, managers and practitioners such as nurses must have access to high quality up-to-date information. This is so children receive the best possible treatment, nurses and other professionals make competent care and treatment decisions and services are delivered that are fit for purpose.

- The notion that nurses should base their decisions on the best available evidence may seem to be common sense. However, consensus has not been reached on what constitutes evidence in CAMHS. New service models are constantly evolving and the effectiveness of many CAMHS interventions has not yet been evaluated.

- It has been suggested that modern CAMHS are preoccupied with risk avoidance. The nurse's duty of care must be brokered with a wider responsibility to enable children to reach their fullest potential. This demands a certain creativity to make informed care and treatment decisions and take calculated, therapeutic risks.

- Each and every nurse in specialist CAMHS should be involved in an active process of continuing professional development (CPD). This is part of the quality improvement process and helps to ensure that nurses keep themselves up-to-date and remain fit for practice. Personal development plans should be used to ensure that the training and CPD needs of nurses are in keeping with the service plan, strategic direction of their host organisation and the wider CAMHS improvement agenda.

Introduction: what is clinical governance?

Accountability and responsibility for the commissioning, organisation, management, delivery and evaluation of CAMHS is multifaceted. The following chapter explores the development of clinical governance in specialist child and adolescent mental health services (CAMHS) and describes some of the key terms, roles and processes that contribute towards clinical governance and quality assurance. Clinical governance is a way of achieving continuous service quality in service performance (Nicholls et al. 2000). Service performance in CAMHS refers to the evaluation of broad outcomes in the context of local, regional and national strategy. Clinical governance is a way of integrating financial control, service performance and clinical quality into the management of health services (Scally & Donaldson 1998; Richardson 2003), and is the overarching principle of the management of CAMHS. Modern concepts of evidence-based practice, values-based practice and clinical governance in CAMHS are related to, and mirrored in, modern policy development and CAMHS implementation (Williams & Kerfoot 2005). Clinical governance first became a mandatory part of health service provision following publication of *A First Class Service* (Department of Health 1998), which described the methods by which the quality of services should be set, delivered and monitored. Nurses in specialist CAMHS must help contribute to service design and evaluation through quality improvement and standard setting (Leighton et al. 2001). In specialist CAMHS this can be achieved by:

- Moving the focus of CAMHS to quality of care, evidence-based practice and supporting the development of staff and services.
- Safeguarding high standards of service delivery by creating an environment in which excellence in clinical care and awareness of current evidence will continue to grow and flourish.
- Continuously improving the quality of CAMHS delivered to children, young people and their families by developing stronger and more effective links with children and young people, their families and carers, by involving them in CAMHS commissioning, planning and evaluation.
- Using complaints and mistakes and the lessons to be learned in order to review CAMHS and to explore how it can improve the quality of care.
- Providing an organisational culture that is blame free and encourages clear role definition within supportive teams.
- Ownership of the clinical governance agenda at a strategic level.
- Competent communication systems and service infrastructure.

Involving children and young people

The involvement of patients, carers and the public in health decision-making is at the heart of the modernisation of the NHS (National Health Service) and its component structures, organisations and services (DoH 2004). *Improvement, Expansion and Reform* sets the context for the delivery of comprehensive CAMHS. As one of its underlying principles, the priorities and planning framework for CAMHS has stated that the commissioning and delivery of services should be informed by stakeholder views, of which children and young people constitute an important group (DoH 2002). Through a series of consultations, surveys and research projects, children and young people have consistently said that they want to be involved in CAMHS (Laws 1999; Street & Svanberg 2003; Street et al. 2005). The participation of children and young people is at the core of the government's *Change for Children Programme: Every Child Matters* (Department for Education and Skills 2003) and the NSF (National Service Framework) for Children, Young People and Maternity Services (DoH 2004). In their strategy, *Learning to Listen*, the government's Children and Young People's Unit (CYPU) made clear its commitment to children and young people involvement in the design, provision and evaluation of policy (DfES 2001).

Systematically involving children and young people in CAMHS design and delivery can be a complex process. There are a number of reasons for this: including a poor track record of user involvement in CAMHS; stigma that is still associated with discussions about mental health which make it hard to engage people; and worries about overloading children who may be seriously unwell, highly vulnerable and already facing many changes and choices (Street & Herts 2005). Notwithstanding these concerns, the benefits of involving children and young people in CAMHS are numerous. If it is undertaken sensitively and with the appropriate consent and support, participation by CAMHS service users can yield vital information and insights to assist nurses and other professionals to plan and provide better, more accessible and appropriate services (Hedges & McKeown 2000). Similarly, involving the parents or carers of children and young people who use specialist CAMHS is likely to reap rewards. Whilst this can be difficult when the views of children and their parents are at odds or issues of confidentiality constrain communication, involving parents may enable them to feel that they have more control over their child's health and welfare, reduce their own levels of stress and improve relationships with CAMHS nurses (Council for Disabled Children 2004).

Before embarking on any user-participation project there are a number of important issues to consider. Nurses should be clear about the aim of user involvement; about the time and resources that will be involved; about support needed to complete the participation exercise; and whether consent and the approval of a local ethics committee is required. Whilst there are many ways to engage children and young people in the planning and evaluation of CAMHS, the following methods, taken from Street & Herts (2005), may be useful for nurses to consider:

- A suggestions box.
- Self-completed questionnaires.
- Questionnaires with drawings or cartoons.
- Computer-assisted packages.
- Telephone or e-mail interviews.
- Face-to-face interviews.
- Focus groups.
- User representation on committees and planning groups.
- User involvement in service evaluation.

Consideration of the views and wishes of children and young people, whether individually or as part of a group, should be a thread that runs through all aspects of CAMHS service commissioning, delivery and evaluation. This process of involving service users at every level should not be thought of as an added extra, but should be an integral component and a major asset to the service. The process of strategically and comprehensively involving service users requires investment with time and energy, enthusiasm and commitment.

Education, training and continuing professional development

It is often the case that the different professionals in specialist CAMHS have different approaches to staff training. To some extent this is to be welcomed. Psychiatrists, psychologists, nurses and other professionals have different foundations in education and training, different philosophies and objectives, and different roles and functions. Nurses who work with children who have mental health problems do so in a multiprofessional and interagency context, and have much to learn from and share with their colleagues. This is part of the rich tapestry of specialist CAMHS and is to be celebrated and embraced by nurses. Like all professionals in CAMHS, nurses should be involved in an active process of CPD. This is part of the quality improvement process and helps to ensure that nurses keep themselves up-to-date with policy and practice changes and remain fit for practice (Nursing & Midwifery Council 2004). Personal development plans (PDPs) should be used to ensure that the individual training and CPD needs of nurses are in keeping with the service plan and strategic direction of their host organisation, and the wider CAMHS improvement agenda.

Brokering individual and team training needs with finance and resource management is a challenge for most CAMHS managers. The training directorates of many provider trusts may be preoccupied with ensuring that their employees meet core or mandatory training needs. It is arguable whether some trusts invest in education, training and CPD opportunities that enable nurses and other professionals to fulfil their registration requirements. Core or mandatory training alone is inadequate to develop the skills base required to maintain excellence in specialist CAMHS. Some professions have training and development written into their employment contracts and timetables, allowing them to programme this into their professional plans and so 'protect time' during their working weeks. With the exception of consultant nurses in CAMHS, this tends not to be the case for most nurses (McDougall 2003). Though nurses have the same commitment to learning and development, there is sometimes an unspoken expectation that nurses work towards fulfilling their CPD requirements and professional aspirations outside work time. The inconsistency between the different professions in this respect appears to emphasise their differences in a negative way. It could be argued that investing in CPD opportunities in this way gives additional value to some professionals over others. Consistency in terms of investing in CPD for nurses in CAMHS would help raise our professional profile, bring greater value to the contribution of each profession to the multidisciplinary team and strengthen team identity and cohesiveness.

Research, audit and outcome evaluation

Those who plan, prioritise and provide mental health services for children with mental health disorders must be able to evidence their decisions. To do this, they must understand which assessment, treatment and management strategies work, and understand where the research is lacking. Policymakers, commissioners and practitioners including nurses must have access to high quality up-to-date information. This is so that children receive the best possible treatment; that nurses and other professionals make competent care and treatment decisions; and that services are delivered that are fit for purpose. The phrases 'research-based practice' and 'evidence-based practice' are often heard in relation to modern public service provision, yet achieving evidence-based practice in CAMHS is far from straightforward. It has been suggested that knowledge is the foundation for effective practice (Sainsbury Centre for Mental Health 2001), but CAMHS does not have a unified knowledge and evidence base. The development of knowledge about childhood mental disorder is rapidly expanding but is still in its infancy (Higgitt & Fonagy 2002). Whilst the cause, effect and outcome of some disorders can be partially understood, our knowledge of what works for other disorders is limited. Many research findings have not been evaluated and the methodological basis for others has been questioned (Whittington et al. 2005). Furthermore, some treatments used in CAMHS have been found to be relatively ineffective or harmful (Fonagy et al. 2002).

Nurses are charged with the responsibility of critically evaluating evidence and translating this into competent decision-making. The notion that nurses should base their decisions on the best available evidence may seem at first to be common sense. However, consensus has not been reached on what constitutes evidence in CAMHS and the majority of interventions with children have not been evaluated. New service models are constantly evolving and have not yet been subject to outcome evaluation to test their effectiveness. Randomised controlled trials (RCTs) are heralded as the 'gold-standard' research method. However, the number of RCTs involving children with mental health problems is very limited, the sample sizes are often small and it is not always clear whether randomisation has been carried out properly. Many children and young people with mental disorders also have complex psychosocial problems and multiple difficulties. Consequently, it may not be possible to conduct the perfect RCT where all variables except the intervention being examined have been fully controlled for (Graham 2000). Inappropriate measures of change are sometimes used in RCTs and there has been a lack of in-depth follow up studies involving children and adolescents. The small amount of studies involving children tend only to report at the end of lengthy trials, not on how children are coping at follow-up intervals. This is important, as some treatment effects may only emerge over time (Fonagy 2003). It could be suggested that RCTs cannot adequately measure and capture the art of CAMHS nursing interventions. Qualitative methodologies may have more to offer nurses in articulating the essence of evidence-based CAMHS nursing. Accessing research, and translating this into practice or service delivery is the key to evidence-based nursing practice in CAMHS. Increasingly, nurses have access to a range of National Institute for Clinical Excellence (NICE) guidelines and evidence-based briefings (Skuse 2004) to inform their practice. Published NICE guidelines that include the care, treatment and management of children and adolescents in their scope include the following:

- OCD (obsessive compulsive disorder) (NICE 2003).
- PTSD (post traumatic stress disorder) (NICE 2004a).
- Self-harm (NICE 2004b).
- Eating disorders (NICE 2004c).
- Depression in childhood (NICE 2005).
- Bipolar disorder (NICE 2006).

In addition, nurses can turn to a wide range of books, journals and web-based resources to access information. However, the relatively recent explosion of evidence has made it difficult for nurses in practice to keep up-to-date with new knowledge about effective treatments and service models. With increased professional networking opportunities available to nurses in CAMHS, the opportunity to update and collect information is now open to all. Many of the quality improvement, nursing development and CAMHS support service web-sites offer e-mail alerts providing quick reminders of changes, information, and audit outcomes. At a time when CAMHS is in a continuous process of change, the need for information becomes essential rather than desirable. Access to the Internet should be available in all CAMHS as the modern alternative to libraries but nurses should remember that information found on the internet will not necessarily be peer reviewed and may well contain inaccuracies.

The NSF for Children, Young People and Maternity Services (DoH 2004) has recommended that all CAMHS services should routinely audit and evaluate their work. The data that is collected should be used to inform service developments and be made available to clinicians, commissioners and children and families themselves. However this is easier said than done and many CAMHS services struggle to do so comprehensively and systematically. There are several reasons for this. There may be more than one perspective about the nature of the outcome to be evaluated. Children and young people, their families or carers, and the multidisciplinary team may each have different priorities in terms of outcomes. CAMHS are also subject to outcome-scrutiny and performance management from their host trust and strategic health authority and local authority. This is to meet government targets and implement social care and education priorities. Outcomes in CAMHS are usually measured in terms of case evaluation, clinician activity and service performance. However, creating a culture of outcome evaluation is quite a challenge. It is the role of CAMHS nurse leaders and managers to foster a climate of innovation so that nurses and other professionals recognise the utility of outcome evaluation. Predictors of success include strong strategic leadership and the empowerment of those involved. Maintaining motivation can sometimes be difficult. Return rates for audit or outcome questionnaires are often low and compliance by nurses and the children and families they work with may be patchy. According to Hoagwood et al. (1996), positive out-comes for children and young people in contact with specialist CAMHS may include the following:

- Changes in the nature or severity of symptoms, perhaps to the extent that a diagnosable mental disorder is no longer present.
- Changes in the child or young person's capacity to adapt to their psycho-social environment and develop according to their expected developmental status.
- Changes in the child or young person's cognitive or emotional capacities.
- Changes in family, social and educational settings that bring about an improvement in the child or young person's mental health problems.

The perspectives of children and families can be measured using a range of evaluation tools such as Section B of the *Health of the Nation* outcome scales for children and adolescents (HoNOSCA). This can be completed by nurses as well as young people themselves (Gowers et al. 1998; Gowers et al. 2002). The views of service-users can also be sought by using the Commission for Health Improvement (CHI) questionnaire. The use of the audit, research and outcome evaluation process in specialist CAMHS can have a number of positive benefits. Not only can it be used to improve the individual and collective service-user experience, but the development of audit and research can have a major influence on service development and expansion. Every CAMHS team should have an active multidisciplinary audit programme, which monitors how the service functions (Richardson 2003). Information and intelligence from these audits can provide the basis on which to establish protocols and standards, and also form the bedrock on which to expand, develop or change the CAMHS service plan. The capacity and capability of CAMHS to audit and evaluate outcomes has been much improved by the recent CAMHS Outcome Research Consortium (CORC) Initiative. This is a collaborative between a number of specialist CAMHS in the UK with the aim of developing and piloting a model of routine evaluation of outcome that can provide high-quality information for service-providers, commissioners and service users (Wolpert et al. 2000). The success of effective outcome evaluation as part of the wider CAMHS clinical governance agenda depends on staff motivation; effective communication systems, including a competent IT (information technology) infrastructure; and adequate administrative support for nurses and other professionals.

Risk management

It has been suggested that modern day policy is preoccupied with risk avoidance (Williams & Kerfoot 2005). Indeed, CAMHS nurses practice in a culture of litigation, and their duty of care must be brokered with a wider responsibility to enable children to reach their fullest potential (DfES 2003). There is now a growing awareness of issues of accountability in relation to treatment decisions and costs. This demands of nurses a certain creativity to make informed care and treatment decisions and to take calculated, therapeutic risks. This is no easy task. Risk management is part and parcel of nursing in specialist CAMHS. Whether this means assessing and managing risks involving individual children or young people, or assessing and managing risk in the working environment, it is a central component of modern nursing practice. In a culture of accountability and responsibility, rising healthcare costs and consumer-led services, all nurses must possess skills to appraise the current evidence in relation to what works for which children and young people with mental disorders. They must then make a reasoned judgement about whether or not to change their nursing practice based on the balance of costs, risks and benefits to the children, families and carers with whom they work.

Methods of recognising, estimating and managing risks are part of everyday work and require increasing formalisation if CAMHS services are not to be found deficient. This raises many issues for the operational management of CAMHS. These include the safety of children and families in community waiting areas, the protection of children and young people as well as staff working in isolation, and the welfare and safety of children and young people who are self harming or engaging in high-risk behaviours. All these risk-laden situations are part of everyday nursing practice in specialist CAMHS, and each needs to be acknowledged, explored and managed as part of the governance process. The need to draw up effective and evidence-based protocols has become part of this management. The risk-management strategy should contain a process for learning from serious incidents, mistakes and near misses. This is to ensure that areas of vulnerability are monitored, and that lessons to be learned are acknowledged and translated into learning opportunities. It is important that this is a blame free process and that risk management is seen as a positive enterprise. Where blame is the exception rather than the rule, new and creative approaches are freely shared and willingly received.

Investing in CAMHS nurses

Clinical governance occurs at a number of clinical, operational and strategic levels. However, whilst it is essential that lines of communication, account-ability and responsibility are clear to CAMHS, their host organisation and partner agencies, accountability and responsibility must also be clear within the CAMHS multidisciplinary team. It is sometimes the case that the energy, commitment and skills shown by nurses is not recognised or acknowledged by their colleagues or managers. Valuing nurses can take place not only through the completion of their PDP but also by recognition and understanding of the nurses' contribution to the CAMHS team which can be made transparent through the service operational policy and clear protocols in relation to account-ability, responsibility, intervention and management. The roles and responsib-ilities of each member of the multidisciplinary team should be clearly identified through his or her job description. This may help clarify the expectations and often competing demands on individual staff members, help the team to under-stand each other, improve role-legitimacy and confidence, and create a stronger team identity (Partridge et al. 2003).

Unlike their psychiatrist and psychologist colleagues, CAMHS nurses do not usually undertake research (Focus 1999). This is likely to result from a com-bination of factors, including lack of research competence, poor confidence and lack of support and commitment in terms of time and resources. This is disappointing since nurses often have much more contact with service users than other CAMHS professionals, and are well-placed to translate this know-ledge and insight into research findings and articulate their interventions in terms of evidence-based practice. It is essential that CAMHS managers and lead nurses invest in this area and improve research capacity and capability. This is in order to raise the profile of nursing research in CAMHS.

Conclusion

Clinical governance aims to ensure that the best possible standards of clinical care are provided throughout the NHS. In specialist CAMHS, nurses and all other professionals should recognise that clinical governance is one of the main vehicles for driving improvements in the quality of NHS care, and pro-vides a comprehensive approach to CAMHS improvement. The way in which CAMHS are planned, commissioned, provided for and evaluated is becoming increasingly systematic. Whilst listening to what children and young people want has previously been a challenge to CAMHS providers, there is good evidence that the rhetoric of user involvement is now being translated into reality. The growing voice of service-providers is bringing welcome pressure to bear on CAMHS, which have a responsibility to ensure that current and future services meet the needs of their local children and families. There is an increasing demand for high-quality, scientific evidence in CAMHS. Children and adolescents, their parents and carers, and the commissioners of relevant services, want to know which treatments are effective. Nurses, like all mental health professionals, have a responsibility to demonstrate that what they do actually works in practice. However, the evidence base for many interventions remains poorly developed. Comprehensive systematic reviews meta-analyses and service-evaluation reports are lacking in the child and adolescent mental health literature. Despite this, there is a growing body of advice about what constitutes good practice in CAMHS. As the evidence base develops, it is important that nurses can apply this to their everyday nursing practice with children and young people, their families and carers.

References

Council for Disabled Children (2004). *Parent Participation: improving services for disabled children (parents' guide).* London: Contact a Family.

Department for Education and Skills (2001). *Learning to Listen: core principles for the involvement of children and young people.* London: DfES.

Department for Education and Skills (2003). *Every Child Matters.* London: HMSO.

Department of Health (1998). *A First Class Service: quality in the new NHS.* London: HMSO.

Department of Health (2002). *Improvement, Expansion and Reform: the next three years priorities and planning framework 2003–2006.* London: HMSO.

Department of Health (2004). *National Service Framework for Children, Young People and Maternity Services.* London: HMSO.

Focus (1999). *Practice and Potential in Child and Adolescent Mental Health: a conference for nurses (conference proceedings).* London: Focus.

Fonagy, P. (2003). *A Review of the Outcomes of all Treatments of Psychiatric Disorder in Childhood: (MCH 17–33).* London: HMSO.

Fonagy, P., Target, M., Cottrell, D., Phillips, J. & Kurtz, Z. (2002). *What Works for Whom?: a critical review of treatments for children and adolescents.* London: Guilford Press.

Goodman, R. (1997). The strengths and difficulties questionnaire: a research note. *Journal of Child Psychology and Psychiatry*, (38), 581–86.

Gowers, S., Harrington, R. & Whitton, A. (1998). *Health of the Nation Outcome Scales for Children and Adolescents (HoNOSCA).* London: Royal College of Psychiatrists Research Unit.

Gowers, S., Levine, W., Bailey-Rogers, S., Shore, A., & Burhouse, E. (2002). Use of a routine, self report outcome measure (HoNOSCA-SR) in two adolescent mental health services. *British Journal of Psychiatry*, (180), 266–69.

Graham, P. (2000). Treatment interventions and findings from research: bridging the chasm is child psychiatry. *British Journal of Psychiatry*, (176), 414–19.

Hedges, C. & McKeown, C. (2000). *Give Us a Voice: consultation and participation in child and adolescent mental health services within the Trent region.* Newcastle: Save the Children.

Higgitt, A. & Fonagy, P. (2002). Clinical effectiveness. *British Journal of Psychiatry*, (181), 170–74.

Hoagwood, K., Jensen, P., Petti, T. & Burns, B. (1996). Outcomes of mental health care for children and adolescents: a comprehensive conceptual model. *Journal of the American Academy of Child and Adolescent Psychiatry*, (35), 1055–63.

Laws, S. (1999). Involving children and young people in the monitoring and evaluation of mental health services. *Healthy Minds*, (6), 3–5.

Leighton, S., Smith, C., Minns, K. & Crawford, P. (2001). Specialist child and adolescent mental health nurses: a force to be reckoned with? *Mental Health Practice*, **5** (2), 8–13.

McDougall, T. (2003). Nurse consultants: children's champions. *Mental Health Practice*, **6** (9), 34–36.

National Institute for Clinical Excellence (2003). *Obsessive-Compulsive Disorder in Adults and Children in Primary and Secondary Care (Scope)*. London: NICE.

National Institute for Clinical Excellence (2004a). *PTSD (Posttraumatic Stress Disorder): The management of PTSD in primary and secondary care (1st draft)*. London: NICE.

National Institute for Clinical Excellence (2004b). *Guidelines for the Short Term Physical and Psychological Management of Self Harm in Primary and Secondary Care*. London: NICE.

National Institute for Clinical Excellence (2004c). *Core Interventions in the Treatment and Management of Anorexia Nervosa, Bulimia Nervosa and Related Eating Disorders*. London: NICE.

National Institute for Health and Clinical Excellence (2005). *Depression in Children and Young People: identification and management in primary, community and secondary care*. London: NICE.

Nicholls, S., Cullen, R., O'Neill, S. & Halligan, A. (2000). Clinical governance: its origins and its foundations. *Clinical Performance and Quality Health Care*, **8** (3), 172–78.

Nursing and Midwifery Council (2004). *The NMC Code of Professional Conduct: standards for conduct, performance and ethics. Protecting the public through professional standards*. London: NMC.

Partridge, I., Richardson, G., Casswell, G. & Jones, N. (2003). Multi-disciplinary team working. In: Richardson, G. & Partridge, I. (Eds). *Child and Adolescent Mental Health Services, an operational Handbook*. London: Gaskell.

Richardson, G. (2003). Clinical governance. In: Richardson, G. & Partridge, I. (Eds). *Child and Adolescent Mental Health Services, an operational Handbook*. London: Gaskell.

Sainsbury Centre for Mental Health & National Institute for Mental Health in England (NIMHE) (2001). *Essential Shared Capabilities*. London: SCMH.

Scally, G. & Donaldson, L. (1998). Clinical governance and the drive for quality improvement in the new NHS in England. *British Medical Journal*, (317), 61–65.

Skuse, D. (Ed.) (2004). *Child Psychology and Psychiatry: an introduction*. London: The Medicine Publishing Company.

Street, C., Stapelkamp, C., Taylor, E., Malek, M. & Kurtz, Z. (2005). *Minority Voices: research into the access and acceptability of services for the mental health of young people from black and minority ethnic groups*. London: YoungMinds.

Street, C. & Svanberg, J. (2003). *Where Next?: new directions in in-patient mental health services for young people*. London: YoungMinds.

Street, C. & Herts, B. (2005). *Putting Participation into Practice: a guide for practitioners working in services to promote the mental health and well-being of children and young people*. London: YoungMinds.

Whittington, C., Kendal, T., Fonagy, P., Cottrell, D., Cotgrove, A. & Boddington, E. (2005). Selective serotonin reuptake inhibitors in childhood depression: systematic review of published versus unpublished data. *Lancet,* (363), 1341–45.

Williams, R. & Kerfoot, M. (2005). *Child and Adolescent Mental Health Services: strategy, planning, delivery an evaluation.* Oxford: Oxford University Press.

Wolpert, M., Tingay, K., Pakes, K. & Stein, S. (2000). *Routine Outcome Measures in a CAMH Service. Paper presented at Association of Child Psychology and Psychiatry Conference.* London: ACPP.

Chapter 16

Education, Training and Workforce Development for Nurses Working in CAMHS

Tim McDougall, Fiona Gale and Barry Nixon

Key points

- It is generally recognised that workforce pressures are key constraining factors in effective delivery of the NHS (National Health Service) plans and the CAMHS (child and adolescent mental health services) agenda.

- Nurses are the single largest professional group in specialist CAMHS and make up a quarter of the current workforce. Preregistration education and training programmes which adequately address child and adolescent mental health issues are lacking. However, the recent growth of multi-disciplinary postgraduate education and training programmes has meant that nurses are increasingly able to access courses to help equip them to work in specialist CAMHS.

- Children and young people, their families and carers, expect nurses to be safe and accountable practitioners. They expect that nurses are adequately trained and possess the necessary knowledge, skills, capabilities and competencies necessary to provide effective care and treatment.

- Nursing children and young people takes place in an interagency context. Education and training programmes should be multiprofessional and interdisciplinary and nurses should have education and training alongside their colleagues in health, education, social services and youth justice agencies.

- Local specialist CAMHS should be supported to create the resources to enable creative CPD (continuing professional development) solutions for all professionals including nurses. Wherever possible, local training activities should be multiprofessional, multiagency and involve practice placements across a range of services.

Introduction

It is generally recognised that workforce pressures are key constraining factors in effective delivery of the NHS plans and the CAMHS agenda. Nurses are the single largest professional group in specialist CAMHS and make up a quarter of the current workforce (Audit Commission 1999). Nurses in Tier 1 CAMHS come from a variety of professional backgrounds and are currently practising as children's nurses, school nurses, registered general nurses and health visitors. Several groups of nurses are working as autonomous practitioners in specialist CAMHS at Tiers 2, 3 and 4 (Leighton et al. 2001). Whilst most are mental health nurses, increasing numbers of children's nurses are entering the speciality, as well as smaller numbers of learning disability nurses (Jones 2004). An increasing number of nurses are also primary mental health workers, practising at the interface between universal first-contact services and specialist CAMHS (Gale et al. 2005).

This chapter is intended to describe the knowledge, skills, competencies and capabilities required of the CAMHS nursing workforce. The chapter is also intended to provide commissioners and providers of nurse education and training with outcome measures and a framework to help prepare nurses for safe and accountable practice in a range of CAMHS settings; it may also have relevance for managers who are charged with the recruitment, development and retention of their workforce. It is important to make clear from the outset that nursing children and young people with mental health problems takes place in an interagency context. The authors agree that education and training programmes should have common currency for nurses and other professionals, and should prepare them with the knowledge, skills and attitudes to work in a range of multidisciplinary and interagency settings. Current education and training programmes for nurses do not necessarily provide nurses with the knowledge, skills and competencies to understand, care for, or treat children and young people with mental health problems (McDougall 2004). In addition, branch programmes in adult, children's, mental health and learning disability nursing do not necessarily produce nurses who are fit for practice in CAMHS settings (Hooton 1999; RCN 2003).

There is currently no nationally recognised prerequisite training required of nurses to practice in CAMHS. As a result, several local and regional education and training programmes have evolved. Many of these training programmes are being modelled on the newly developed capability frameworks, and are currently being reviewed in the context of their fitness for purpose and impact on CAMHS service delivery. Various unpublished projects, initiatives and training analyses have attempted to define the skills and competencies required by nurses to work in specialist CAMHS. As well as attempting to address core competencies that have common currency across universal CAMHS, this chapter will also attempt to define some of the additional competencies, for nurses and other professional groups working in specialist CAMHS in health, education, social services and youth-justice settings. It will attempt to differentiate between working in universal or primary services and working in specialist CAMHS. Distinctions will also be made between working with different age-groups of children and young people.

Background: policy and workforce development

The importance for all professionals who work with children and adolescents to have a basic understanding of child and adolescent mental health is now widely acknowledged and well-documented (National Assembly for Wales 2001; Department for Education and Skills 2003; Public Health Institute for Scotland 2003; Department of Health 2004; NHS Education for Scotland 2004). Few would disagree that all professionals who are responsible for the health, education and welfare of children and young people should possess the knowledge, skills, competencies and capabilities needed to address the mental health needs of those for whom they are professionally responsible. A broad array of policy and practice guidance, strategy and public inquiries have set the context for a review of the training needs required by professionals working with children who have mental health problems. *Improvement, Expansion and Reform* (DoH 2002) identified a public service agreement (PSA) target for CAMHS which set the expectation that comprehensive CAMHS must be in place by 2006. Successful implementation of PSA targets set for CAMHS depends crucially on a comprehensive and competent workforce. In addition, the government's interdepartmental *Change for Children Programme: Every Child Matters* (DfES 2003) and the NSF (National Service Framework) for Children, Young People and Maternity Services (DoH 2004) each recommend that all child healthcare staff, including nurses, should have education and training to meet the mental health needs of children and young people in their care. In addition to key government policies, there have been a number of children's and mental health workforce strategies that have been important for nurses in CAMHS.

The Chief Nursing Officer (CNO) review of the nurses' midwives' and health visitors' contribution to vulnerable children (DoH 2004); the CNO reviews of mental health nursing underway in England and Scotland; and the CNO review of school nursing in England; all signal important roles for nurses in safeguarding children and young people which includes meeting their mental health needs. Professional organisations have also highlighted the important part that CAMHS nurses play in meeting the mental health needs of children and young people. The Royal College of Nursing (RCN) in particular has consistently attempted to raise the profile of CAMHS nursing and strengthen the nursing contribution to CAMHS. They have focused on preparing nurses to care for children and young people (RCN 2003); the post-registration education and training needs of nurses working with children and young people with mental health problems in the UK (RCN 2004); and making children and young people's mental health every nurse's business (RCN 2004).

Preparing the current and future workforce

More than 4 million people in England work with children, or support those working with children. This includes 2.4 million paid staff and 1.8 million unpaid staff and volunteers. The children's services workforce is diverse, with people entering at various stages in their lives, and includes workers who will have little or no specific training for working with children who have mental health problems. The needs of children and young people are different from those of adults. Nurses and other professionals will require particular skills, knowledge and competencies to meet these needs. Despite this, much education and training for nurses and other key professionals continues to neglect child and adolescent mental health (National Assembly for Wales 2001). The need to improve the experience and outcomes for children and young people has led to the development of various standards against which the quality of care being delivered and services themselves can be measured. At the time of writing this chapter, various competency frameworks are being developed, including the recently launched competency and capability framework for primary mental health workers in CAMHS (Gale et al. 2005). The development and implementation of this framework is discussed later in the chapter.

Before going further, it is worth exploring the links and differences between national service standards, occupational standards and competency frameworks. NSFs detail minimum standards at which service providers should be expected to operate. They are designed to ensure the protection of service users; to safeguard and promote the health, wellbeing and quality of life for service users; and to provide standards which are robust, measurable and enforceable. Education and training for nurses in CAMHS should be underpinned by occupational standards. These describe the best practice in particular areas of work and are statements of competence. Occupational standards can also be used as a tool for workforce management, and for specification tasks such as appraisal, personal development planning and performance management. National occupational standards for mental health have been published elsewhere (National Institute for Mental Health in England 2003). In addition, social care services currently have a variety of occupational standards relating to the care of children and young people (DfES 2003).

A competency framework broadly describes a range of work activities, which need to be carried out in order to achieve the objectives of part or all of an occupational sector or organisation. They usually cover the work activities which need to be undertaken to achieve a particular purpose and the quality standards to which the activities should be performed. Competencies do not refer to outstanding achievements or performances, but stipulate the basic requirements to deliver core interventions. Competency for the purposes of CAMHS nursing can be defined as the knowledge, skills and attitudes required to undertake the nursing role in CAMHS. Ensuring competency in nursing practice presents a particular challenge due to its potentially subjective nature. Competency requires knowledge, appropriate attitudes and observable skills, either practical or intellectual, which account for the delivery of specified tasks, interventions or services. Competency frameworks are increasingly being developed across children's services in health, social care and education (DfES 2003). Most of the generally accepted frameworks are based on a common principle that there is a need for a universal and generic service for all children and young people, and that the complexity of service-level provided will increase as does the child's need level. The Sainsbury Centre report, *The Capable Practitioner* (Sainsbury Centre 2001), introduced the concept of an increasingly specialised level of service and used it to provide a framework and list of practitioner capabilities required to implement the NSF for Mental Health (DoH 1999). The capability framework, summarised in the following section, combines the notion of the reflective practitioner with that of the effective practitioner. This framework may be useful in looking at the competencies needed by the workforce across sectors, responsible for delivering the NSF for Children, Young People and Maternity Services and *Change for Children Programme: Every Child Matters*.

Competencies, capabilities and occupational standards

The Sainsbury Centre (2001) suggests that a competency describes the level of expertise expected within a particular domain of capability. This is usually expressed through occupational standards and more clearly outlines the boundaries between the core and specialist skills of various professional and professionally non-affiliated groups. There is sometimes confusion about the relationship between occupational standards and competencies. The Sainsbury Centre report (2001) argues that the concept of capability can help by providing an organising framework which begins the process of describing the inputs, through curriculum development, to becoming competent; whereas occupational standards act as a performance measure of competence within the work environment. Indeed, national occupational standards define the level of performance required for the successful achievement of work expectations. They are described as benchmarks of workplace performance and can be used to ascertain and to determine fitness for practice (Storey 1998), as well as to assist employers in the recruitment, strategic planning, development and retention of the CAMHS workforce.

In order to look at the competency framework of a particular capability, the expected level of expertise within that particular domain of capability needs to be described. Competencies should be viewed in terms of a continuum, and from a variety of professional and organisational perspectives. In thinking about the development of core competencies in CAMHS it is acknowledged that not all professionals need them at the same level. For example, a Connexions worker will require basic understanding of mental health and knowledge of common mental health problems, whereas a more in-depth understanding will be required by a specialist nurse, psychologist or psychiatrist. It is generally agreed that education and training courses to enable nurses to develop capabilities should be multidisciplinary, modular and defined along pathways to competence. A variety of continuums for considering nursing competencies are currently available. Examples include the *Admiral Nurse's Competency Framework* (RCN 2002); the *Scottish Framework for Nursing in Schools* (Scottish Executive 2003); and a competency framework for acute in-patient mental health nurses (Evans & Spencer 2003). As nurses enter a particular speciality it is likely that they will become more knowledgeable and proficient in that area. It is acknowledged that different levels of capability are appropriate between the different service providers. For example, the knowledge that a school nurse may have of mental health problems and disorders will develop as their experience does. However it would be inappropriate for them to develop it to a level of, say, a nurse specialist working in a Tier 3 CAMHS.

A capability framework

A report published by the Social Exclusion Unit (2000) recommended that the government should improve the coordination of policies affecting children and families, improve services for young people and reduce social exclusion. As a result, a Cabinet Committee of Children and Young People's Services was established, the post of Minister for Children was created and the Children and Young People's Unit (CYPU) was set up. This was an interdepartmental group charged with linking up policies and strategies across government offices. In 2001 the CYPU published *Building a Strategy for Children and Young People* (DfES 2001). This set out proposed capabilities for those working with children, young people and their families or carers, and is consistent with workforce recommendations in the NSF for Children, Young People and Maternity Services (DoH 2004), the *Change for Children Programme: Every Child Matters* (DfES 2003) and the recently published youth Green Paper, *Youth Matters* (DfES 2005). The CYPU strategy proposed that these capabilities should help ensure that services are:

(1)   *Centred on the needs of the child or young person*: the best interests of the child or young person should be paramount, taking into account their wishes and feelings.

(2)   *High quality*: policies and services should aspire to reach high standards of quality for the benefit of the children and young people they serve.

(3)   *Family-orientated*: full recognition should be given to family members, including extended family members who contribute to the wellbeing of the child or young person.

(4)   *Equitable and non-discriminatory*: all children and young people should have access to the services they need, when they need them and in a way which respects diversity, equality and individuality.

(5)   *Inclusive*: policies and services should be sensitive to the individual needs and aspirations of every child and young person, taking full account of their race, ethnicity, gender, sexual orientation, and ability or disability.

(6)   *Empowering*: children and young people should be given the opportunity to play an effective role in the design and delivery of policies and services.

(7)   *Results-orientated and based on evidence*: high quality research, evaluation, monitoring and review should ensure that decisions that affect children and young people are well-informed.

(8)   *Coherent service design and delivery*: services should work together in a coherent, comprehensive and integrated way.

(9)   *Supportive and respectful*: policies and services should be delivered in a manner that is respectful and supportive of children and young people.

(10)   *Community-enhancing*: communities should be empowered to make positive changes for their children and young people, so that improvements can be owned and sustained locally.

CAMHS nurses: ten essential shared capabilities

Any capability model for those working with children, young people and their families in relation to issues of mental health should be considered alongside a number of other important overarching frameworks. These include the *Ten Essential Shared Capabilities* for the whole of the mental health workforce (NIMHE 2004) and the *Common Core of Skills and Knowledge for the Children's Workforce* (DfES). The development of essential capabilities for all mental health workers, including nurses, builds on the work of the Sainsbury Centre's *Capable Practitioner Framework*. This outlines the capabilities that all professionals should have as a minimum part of their basic training. These capabilities should form the core building blocks for the education, learning, teaching and training of all staff working in children and young people's services in the public, independent and voluntary sectors. The authors agree that the following capabilities (see list below) are fundamental and should form the bedrock for effective and high-quality nursing practice across all areas of CAMHS. However, the level of skills and competencies will of course vary depending on whether nurses work in mainstream or specialist CAMHS:

(1)   Working in partnership.
(2)   Respecting diversity.
(3)   Practising ethically.
(4)   Challenging inequality.
(5)   Promoting recovery.
(6)   Identifying people's needs and strengths.
(7)   Providing child and family-centred services.
(8)   Making a difference.
(9)   Promoting safety and positive risk-taking.
(10)   Personal development and learning.

Working in partnership

Partnership-working is part and parcel of modern nursing practice. A variety of creative approaches are needed if we are to improve participation and user-involvement, and enhance partnership working in CAMHS. Failure to place a child or young person, their family or carers firmly at the centre of the care and treatment we provide may lead to service users feeling stigmatised, excluded and lead to problems in engaging with CAMHS. A review of the research about engagement with children and young people in CAMHS concluded that interventions should generally be informed by choice and a determined effort to engage the child or young person and their family of carers at every stage of the assessment and treatment process (Griffiths 2003). Designing care and treatment interventions in collaboration with children and young people, their families and carers may do much to improve 'did-not-attend' (DNA) rates and demands on out-of-hours services (Mental Health Foundation 2002). All nurses should aim to develop and maintain constructive working relationships with children and young people, their families and carers. In addition, nurses increasingly work across a range of multidisciplinary and interagency teams and networks, and rarely practise in isolation from other children's service providers. This means that the need to strengthen links with their multidisciplinary and multiagency colleagues, and with wider children's and young people's service networks, is crucially important. All core training for nurses should facilitate skills for effective and creative partnership working.

Respecting diversity

Nurses practice in a diverse society and it is essential that they possess the knowledge, skills and attitudes to respect such diversity, provide choice and deliver child or young person-centred services. Through core education and training, nurses should be supported with the skills to meet the mental health needs of a diverse group of children, families and carers. This is in terms of ensuring that nursing interventions are appropriate to the child or young person's age, race, culture, disability, gender, spirituality and sexuality. By respecting diversity, nurses can help contribute to flexible and responsive services where children and young people, their families and carers can enjoy ready access and make meaningful choices about the mental healthcare and treatment interventions they receive.

Practising ethically

In order to practise ethically and fulfil their professional obligations, nurses must be able to recognise the rights and responsibilities of service users and their families and carers. This requires them to recognise and acknowledge power differentials and minimise them whenever possible. Nurses are accountable for all nursing care and treatment that they provide to service users and carers (Nursing and Midwifery Council 2004). Wherever possible, nursing interventions should be evidence based, and nurses should be able to demonstrate the knowledge, skills and attitudes to use research and evidence to inform their practice. It is essential that nurses understand their professional duties in relation to confidentiality, consent and the rights of children and parents in the context of providing mental health services for children and young people. It is incumbent on nurses who work with children and young people who have mental health problems and disorders to provide interventions that are lawful. This means that they must have a good understanding of children's legislation and mental health law, and must know how to interpret the relevant provisions of these legal frameworks in their daily nursing practice.

Challenging inequality

It is generally agreed that social adversity is both a contributory and maintaining factor in childhood mental disorders (Social Exclusion Unit 2004). Addressing the causes and consequences of stigma, discrimination, social inequity and exclusion on children, young people, their families and carers is fundamental to the prevention of mental ill-health. Helping to create, develop and maintain valued social roles for children, young people and their families is essential to the mental health prevention agenda, and an important part of social inclusion, recovery and normalisation for those who are already receiving mental health services. As well as skills and competencies to ensure their individual nursing practice is not oppressive, discriminatory or prejudiced, nurses also share a responsibility for challenging attitudes and practices within their service or agency settings which may serve to exclude particular groups of children or young people on the grounds of their age, race, culture, disability, gender, religion, spirituality or sexuality. Particular groups of children and young people have previously received a poor CAMHS service. As well as minority ethnic groups (Mental Health Act Commission 2004), young people aged 16 and 17, and those with a learning disability or pervasive developmental disorder have previously been excluded and marginalised, with CAMHS being at best patchy and variable. Challenging inequality is no straightforward task. Nurses, like all children's professionals, will need to be supported through education and training to develop the skills to help challenge inequality in CAMHS effectively.

Promoting recovery

It is essential that nurses are supported to work in partnership to provide care and treatment that enables children and young people, their families and carers to tackle mental health problems with hope and optimism. By assisting young people to work towards a valued lifestyle within and beyond the limits of their mental health problems, nurses can help enhance the social functioning, inclusion and overall quality of life for children and young people with mental health problems. To do this effectively, nurses must provide children, young people and their families with appropriate psychoeducational support to manage transitions, to access services and to utilise support systems to sustain recovery and prevent relapse.

Identifying people's needs and strengths

Working in partnership to gather information to agree health and social care needs in the context of the preferred lifestyle and aspirations of service users and their families, carers and friends, is at the heart of child and young person-centred care and treatment. Since the core business of CAMHS is to develop mental health and psychological wellbeing, prevent mental disorder and provide support when children and young people suffer mental health problems and disorders, it is essential that nurses can recognise and build on strengths and resilience factors in the child or young person, their family or carers. Core education and training should help equip nurses with the knowledge, skills and attitudes to comprehensively and sensitively identify young people's needs and strengths.

Providing child and family-centred services

Negotiating meaningful and achievable goals is fundamental to successful assessment and treatment and is essential from the perspective of service users and their families. Nurses must be supported to identify treatment outcomes for children and young people, their families or carers. To do this systematically, they must develop the skills and competencies to assess, plan, implement and evaluate intervention or treatment goals alongside service users and their families.

Making a difference

Nurses are highly valued and trusted by service users (Healthcare Commission 2005). Facilitating access to and delivering the best quality, evidence-based, values-based health and social care interventions to meet the needs and aspirations of service users and their families is central to the role of nursing in CAMHS.

Promoting safety and positive risk-taking

Depending on the age, maturity and understanding of young people, promoting safety and therapeutic risk-taking requires nurses to empower children and young people and their families and carers. This includes working with the tension between promoting safety and positive risk-taking.

Personal development and learning

Keeping up-to-date with changes in practice and taking part in personal development through supervision, appraisal and reflective practice is essential for nurses to remain on the professional register (Nursing and Midwifery Council 2004).

A competency framework for children's services

The children's competency framework forms part of a series commissioned by the Department of Health in England. The Children's Skills and Competency Framework was developed by the government's Children Care Group Workforce Team (CGWT). The CGWT's strategic aim is to support service-improvement for children, young people and expectant mothers through integrated workforce-planning and development across health, social care and education agencies. Its desired strategic outcome is to see more staff working in different ways to deliver quality person-centred care to children, young people and expectant mothers. The CGWT covers all health and social care services to children from birth to transition to adult services. This Children CGWT and Skills for Health has identified a range of work activities, quality standards and core competencies required to deliver safe and effective children's services. These have been designed to span professional boundaries, organisations and locations, and to be child-focused and based on the best available evidence. At the time of writing, this framework covers the competencies for working with acutely ill children and children at risk of significant harm. However, the competencies are also intended to be applicable to a range of settings and professional groups and are related to:

- Communication.
- Assessing health and wellbeing needs.
- Improving health and wellbeing.
- Safeguarding children and young people from harm.
- Supporting children, young people and their family and friends during change and difficult situations.
- Care for expecting and new parents and families, and their babies.
- Provision of support services for the delivery of care for children and young people.
- Personal and people development.
- Health, safety and security.
- Service development.
- Equality, diversity and rights.
- Production and communication of information.
- Partnership.
- Management of people.
- Management of physical and financial resources.
- Research and development.

Common core skills, knowledge and competencies

The *Common Core of Skills and Knowledge* prospectus sets out the basic skills and knowledge needed for the children's mental health workforce to work together effectively in the best interests of the child. The Green Paper, *Every Child Matters* proposed the implementation of a common core of skills, knowledge and competence for the 'widest possible range of workers in children's services' (DfES 2003). This proposal drew on earlier work which suggested that a common core of skills, knowledge and competence would support the development of more effective and integrated services; introduce a common language amongst professionals and support staff; and start the process of breaking down some of the cultural and practice barriers that have previously failed children. Allied to a single framework of qualifications, this would also promote a more flexible development of career progression within the children's workforce. The *Common Core* prospectus outlines the skills and knowledge that nurses and all other practitioners working with children and young people should possess. Its aim is to ensure that those working with children and young people demonstrate that they are doing so with a shared set of knowledge, skills and behaviours. These relate to effective communication with children and young people; child and young person development; safeguarding and promoting the welfare of the child; supporting transitions; multiagency working; and sharing information. It is anticipated that many nurses in the children's mental health workforce will already have a range of skills and knowledge contained in this common core. However some may not and may need additional training and support to enable them to develop the baseline level. Although the following capabilities are not exhaustive, the following range of skills, knowledge and competence can be described as essential for CAMHS nurses and are described below.

Core capabilities for all nurses and other professionals who work with children

Understanding mental health and psychological wellbeing

All nurses who have a responsibility for the mental health and psychological wellbeing of children and young people should be capable of understanding how mental health and emotional wellbeing relates to children, young people and their families or carers. Education and training should promote understanding of the different approaches for those with physical and mental health difficulties. Nurses and other professionals should be able to recognise and understand a wide range of different behaviours and know when to ask for assistance from colleagues in specialist CAMHS. As a minimum, education and training for nurses to understand issues in relation to mental health and psychological wellbeing should include opportunities to develop the awareness, knowledge, skills, attitudes and strategies in relation to the criteria in Box 16.1.

For nurses working with children and young people in specialist CAMHS, a systematic and critical understanding of child and adolescent developmental theories, including a critical overview of notions of 'normal' development, is

Box 16.1   Mental health and psychological wellbeing.

- Biopsychosocial development of children and young people.
- Factors and processes that promote positive mental health and wellbeing.
- Risk and resilience factors in relation to the mental health and emotional wellbeing of children, young people and their families.
- The family as a concept and a system, and its influences and dynamics on the child or adolescent.
- Reflect the nurse's own childhood, adolescence and family life and their own values regarding particular life stages, and the impact this has on the nurse's work with children, young people and families.

of fundamental importance. This is alongside a comprehensive and critical understanding of childhood mental health disorders and the experience of mental distress in children and young people. To provide competent care and treatment interventions, nurses should be able to analyse critically and use the knowledge base of the range of factors that influence the mental health of children and young people in care-planning, and service delivery and evaluation. This will require a good overview of the evidence base and range of therapeutic interventions used to assess, treat and care for children and young people with mental health problems and disorders.

Mental health promotion, illness prevention and early intervention

The NSF for Children, Young People and Maternity Services states that within primary level services, those in contact with children need to be able to have sufficient knowledge of children's mental health to identify those who need help; to offer advice and support to those with mild or minor problems; and to have sufficient knowledge of specialist services to be able to refer on appropriately when necessary (DoH 2004). All nurses should possess the knowledge, skills and attitudes relevant to mental health-promotion, education, prevention and early intervention strategies for child and adolescent mental health (DoH 2004). They should be able to recognise the factors that lead to good mental health and psychological wellbeing. Nurses should also know how to help children develop resilience and develop positive strategies to cope in the face of stress and adversity. As a minimum, their education and training should include opportunities to develop the awareness, knowledge, skills, attitudes and strategies to achieve the aims in Box 16.2.

Communication

All nurses should have an understanding of appropriate communication strategies with children, adolescents and their families, as well as carers, community members and other children's professionals. This should include skills for engaging, motivating, listening and reflecting during assessment and treatment with children and young people. Communicating at a level which is

Box 16.2 Mental health promotion and early intervention.

- Promote mental health at various levels of intervention (individual, family or group and community, within the relevant cultural or ethnic context).
- Promote the emotional health of children, young people and families in the community.
- Raise awareness of issues affecting children's mental health and promote ideas about child mental health and its effect on resilience.
- Liaise with health promotion workers and help develop community-based mental health promotion programmes.
- Identify universal and targeted clinical interventions.
- Identify and appropriately apply knowledge about vulnerability and risk of the development of child mental health problems by developing targeted programmes.
- Identify gaps in the provision of services for children and young people at risk of mental health difficulties and their families.

Box 16.3 Communication strategies.

- Engage and motivate children, young people and their families in order to facilitate access to appropriate services to meet their mental health needs.
- Listen and understand effectively.
- Apply a range of engagement–negotiation models which respect autonomy and promote a child - or young person-centred approach.
- Provide effective liaison and consultation to a range of professionals and agencies involved in the child or young person's care.
- Create an appropriate therapeutic setting for the child or young person, their families or carers to engage in assessment or treatment.

appropriate to the child or young person's age, development and understanding requires nurses to have a broad range of communication skills and strategies. As a minimum, communication skills for nurses working with children and young people with mental health problems should be based on the awareness, knowledge, skills, attitudes and strategies in Box 16.3.

Understanding mental ill-health

All nurses should be able to assess the mental health needs of children, young people and their families or carers. This should include the ability to recognise mental ill-health and mental health problems and disorders. As a minimum, education and training for nurses to fulfil this capability should include opportunities to develop awareness, knowledge, skills, attitudes and strategies in relation to the criteria in Box 16.4.

Knowledge of current legislation and policy

Nurses in CAMHS must keep up pace with the changing face of service provision, legislation and best practice as it affects children and young people. All nurses should have knowledge of relevant legislation and the national policy

Box 16.4 Understanding mental ill-health.

- Early identification of mental health problems in children and young people.
- Factors and processes that can lead to mental ill-health.
- Diagnosis of mental illness and its stigma, especially as they relate to children and young people.
- The various models of understanding mental health and illness (e.g. the medical perspective, social perspective).
- Child and adolescent psychiatric disorders and skills to assess needs and identify appropriate ways to meet these needs.
- Transition needs of children and young people with mental health needs (e.g. from CAMHS to adult mental health, access at different tiers, out-patient to in-patient) and skills to liaise and coordinate services to facilitate smooth transitions between episodes of care.
- The nurse's own values and attitudes about, and models for understanding, mental ill-health and how this impacts on the nurse's own practice.

Box 16.5 Legislation and policy.

- Childcare law (see Children Acts 1989 and 2004) and the mental health act legislation.
- Current developments in terms of policy and strategy relevant to multiagency, comprehensive CAMHS provision.
- Translating and implementing legal and strategic frameworks in order to help delivery comprehensive CAMHS.
- Relevant policy developments in health, education, social services that have an impact on CAMHS provision. For example, disability, race relations, youth offending, fostering and adoption, domestic violence etc.

---

context for multiagency comprehensive CAMHS, and how this applies to their professional practice and organisation in which they work. They should understand and know how to use policies and procedures in relation to safeguarding children, consent to treatment, confidentiality and information-sharing. This means that their core education and training should facilitate learning in relation to the legislation and policies in Box 16.5.

Knowledge about children's and young people's services

It is important that CAMHS nurses understand the strategic context in which they work. A better understanding of strategy enables nurses to recognise that their colleagues in education, social services and youth justice often have different pressures and targets to work towards. Nurses must factor this into their multiagency working relationships to avoid parochialism and bunker mentality. All nurses should have knowledge of services provided to children by health, social services, education, youth justice and the voluntary sector. In order to work effectively across professional boundaries, nurses must understand the role, purpose, function, values and limitations of all agencies that provide services for children and young people. At an individual professional

Box 16.6   Service provision.

- Knowledge of local multiagency comprehensive CAMHS, what is provided and how, to whom and accessing the services.
- Ability to assess level of mental health need and identify the appropriate services and level required to meet those needs.
- When it is appropriate to work across boundaries to develop a coordinated response to children and young people's mental health between agencies, and within professional and clinical governance boundaries.

level, nurses should understand the different professional roles and ways of working in multiagency CAMHS. They should also be aware of, and knowledgeable about, different cultures, values and beliefs when working with other agencies (Leighton et al. 2001). This is in order to work collaboratively, overcome the barriers to effective joint-working and avoid 'us and them' discussions. As a minimum, their education and training should address the points in Box 16.6.

For nurses working in specialist CAMHS, their understanding of the multiagency context in which services are commissioned, planned and delivered needs to be more sophisticated. A systematic understanding of the matrix of service delivery in CAMHS will require an in-depth and critical awareness of the nature of multiprofessional and interagency working. This should be underpinned by a critical understanding and knowledge of the legal, ethical and moral issues with regard to practice in multiagency CAMHS.

Understanding the context and impact of socioeconomic, cultural, ethnic and gender issues

All nurses should have an understanding of the context and impact of socioeconomic, cultural, ethnic and gender issues on the mental health of children, adolescents and their families. They should have knowledge about equality and diversity to ensure that their practice, and the services in which they work, do not exclude or discriminate against any group of young people on the basis of their ethnicity and culture, or gender or disability (see Box 16.7). This is to help ensure that services are respectful and non-stigmatising.

Improving access to CAMHS

Improving access to comprehensive CAMHS for all children and young people who require them is an integral part of the wider children's services modernisation agenda. The 2003 follow-up to the Office for National Statistics (ONS) survey showed that almost one-third of parents of children with mental health problems had not sought help because they feared being blamed or seen as a failure (Meltzer et al. 2003). Through their core education and training, all nurses should have opportunities to develop their awareness, knowledge, skills, attitudes and strategies in relation to the identification, assessment, intervention

Box 16.7   Socioeconomic, cultural, ethnic and gender issues.

- Social inequalities and social exclusion and how these affect mental health and other developmental processes.
- Differences in terms of access to resources and opportunities according to socioeconomic status.
- Engaging children, young people and families from black and minority ethnic groups.
- Engaging children and young people from vulnerable groups, ensuring the promotion of social inclusion (e.g. young offenders, looked-after children, those with learning disabilities etc.).
- Enhancing accessibility and equity for children and families to comprehensive CAMHS, especially those who would not ordinarily have opportunities to seek help from statutory and non-statutory agencies (for example, asylum seekers, refugees and homeless families etc.).
- Reflecting on how one's own biases relating to issues of socioeconomic, cultural, ethnic and gender issues impact on one's own practice.

Box 16.8   Improving access.

- A range of appropriate assessment, identification and screening tools.
- Different treatment strategies in primary, secondary and specialist CAMHS.
- Knowledge of the referral system and ability to make appropriate referrals on behalf of the child or young person, their families and carers.
- Planning interventions appropriate to the nurse's level of knowledge, skills and experience, and the availability of support.
- A range of techniques to intervene with children, young people and their families in a variety of ways appropriate to the nurse's level of work (e.g. behavioural programmes, anxiety-management programmes, CBT; setting up and running parenting programmes; basic counselling skills; brief psychotherapy; solution-focused approaches, etc.).
- Direct work with children and young people, their families and carers according to their identified mental health needs.
- Ensuring that children and young people can access the level of service provision and therapeutic intervention relevant to their mental health need.
- Identifying opportunities for providing a direct service to children and young people and their families, in an accessible and least stigmatising environment.
- Assessing when to intervene and in what situations it is not appropriate to intervene and ability to justify action taken.

and referral strategies for children and young people, their families and carers and communities as they relate to mental health and emotional wellbeing. As a minimum, their core education and training should include opportunities to develop the awareness, knowledge, skills, attitudes and strategies in relation to the situations in Box 16.8.

Strategic problem-solving and care-planning

All nurses should understand assessment frameworks and develop aware-ness of the law, code of professional conduct and other guidance applicable to information-sharing. Their core education and training should enable nurses to:

- Demonstrate knowledge and skills to anticipate and identify challenges to delivery of CAMHS, and develop strategies for creative problem solving and local solutions.
- Demonstrate knowledge and skills to plan, implement and critically evaluate nursing interventions with children and young people with mental health problems and disorders.

Challenging inequality

A key theme which runs through the government's *Change for Children Programme: Every Child Matters* and the NSF for Children, Young People and Maternity Services is the need to reduce inequalities in access to appropriate healthcare services. Working with diversity, providing choice and delivering child or young person-centred services is a core function of modern nursing care. Concepts of mental health and illness, and beliefs about the origins of mental health problems in children and young people vary across cultures. All nurses working in CAMHS need to be sensitive to the particular needs of children and young people from minority ethnic groups. Developing competence in nursing practice is not only about culturally sensitive care and treatment, but also includes a broad range of activities including collaboration, administration and service planning (Malek & Joughin 2004). As a minimum, education and training within this area should include opportunities to develop the awareness, knowledge, skills, attitudes and strategies in relation to inequality (see Box 16.9).

Box 16.9 Challenging inequality.

- Demonstrate knowledge and skills to establish and maintain dialogue with regard to difference and diversity in terms of age, race, culture, disability, gender, religion, spirituality and sexuality.
- Demonstrate knowledge, skills and attitudes for working in partnership with children and young people, their families and carers to provide nursing care and treatment interventions which respect and value diversity.
- Demonstrate knowledge of causes and consequences of stigma, discrimination, social inequality and exclusion as it impacts on the mental health and psychological development of children and young people.
- Demonstrate knowledge in relation to the context and impact of socioeconomic, cultural, ethnic and gender issues on children and young people, their families and carers.
- Demonstrate knowledge about differences and power inequalities between communities and groups who may be socially excluded.
- Demonstrate the knowledge and skills to create, implement and evaluate strategies to enable children and young people to adopt and maintain valued social roles, which promote and sustain their mental health and psychological wellbeing.
- Demonstrate knowledge, skills and attitudes to engage in active dialogue with minority ethnic groups and local communities.
- Demonstrate knowledge, skills and attitudes to engage in reflective practice to recognise and address personal, service and agency biases in relation to socioeconomic, cultural, ethnic and gender issues.

Recovery and rehabilitation

Working in partnership with children and young people and their families and carers is essential if nurses are to promote recovery and rehabilitation and enhance social functioning and quality of life. To do this effectively, nurses should be able to:

- Demonstrate knowledge and skills to enable children and young people, their families and carers to manage transitions and access aftercare services.
- Demonstrate knowledge and skills to identify appropriate community-based support and aftercare systems.
- Demonstrate knowledge and skills to provide effective psychoeducation and family support interventions.

Safety and positive risk-taking

Education and training in this area should focus on understanding protocols for promoting and safeguarding the welfare of children and young people, knowing who to contact to express concerns, understanding protective factors and understanding how children and young people themselves manage risk. As a minimum, nurses should be able to:

- Demonstrate the knowledge and skills to safeguard and protect the safety and welfare of children and young people, in line with the requirements of the Children Act 2004.
- Demonstrate the knowledge, skills and strategies to recognise, identify and assess risk factors.
- Demonstrate the knowledge and skills to develop effective risk-management strategies with other professionals and agencies, as well as with children and young people, their families and carers.
- Demonstrate the knowledge, skills and attitudes to promote safe practice for themselves and others.

Continuing professional development

CPD and continued learning are necessary for nurses to remain on the professional register (Nursing and Midwifery Council 2004). Keeping up-to-date with changes in practice and participating in lifelong learning involves personal and professional development for nurses and their colleagues through supervision, appraisal and reflective practice. It is also an essential part of the CAMHS clinical governance agenda and the service quality framework within which nurses practice (Leighton et al. 2001). Nurses working in specialist CAMHS should be required to fulfil their CPD requirements in a systematic and transparent way. All nurses who work in CAMHS should be able to:

- Demonstrate awareness, knowledge, skills and attitudes to reflect on nursing practice and to identify strengths and weaknesses in their own practice.
- Demonstrate knowledge and skills to evaluate personal and professional development needs in relation to the needs of CAMHS provision and the organisation within which they work.

Age-related core capabilities

Many of the skills required by nurses working with infants, pre-school or primary school children will be different to those needed by nurses who work with adolescents or young adults. Indeed, the Children's Commissioner for England, Al Aynsley-Green once famously suggested that there is no such thing as a child. By this he meant that there are seven stages of childhood: the fetus, the neonate, the infant, the preschool child, the school age child, the adolescent and the transition to adulthood. To meet the mental health needs of children at different ages, nurses should have a good understanding of developmental theory and of physical, psychological and social developmental milestones. They should also understand the impact of trauma and adversity, abuse and other acute or chronic life stresses on the development and mediation of mental health and illness in children of different ages. There are a number of specific capabilities that nurses working with particular age groups should possess.

Working with expectant parents and their infants

Pregnancy brings many emotional, physical and social changes for the mother, her partner and the rest of the family. While many women and their families find pregnancy and the addition of a new member to their family joyous, some do not experience this period of change as positive and may undergo severe biopsychosocial distress (Currid 2004). The perinatal period, from conception until two years after childbirth, places the mother at heightened risk of mental health problems, including postnatal depression (Royal College of Psychiatrists 2000). For nurses working with expectant parents and preschool children, knowledge of prebirth development and factors that impact on the perinatal period are of central importance. This is to help promote the physical, social and emotional development of babies and infants. As a minimum, capabilities to work with expectant parents and infants should address the criteria in Box 16.10.

Working with children from birth to four years-old

For nurses who work with children during the early years it is important to understand the needs of infants as well as the role of the parental relationship and the impact of this on the development of the child. Nurses will also need to understand the processes involved in parenting, the needs of parents and

Box 16.10 Working with expectant parents.

- An understanding of the development of the unborn child (e.g. understanding the nature/nurture debate and developmental phases of the fetus).
- An understanding of the impact of the expectant mother and the environment on the development of the unborn child (e.g. knowledge of the impact of the mother's health and mental health on the unborn child, and knowledge of other environmental issues such as drug or alcohol use and stress, that can impact on the health of the unborn child).
- A knowledge of the stages of pregnancy.
- Understanding the impact the process of birth has on the mother and those in her environment (father, siblings, grandparents, etc.) and the impact this has on the baby.
- Understanding the importance of the relationship between mother and child through attachment, mothering and nurturing.
- Understanding the role of the father and others in the environment and understanding the impact of the birth process on the family and carers.
- Understanding the process of adjustment to motherhood (e.g. issues associated with loneliness, dependency, self-esteem, tiredness, body image, expectations, and role-change).
- The knowledge and skills to identify those mothers and fathers during the antenatal period who may be vulnerable themselves to mental health problems or disorders during the postnatal period.
- The knowledge and skills to identify carers who are at risk or vulnerable.
- The ability to intervene in an appropriate manner to prevent carer-vulnerability from impacting on the child.
- The identification of other risk factors in the environment that may put the unborn child at risk (for example socioeconomic factors; or the impact of premature birth on the infant).

the impact of parenting on the development of the child. Education and training programmes to help prepare nurses to meet the mental health needs of children during the early years should address key aspects of attachment theory, the development of parent–child relationships and normal expected milestones in relation to physical, psychological and social functioning. As a minimum, education and training for nurses to work with infants and their parents or carers should include the criteria in Box 16.11.

Working with primary school-aged children

For nurses working with children aged between 5 and 11 years, an understanding of the role of the school and the family in the development of the child becomes increasingly important. An understanding of the development, purpose and function of social and peer relationships, and the beginning of independence and separation from the child's family or carers is also essential. In relation to children within their families, an understanding of the impact of siblings, sibling relationships, birth position, single parenthood and the different sorts of family and kinship structures, is crucially important in understanding mental health risk and resilience factors. Life-events affect children differently according to their age, and the nature and degree of supportive and protective

Box 16.11   Working with babies and infants.

- Understanding issues related to attachment, bonding and 'good-enough' parenting.
- Understanding the impact of the mother's mental health on attachment and the development of the child.
- An ability to identify different parenting styles.
- An ability to specify how different parenting styles may affect the infant or child's wellbeing and problem behaviours, and their impact on the child's development.
- An understanding of the impact of the parent's parenting experience on their parenting i.e. understanding of cycles of behaviour across generations.
- Understanding the impact of issues related to parents' own lives on the development of the child e.g. any parental mental illness, drugs and alcohol use, domestic violence.
- An ability to reflect on how the nurse's own biases due to culture, socioeconomic status, etc., impact on perceptions of good and bad parenting.

factors. Not only do separations, bereavements, disruption, abuse and trauma affect some children more than others, parents too vary in their abilities to contain, support and effectively manage their children as they grow up and approach adolescence.

Working with young people aged between 12 and 16 years

During the adolescent period, the role of friends and the influence of the media becomes increasingly important. Nurses working with this age-group should have knowledge of the 'peer group' as a concept and its positive and negative influences on the young person's mental health and emotional resilience. They should also understand the nature of exploratory and risk-taking behaviours, and be able to recognise and help develop factors and influences that may be protective during the teenage years (see Box 16.12).

Box 16.12   Working with adolescents.

- Understanding the concept of the peer group and its role in adolescent development.
- Understanding how mental healthcare providers can make use of the strengths within the peer group to support the adolescent.
- Identifying different peer settings and their impact on the adolescent's emotional wellbeing and problem behaviours.
- Understanding the concept of exploratory behaviours, risk behaviours and resilience and protective factors in the context of biopsychosocial development.
- Developing skills in recognising risk factors.
- Developing skills in applying a resilience-based framework to the nurse's work setting.
- Applying a resilience-based framework to preventive interventions at community-level, taking into account the ethical limits of this concept.
- Clarifying the nurse's own attitudes towards young people demonstrating exploratory or risk-taking behaviours.

Nursing in specialist CAMHS

The majority of this chapter has focused on the education and training needs of nurses in non-specialist CAMHS. Only a few years ago, nurses experienced significant difficulty in accessing education and training opportunities to prepare them for work in specialist CAMHS (Royal College of Nursing 1998; McDougall 2000; Townley 2002). However, there is now evidence that this picture is changing. A growing number of higher education institutions (HEIs) are delivering multidisciplinary CAMHS training, accessible to nurses and other professionals, and it is now generally agreed that specialist CAMHS training should be multiprofessional and multiagency-based (Jones 2003). The quality of the former ENB 603, a so-called specialist CAMHS training award for many years, was highly variable (Symington 1997; Heimann 2000) and is now considered to be inadequate in meeting the training needs required to work in modern multiagency CAMHS (Joughin 2000). It has been replaced by a growing number of multiprofessional postgraduate certificates, diplomas, degrees and higher-degree CAMHS courses, accessible to nurses alongside their CAMHS colleagues. Many of these courses have their origins in CAMHS primary mental-health worker training (Gale 2003) and provide a sound bed-rock for specialist CAMHS nursing. However, additional competencies need to be developed for nurses to assess and treat children and young people with complex, severe or persistent mental health problems and disorders. Although these competencies could be developed in the practice setting, systems for appraisal, preceptorship, supervision, and CPD for nurses in specialist CAMHS are currently poorly defined and under-utilised in terms of their potential to improve education and training opportunities.

Nurses who work in advanced, specialist or expert roles in CAMHS must possess advanced, specialist or expert practice knowledge, skills and competencies. Education and training should be provided by higher education institutions and academic centres, and the role and profile of lecturer–practitioners and link tutors should be maximised, in order to support CAMHS nurses in linking theory and practice. Locally-provided education and training is currently patchy and not universally recognised as valid and beneficial in terms of service quality. Many nurses who work with children have broad-based experience, which enhances the service they can offer children, their families and carers. However, currently there exists no process to translate relevant experience into academic currency. A flexible system to accredit and validate prior learning by nurses who want to work in specialist CAMHS should be developed. In addition, all nurses who enter specialist CAMHS should have access to a period of supervised practice. This should be similar in structure and process to that of preceptorship and should be competency based.

Nurses are in key positions to receive and provide education and training from and to their CAMHS colleagues. Indeed, specialist CAMHS nurses are often involved in teaching and training other professionals in relation to mental health and disorders (McDougall 2000; McDougall 2003). A range of teaching and learning strategies should be available to enable CAMHS nurses to access creative training solutions. A coherent career pathway for nurses in specialist CAMHS should be defined. This should be flexible enough for nurses to embrace new ways of working and develop advanced and specialist roles. A CAMHS nursing recruitment, retention and career framework strategy should also be developed.

Conclusion

Children, their families and carers expect nurses to be safe and accountable practitioners. They expect that nurses, like all other professionals, are adequately trained and possess the necessary skills, competencies and knowledge to provide effective care and treatment. It is now widely recognised and acknowledged that the development of a competent and capable children's workforce must be a long-term strategy. Education and training for nurses who work with children must be consistent with the wider children's workforce strategy. CAMHS nurse education and training should be commissioned and provided and evaluated in an interagency context. Wherever possible, education and training to prepare nurses to work in specialist CAMHS should fit seamlessly with broader children and young people's workforce training initiatives. Workforce development in CAMHS is not only about skills and competencies, but also about creating a shared understanding, shared vision and effective partnerships.

References

Audit Commission (1999). *Children in Mind: child and adolescent mental health services.* Oxford: Audit Commission.

Currid, T. (2004). Improving perinatal mental health care. *Nursing Standard*, **19** (3), 40–43.

Department for Education and Skills (2003). *Every Child Matters.* London: HMSO.

Department for Education and Skills (2005). *Youth Matters.* London: The Stationery Office.

Department of Health (1999). *National Service Framework for Mental Health.* London: HMSO.

Department of Health (2004). *National Service Framework for Children, Young People and Maternity Services.* London: HMSO.

Department of Health (2005b). *National Child and Adolescent Mental Health Service Mapping Exercise.* London: HMSO.

Durlak, J. & Wells, A. (1997). Primary prevention mental health programmes for children and adolescents: a meta-analytic review. *American Journal of Community Psychology*, **25** (2), 115–152.

Evans, R. & Spencer, J. (2003). Developing a clinical competency framework for acute inpatient mental health nurses. *Mental Health Practice*, **6** (5), 33–37.

Gale, F. (2003). When tiers are not enough: developing the role of the child primary mental health worker. *Child and Adolescent Mental Health in Primary Care*, **1** (1), 5–8.

Gale, F., Hassett, A., & Sebuliba, D. (2005). *The Competency and Capability Framework for Primary Mental Health Workers in Child and Adolescent Mental Health Services (CAMHS)*. London: National CAMHS Support Service.

Griffiths, M. (2003). Terms of engagement: reaching hard to reach adolescents. *Young Minds Magazine*, (62), 23.

Healthcare Commission (2005). *Survey of Users 2005: mental health services*. London: Commission for Healthcare Audit and Inspection.

Heimann, M. (2000). The nurse's role in the multi-disciplinary team. In: FOCUS (2000). *Practice and Potential in Child and Adolescent Mental Health: a conference for nurses (conference proceedings)*. London: Royal College of Psychiatrist's Research Unit.

Jones, J. (2004). *The Post-registration Education and Training Needs of Nurses Working with Children and Young People with Mental Health Problems in the UK: a research study conducted by the Mental Health Programme, Royal College of Nursing Institute, in collaboration with the RCN Children and Young People's Mental Health Forum*. London: RCN Institute.

Jones, N. (2003). Training. In: *Child and Adolescent Mental Health Services: an operational handbook*. London: Gaskell.

Joughin, C. (2000). The nurse's role in the multi-disciplinary team. In: FOCUS. (2000). *Practice and Potential in Child and Adolescent Mental Health: a conference for nurses (conference proceedings)*. London: Royal College of Psychiatrist's Research Unit.

Leighton, S., Smith, C., Minns, K. & Crawford, P. (2001). Specialist child and adolescent mental health nurses: a force to be reckoned with? *Mental Health Practice*, **5** (2), 8–13.

McDougall, T. (2000). The role of the nurse specialist in raising the profile of children's mental health. *Nursing Times*, **96** (28), 37–38.

McDougall, T. (2003). Nurse consultants: children's champions. *Mental Health Practice*, **6** (9), 34–36.

Malek, M. & Joughin, C. (2004) *Mental Health Services for Minority Ethnic Children and Adolescents*. London: Jessica Kingsley.

Meltzer, H., Gatward, R., Corbin, T., Goodman, R. & Ford, T. (2003). *Persistence, onset, risk factors and outcomes of childhood mental disorders*. London: HMSO.

Mental Health Act Commission (2004). *Safeguarding Children and Adolescents Detained under the Mental Health Act 1983 on Adult Psychiatric Wards*. Nottingham: MHAC.

Mental Health Foundation (2002). *Turned Upside Down: developing community-based crisis services for 16–25 year-olds experiencing a mental health crisis*. London: Mental Health Foundation.

National Assembly for Wales (2001). *Child and Adolescent Mental Health Strategy: everybody's business*. Cardiff: National Assembly for Wales.

National Assembly for Wales (2001). *Everybody's Business: improving mental health in Wales – a CAMHS strategy*. Cardiff: National Assembly for Wales.

National Institute for Mental Health in England (2003). *Raising the Standards: national occupational standards: what they mean for you as a practitioner, manager, leader or HR personnel*. London: NIMHE.

National Institute for Mental Health in England (2004). *The Ten Essential Shared Capabilities: a framework for the whole of the mental health workforce*. London: HMSO.

NHS Education for Scotland (2004). *Promoting the Well-being and Meeting the Mental Health Needs of Children and Young People: a development framework for communities, agencies and specialists involved in supporting children, young people and their families*. Edinburgh: NHS Education for Scotland.

Nursing and Midwifery Council (2004). *The NMC Code of Professional Conduct: standards for conduct, performance and ethics. Protecting the public through professional standards.* London. NMC.

Public Health Institute of Scotland (2003). *Scottish Needs Assessment Report on Child and Adolescent Mental Health.* Glasgow: PHIS.

Royal College of Nursing (2002). *The Admiral Nurse's Competency Framework.* London: RCN.

Royal College of Nursing (2003). *Preparing Nurses to Care for Children and Young People: summary position statement by the RCN Children and Young People's Field of Practice.* London: RCN.

Royal College of Nursing (2004). *Children and Young People's Mental Health: every nurse's business.* London: RCN.

Royal College of Nursing (2004). *The Post Registration Education and Training Needs of Nurses Working with Children and Young People in the UK: a research study conducted by the Mental Health Programme, RCN Institute, in collaboration with the RCN Children and Young People's Mental Health Forum.* London: RCN Institute.

Royal College of Nursing Child and Adolescent Mental Health Forum (1998). *Report of Sub-committee on Education and Training: a review of post registration education and training for CAMH nurses* (unpublished). London: RCN.

Royal College of Psychiatrists (2000). *Perinatal Maternal Mental Health Services. Council Report: CR88.* London: Royal College of Psychiatrists.

Sainsbury Centre for Mental Health & National Institute for Mental Health in England (NIMHE) (2001). *Essential Shared Capabilities.* London: SCMH & NIMHE.

Scottish Executive (2003). *Scottish Framework for Nursing in Schools.* Edinburgh: Scottish Executive.

Social Exclusion Unit (2004). *The impact of government policy on social exclusion among children aged 0–13 and their families: a review of the literature for the Social Exclusion Unit in the Breaking the Cycle series.* London: Social Exclusion Unit.

Symington, R. (1997). Mental health services for young people: inadequate and patchy. *Paediatric Nursing,* **9** (7), 6–7.

Townley, M. (2002). Mental health needs of children and young people. *Nursing Standard,* **16** (30), 38–45.

Wells, J., Barlow, J. & Stewart-Brown, S. (2001). *A Systematic Review of Universal Approaches to Mental Health Promotion in Schools.* Oxford Health Services Research Unit: University of Oxford Institute of Health Sciences.

Chapter 17

The Legal Context in which Nurses Work with Children and Young People with Mental Disorders

Tim McDougall and Augustine Sagoe

Key points

- All public authorities and service providers in the NHS (National Health Service) and independent sector have an obligation to ensure that respect for human rights are at the core of day to day work with all people.

- The Children Act (2004) compliments the Children Act (1989), and makes new provisions to help ensure interagency cooperation between children's trusts, local authorities and other partner organisations to safeguard, promote the welfare of and improve the wellbeing of children and young people.

- Nurses who work in in-patient and forensic settings should understand the range of Mental Health Act provisions. This is in order to ensure that their practice is lawful and so that they can inform children and young people about the purpose of their detention and their rights of appeal.

- Generally speaking, children's rights to confidentiality should be strictly observed. It is important that all nurses have a clear understanding of their duties of confidentiality to children and young people. Any limits to such an obligation should be made clear to the child or young person who has the capacity to understand them.

- Nurses should always give children and young people a clear explanation of any treatment that is being prescribed. The information provided should be culturally competent, gender-sensitive and at a level that is appropriate to the age, developmental status and understanding of the child or young person.

- Advocacy by nurses on behalf of children and young people can occur at a range of different levels. This can be through representing the views of the child or young person at a review or case conference; informing them of their rights; and making their voice heard throughout the care and treatment process. Nurses also share a responsibility to speak on behalf of children and young people at a strategic level. This may be in relation to CAMHS (child and adolescent mental health services) service-planning, or by representing the views and wishes of children and young people to CAMHS service managers and commissioners.

Introduction

The legal framework in which child and adolescent mental health services (CAMHS) are delivered is complex and the numerous legal provisions as they apply to each of the UK countries may at first appear daunting for nurses. This can create uncertainty about professional authority and the legal and ethical context in which nursing practice with children takes place. Nurses therefore require access to clear information in relation to the legal basis for intervention and treatment. This is both to ensure clarity about their professional responsibilities and also to ensure that children are properly advised of their rights. The following chapter considers the implications of a range of legislative frameworks and considers how they impact on the care and treatment of children and young people with mental health problems. Consent to treatment and advocacy for children will also be discussed.

Human Rights

The United Nations (UN) Convention on the Rights of the Child was ratified by the UK in 1991 and by Ireland in 1992. The Convention, containing 54 articles, puts children first and sets internationally accepted minimum standards on key areas relating to children's rights (see Box 17.1). For example, state parties recognise the right of a child who has been placed in care by competent authorities for the purposes of care, protection or treatment of his or her physical or mental health, to a periodic review of the treatment provided to the child and all other circumstances relevant to his or her placement (United Nations Convention on the Rights of the Child). The European Convention on Human Rights, now part of English law, was not specifically designed to protect the rights of children and young people. Consideration of the Convention is, however, central in determining the lawfulness of psychiatric treatment of children and young people. For example, if a child or young person is being treated against their wishes, their rights under Article 5 of the Convention must be considered alongside the Article 8 rights of their parents to seek medical treatment on their child's behalf. The deprivation of liberty for a child or young person on the basis of parental consent must now be reconsidered in the light of a recent judgement in the European Court of Human Rights. All public authorities and service providers in the NHS and independent sector have an obligation to ensure that respect for human rights are at the core of day-to-day work with all people. A claim can be brought against any public authority that breaches human rights. Children and young people who come into contact

Box 17.1   United Nations Convention on the Rights of the Child.

Article 2
This refers to the child or young person's right to life. This article can be used to argue that a patient should be able to get treatment that would save their life.

Article 3
This article refers to the right to freedom from torture or inhuman or degrading treatment. Children have a right to complain when they are subjected to restraint, detention or seclusion. Inhuman treatment can include failing to provide medical or nursing treatment to a child with a serious physical illness or mental disorder or withdrawing such treatment.

Article 5
This article makes clear that no-one should be deprived of their liberty and security. However, certain provisions of the Mental Health Act 1983 and Children Act 1989 allow for children to be detained in hospital or a local authority secure children's home. According to the European Court of Human Rights such detention in a mental health setting must be based on medical opinion, be for a serious mental disorder and continue only as long as the mental disorder persists.

Article 6
This article provides an entitlement to a fair trial and the right to a fair hearing. For nurses this is relevant when a child is detained within a section of the Mental Health Act or in the youth justice system when children are entitled to appropriate legal assistance.

Article 8
This article involves the right to privacy and family life. It covers a range of issues including consent to medical treatment and the right to have information kept private and confidential.

Article 10
This article relates to basic rights of freedom of expression. In the context of nursing practice, children should be actively encouraged to express their views about the service they receive.

Article 12
This article emphasises the rights of children to express their views, and have their views taken into account, in any matter affecting them.

Article 14
This article relates to freedom from discrimination, and may be used to argue for equality of access and non-prejudicial care and treatment provision.

---

with specialist mental health services should receive recognition of their basic human rights under both UN and European Conventions. Even though there are 54 human rights articles, the articles in Box 17.1 have direct relevance for nurses who work with children.

Children's law

The Children Act 1989

The Children Act 1989 was implemented in England and Wales in 1991. The primary purpose of the Act was to bring together private and public law affecting children and young people and to achieve a balance between protecting children and enabling parents to challenge state intervention. This was through legislation to protect children who may be suffering or are likely to suffer significant harm, reinforcing the autonomy of families through definition of parental responsibility and providing for support from local authorities, in particular for families whose children are in need (White et al. 2004).

The Children Act 2004

The Children Act 2004 does not replace the Children Act 1989, but compliments it. New provisions have been made in order to deliver the government's *Change for Children Programme: Every Child Matters* (Department for Education and Skills 2003). This is to ensure interagency cooperation between children's trusts, local authorities and other partner organisations to safeguard, and promote the welfare and improve the wellbeing of children through a strategic Children and Young People's Plan (CYPP). The Act sets out new responsibilities for directors of children's services and lead council members which includes statutory guidance on establishing Local Safeguarding Children's Boards (LSCBs).

The Children (Scotland) Act 1995 .

This sets out the duties and powers available to public services to support children and their families in the interests of the child's welfare. The needs of the child are central to this Act and specific provisions are made to support and protect the interests of looked-after and accommodated children, and those who have been in public care.

The Children (Northern Ireland) Order 1995

Under Article 18 of the Children (Northern Ireland) Order, each authority has a general duty to safeguard and promote the welfare of children in need within its area. There are additional responsibilities for children who are looked after by an authority. The respective duties and responsibilities for health and social services boards and trusts for children are set out in the Children (NI) Order and its associated regulations and guidance. The main legislation relating to the treatment of children and young people with mental disorders in Northern Ireland is the Children Order 1995. Part 1 of that order provides core principles for legal decision-making as it affects children and young people. In addition, the principles in the Children Order provide the legislative framework for planning and delivering all children's services in Northern Ireland. Relatively few children are made the subject of compulsory care and treatment under the powers provided by the current Mental Health (NI) Order (1986).

Mental Health Law

Nurses who work in in-patient and forensic settings should understand a range of the Mental Health Act (1983) provisions. This is in order to ensure that their practice is lawful, ethical and so that they can inform children and young people about the purpose of their detention and their rights of appeal.

England and Wales

Although the current Mental Health Act (1983) applies to children as well as adults, there are particular considerations for mental health professionals who work with children and adolescents. The welfare of the child and young person with a mental disorder should be paramount in any interventions imposed on the child or young person under the Act. The child and young person's views, wishes and feelings should always be given due consideration, having due regard to their competence and capacity. Any intervention in the life of a child considered necessary by reason of their mental disorder should be the least restrictive and least stigmatising option consistent with effective care and treatment, and should result in the least possible separation from family or carers, friends, community and education. All children and young people who are in hospital for treatment of a mental disorder should be accommodated in age-appropriate facilities and receive appropriate educational provision, subject to the rights of young people to opt out of such provision.

Children and young people should always be kept as fully informed as possible, and should receive clear and detailed information concerning their care and treatment. The privacy, dignity and confidentiality of all children and young people should be respected. Formal powers within the Mental Health Act should only be used if there is a good prospect of benefit and if informal care and treatment within the community has failed, is impractical or is associated with unacceptable risks to the child or others. There are at least four key reasons why the provision of mental healthcare for children differs from that for adults:

- For children under 16, the role and the views of parents or those with parental responsibility must always be taken into account.
- There are particular responsibilities to ensure that children are protected from abuse of any kind and that their interests and welfare are safeguarded.
- Other legislation, particularly the Children Acts of 1989 and 2004, is applicable to children and may need to be considered in parallel or as an alternative to the Mental Health Act (1983) when determining how best to meet the needs of a child.
- The Human Rights Act contains specific articles in relation to children.

At the time of writing this chapter, the Mental Health Act in England and Wales is under review. A new mental health act is expected to be published in 2007 and, if so, many of the principles outlined in this section will become obsolete and be replaced. The current Mental Health Act (1983) applies to all patients, including children and young people, in England and Wales. The 1983 Mental Health Act is primarily concerned with treatment in hospital.

In July 1998 the Secretary of State for Health in England announced a wide ranging review of the Mental Health Act. This was aimed at producing new legislation to reflect care and treatment moving away from hospital to community settings and incorporate developments such as the European Convention on Human Rights. A White Paper called *Reforming the Mental Health Act* was published in 2000 and consultation on a new Mental Health Bill started in 2002.

The Mental Health Bill (2002) sets out particular provisions for children and young people. These provisions differ from the 1983 Mental Health Act in two main ways. First, young people aged 16 and 17 will be able to agree to or refuse treatment for mental disorders, and their decisions cannot be over-ridden by someone with parental responsibility. If enacted, mental health nurses working with children and young people with mental disorders will be given new powers under the new Mental Health Bill. They will be able to act as approved mental health professionals (AMHPs), and will be responsible for coordinating the assessment of the child or young person to see if they can be subject to formal powers. In their role as the AMHP they will also be responsible for registering the child or young person, appointing a nominated person and keeping those with parental responsibility fully informed during the care and treatment process. Nurses acting as AMHPs will also be responsible for notify-ing the hospital manager when a tribunal is unable to approve a mental health act treatment plan. Nurses who are AMHPs for children and young people should have specialist training and should be attached, wherever possible, to specialist CAMHS. Consultant nurses who work in specialist CAMHS may also be in a position to act as approved clinicians and clinical supervisors. The role of a clinical supervisor is similar to that of the current responsible medical officer and will include responsibility for coordinating and regularly evaluating the Mental Health Act treatment plans for a child or young person who is sub-ject to the formal powers of the Act. These supervisors must also keep under review the question of whether the child or young person needs to remain detained in hospital or whether their care and treatment could continue at home or in the community.

Scotland

The Mental Health (Scotland) Bill was introduced to the Scottish Parliament in September 2002 and became the Mental Health (Care and Treatment) Scotland Act in 2003. This replaced the Mental Health (Scotland) Act (1984) and made provisions to protect the rights of all people with mental disorders, defined in the Act as including any mental illness, personality disorder or learning disability. The Act's primary objective is to ensure that all people with mental disorders, including children, receive care and treatment that is lawful and effective. The Act makes particular provisions to protect the specific interests of children and young people. Section 23 of the Act places a duty on NHS boards to ensure that, on those occasions when a child or young person requires in-patient treatment, that this is provided in a way that is appropriate to their particular needs. The Act came into force in October 2005.

Northern Ireland

The Mental Health (Northern Ireland) Order (1986) is the principal act governing the treatment of people with mental disorders. In October 2002, the Department of Health, Social Services and Public Safety announced a major independent review of the law, policy and provision affecting people with a mental disorder or learning disability in Northern Ireland. This is a process similar to the reviews of mental health legislation in England and Scotland and is intended to take account of the need to recognise, preserve and promote the personal dignity of people with mental health problems; to incorporate human rights obligations; and to make recommendations for future mental health policy, strategy and guidance.

Consent to treatment

Children's rights are central to issues of consent to treatment and the term is used to denote where a claim can be made for treatment, either by the child or on their behalf, based on established legal or quasi-legal authority such as an act of Parliament, international convention, code of practice, case law or official policy document. Consent to medical treatment by or for children can be complex and requires a balance between preserving the principle of legal autonomy for children, while providing protection to safeguard their physical and mental health. Medical treatment for the purposes of this chapter includes psychiatric, psychological and psychotherapeutic intervention including creative therapy using art, music, drama or play etc. Before examining, treating or caring for a child, consent must be given (Department of Health 2001). Young people aged 16 and 17 are presumed to have the competence to consent for themselves. Children under 16 who fully understand the nature of treatment can also give consent; however, it is good practice to involve parents in such treatment decisions. In order for consent to be valid, the child or young person must be capable of consenting, the consent must be freely given and the child or young person involved must be given appropriate information.

Treatment without consent using the common law can only be given in emergencies (Fennell 1996). This is when immediate action is needed to either save life, protect the young person from serious harm, or prevent a serious and immediate danger to the public. In such cases the treatment must be reasonable and limited to whatever appears necessary to resolve the emergency. The Children Act (1989) refers to circumstances where a child can refuse to be assessed, examined or treated. The provisions state that, notwithstanding any court direction, a child with sufficient understanding to make an informed treatment decision can refuse to be assessed, examined or treated. However, in rare circumstances the court can override such a refusal if it is deemed to compromise the best interests of the child.

Capacity and competence

Children's competence is determined by their maturity and understanding rather than their fixed chronological age. This means that they may be competent to make one treatment decision but not another. A person with the capacity to consent should be able to:

- Understand in broad terms what the treatment is, what it is for and why it is being proposed.
- Understand the principle benefits, risks and alternatives to the treatment being proposed.
- Understand the likely consequences of not receiving the treatment being proposed.
- Retain the above information for long enough to make an informed decision.
- Make a choice that is free from external pressure and secondary gain.

A person can be said to lack capacity if they are incapable of understanding or retaining information relevant to making the treatment choice, or if they are incapable of using this information to arrive at a choice (Green 2000). Where children are incapable of consenting to treatment themselves the consent of their parents or those with parental responsibility must be obtained except in emergencies. It may be appropriate to involve a court to intervene where parents refuse to consent for treatment (considered by a physician to be necessary) to be given to their child; or where there are child protection concerns that impact negatively or parental ability to act in the best interests of their child. Evaluating competency is an essential part of the assessment process prior to the provision of any treatment for mental disorder for a child or young person.

Involving parents in treatment decisions

The Children Act 1989 uses the term 'parental responsibility' to describe the duties, rights and authority which a parent has in respect of a child. Wherever the care and treatment of a child is being considered the person, or persons with parental responsibility, must be identified, and their views sought as appropriate. If the child is subject to a care order, the local authority and parents share responsibility for the child, subject to the local authority's power to limit the exercise of such responsibility by the parents in order to safeguard the child's welfare. Where more than one person has parental responsibility for a child, each of them may act alone, and without the other, in meeting that responsibility. This means that, for example, nurses can lawfully provide treatment to the child with the authority of one parent, even though both parents may have parental responsibility. A person who does not have parental responsibility for a child but has care of the child may do what is reasonable under the circumstances to safeguard or promote the child's welfare. This provision will, for example, allow nurses to act in emergencies.

Ideally, treatment decisions involving children and young people will involve people close to them. Indeed, more often than not, children and young people may want decisions concerning their health and welfare to include those with parental responsibility. However, the Gillick ruling (1985) established that advice and treatment by a physician could be given to a competent child without their parents being consulted or consenting. This is where the child understands the treatment being proposed; where the physician is unable to persuade the child to inform their parents of the treatment being proposed; or where the child's best interests require the treatment to be given. However, it is not necessarily the case that a child considered competent by the standards of the Gillick case can both legally refuse treatment as well as consent to be treated. A child's refusal to be treated can be vetoed. Therefore, in most cases medical treatment which a child is refusing can in fact be given with the consent of those with parental responsibility. Although the Gillick ruling referred to contraceptive advice, the principles can be applied to other forms of medical treatment, including psychiatric treatment and nursing interventions.

A new Mental Capacity Act is likely to come into force in 2007 and is intended to establish a comprehensive framework for decision-making in relation to young people aged over 16 who lack capacity to make their own decisions. This is to regulate decisions about a range of matters including medical treatment and residency. If there is no person with parental responsibility, or those with parental responsibility disagree or do not act in their child's best interests, the Mental Capacity Act will provide those who must make such decisions with a statutory framework. Court proceedings may be transferred from the children's courts to the Court of Protection. For example, if the parents of a 17 year-old who has severe learning disabilities cannot agree on residence or contact arrangements, it may be more appropriate for the Court of Protection to adjudicate the disputed issues, as any orders made under the Children Act will expire on the young person's eighteenth birthday.

Distinctions between the Children Act and the Mental Health Act

Debate exists among CAMHS professionals about which legal framework should be used to enforce treatment decisions. Given the complex relationship between the Children Act, the Mental Health Act and evolving case law, it is only possible to provide general pointers for CAMHS professionals to take into account. Consideration should be given to a number of important factors. The Children Act may appear to be less stigmatising since its use may be seen as a reflection of social and family breakdown rather than a problem associated with an individual child's mental health. By comparison, detention within the Mental Health Act may be regarded as carrying discrimination and stigma. The Children Act, unlike Part 4 of the Mental Health Act, does not provide specific powers to enforce medical treatment, or to safeguard the rights of detained patients. These safeguards are provided by the Mental Health Act and include the review of detention by hospital managers, the Mental Health Review Tribunal and the general oversight of the Mental Health Act Commission. Notwithstanding these factors, although the Mental Health Act can be applied to children, it is not specifically orientated towards the needs and circumstances of children. It may therefore be argued that the underlying principles and safeguards of the Mental Health Act are not sufficient to protect adequately the best interests of children.

Many professionals argue that detention under the Mental Health Act provides a legal framework which protects the rights of the child or young person more effectively than using parental authority. In these latter circumstances there is a lack of procedural and legal safeguards. The provisions of Part 4 of the Mental Health Act afford safeguards when a child's refusal of treatment for mental disorder is being overridden. These safeguards apply to the provision of certain forms of treatment, particularly the administration of medication for mental disorder after three months and the use of ECT (electro-convulsive therapy). Treatment of 16 and 17 year-olds on the basis of parental authority alone will not be permitted within the new Mental Health Act. An additional point for consideration is that most lasting powers under the Children Act are consequent on court decisions, unlike the powers of the Mental Health Act, which are exercised on the basis of professional judgement and do not involve court review. If a child is detained under the Mental Health Act, their consent is not required for any medical treatment which falls outside Part 4 of the Act (DoH & Welsh Office 1999). Treatment within the provisions of Section 63 of the Act has been given a wide interpretation and can include nasogastric tube feeding. However, good practice would require that consensus is achieved wherever possible.

Parental responsibility is another important factor. If a child is detained under the Mental Health Act, the parent will usually be the nearest relative and must be consulted about treatment. If the parent holds parental responsibility, the child can be treated with the consent of the parent. Professionals should consider whether this is appropriate if abuse by the parent is alleged and when consulting the relative may not be considered desirable or therapeutic. In such circumstances it may be necessary to obtain a court direction to dispense with the parent's consent. When considering the most appropriate legal framework it is important to consider the purpose of the intervention in the child's life. Relevant considerations include the length of time a child may require treatment and detention, and how serious or chronic their illness is likely to be. Finally, the involvement of the child in any legal process requires legal representation. Within the Children Act, the guardian *ad litem* is appointed by the court, may be represented by a solicitor, and the application is audited and reviewed in a court setting. External review in relation to detention under the Mental Health

Act has caused debate. Whilst admission using the Act can only take place according to specific legal criteria, this can still be a highly subjective process and there is no external audit of that process. However, the continuing need for detention is externally reviewed by the Mental Health Review Tribunal.

Good practice guidance for nurses

The following guidance applies to both children who are the subject of care orders within the Children Act or detained under the Mental Health Act. Care and treatment plans for medical treatment must be reviewed on a regular basis. Any plan should reflect partnership between the local authority, those with parental responsibility and the child or young person concerned. Wherever possible, the care or treatment plan should be established prior to the prescription of medical treatment and will be reviewed regularly by the multidisciplinary team, parents and child or young person themselves. Nurses and all other professionals involved in the treatment should ensure that valid consent is sought and established, recorded and regularly evaluated. Withdrawal of consent at any stage during the treatment process should be addressed by the multidisciplinary team. Nurses should ensure that information in relation to care and treatment is relevant and accurately recorded. This is to ensure that issues in relation to consent and treatment are regularly reviewed and audited.

Nurses, along with other members of the CAMHS multidisciplinary team should always give children and young people a clear explanation of any treatment that is being prescribed. The information provided should be culturally competent, gender-sensitive and at a level that is appropriate to the age, developmental status and understanding of the child or young person. The child or young person should be advised of their rights in relation to withholding consent to treatment. Where consent is withheld, the child should receive a clear explanation of the implications of the refusal decision and the likely consequences of not receiving treatment. Nurses administering medication as part of a child or young person's treatment plan must ensure that they are legally entitled to administer that medication. Nurses must act in accordance with the Nursing and Midwifery Council's standards on professional conduct (Nursing & Midwifery Council 2004); and with guidance on the administration of medicines (Nursing & Midwifery Council 2004); and with guidance on records and record-keeping (Nursing & Midwifery Council 2005). Where the nurse has concerns about consent to treatment or withdrawal of consent to treatment using medication this should be reported to the responsible medical officer.

Confidentiality

During the course of their work with children and young people, nurses are often recipients of confidential information. Information provided in the context of the therapeutic relationship may generate complex moral, ethical and legal dilemmas. Generally speaking, children's rights to confidentiality should be strictly observed. It is important that all nurses have a clear understanding of their duties of confidentiality to children and young people. Any limits to such an obligation should be made clear to the child or young person who has the capacity to understand them. Young people aged 16 and 17 are entitled to the same duty of confidentiality as adults. This means that information cannot be shared without their explicit consent, or if a failure to share information is likely to lead to harm to others. Nurses should be aware of current guidance on information-sharing and confidentiality and the application of this guidance to children and young people. This is contained in *Working Together to Safeguard Children*, currently being reviewed by the DoH, which is a guide to interagency working to safeguard and promote the welfare of children (DoH 2003).

Children under the age of 16 who have the capacity and understanding to take decisions about their own treatment are also entitled to make decisions about the use and disclosure of information they have provided in confidence. For example, they may be receiving treatment or counselling that they do not want their parents to know of. The nurse may try to persuade the child or young person to allow their parents to be informed about the treatment. There are two situations when a child's confidentiality may need to be breached. The main indication for breaching confidentiality is where information is disclosed that suggests that the child may be at significant risk of harm or abuse. In these circumstances it is good practice for the nurse to support the child or young person to make the disclosure themselves. However, if the child is unable or unwilling to make the disclosure themselves, the nurse is professionally obliged to report the disclosure on their behalf. In addition, where a competent young person or child is refusing treatment for a life-threatening condition, the duty of care would require confidentiality to be breached to the extent of informing those with parental responsibility for the child who might then be able to provide the necessary consent to the treatment. In both scenarios, nurses must have a clear understanding of their duties and have ready access to service policies on confidentiality and information sharing.

Advocacy

Advocacy by nurses on behalf of service users is vitally important. It involves helping children and young people navigate the mental health system, and to access independent and confidential information, culturally sensitive advice, representation and support (Valentine 2004). Advocacy by nurses on behalf of children and young people can occur at a range of different levels. This may be through representing the views of the child or young person at a review or case conference; informing them of their rights; or making their voice heard throughout the care and treatment process. Nurses also share a responsibility to speak on behalf of children and young people at a strategic level. This may be in relation to CAMHS service-planning or by representing their views and wishes to CAMHS service managers and commissioners. It is not always appropriate or possible for nurses to advocate on behalf of a particular child or adolescent. The young person may, for example, have a complaint that they do not want the nurse or service provider to know about. Independent advocacy services are therefore very helpful and can also help children and young people to understand their rights, make complaints about their care, treatment or detention and provide confidential advice. In 2002, the Department of Health published national standards for the provision of children's advocacy services (DoH 2002).

References

Department for Education and Skills (2003). *Every Child Matters*. London: HMSO.

Department of Health (2001). *Seeking Consent: working with children*. London: HMSO.

Department of Health (2002). *National Standards for the Provision of Children's Advocacy Services*. London: HMSO.

Department of Health (2003). *Working Together to Safeguard Children: a guide to interagency working to safeguard and promote the welfare of children*. London: HMSO.

Department of Health & Welsh Office (1999). *Mental Health Act 1983: Code of Practice*. London: HMSO.

Fennell, P. (1996). *Treatment Without Consent: law, psychiatry and the treatment of mentally disordered people since 1845*. London: Routledge.

Green, C. (2000). Mental health care and human rights. *Mental Health Practice*, **4** (4), 8–10.

Nursing and Midwifery Council (2004a). *The NMC Code of Professional Conduct: standards for conduct, performance and ethics. Protecting the public through professional standards*. London: NMC.

Nursing and Midwifery Council (2004b). *Guidelines for Records and Record Keeping*. London: NMC.

Nursing and Midwifery Council (2004b). *Guidelines for the Administration of Medicines*. London: NMC.

Valentine, F. (2004). 'Skilling up' to influence commissioning. *Nursing Management*, **11** (8), 22–25.

White, R., Harbour, A. & Williams, R. (2004). *Safeguards for Young Minds: young people and protective legislation*. (2nd edn). London: Gaskell.

Chapter 18

Ten Practical Tips for Nursing Children and Young People with Mental Health Problems

Tim McDougall

Practical tips for nurses

(1) *Champion the children you work with*: get involved in local strategic part-nerships and take every opportunity to raise the profile of their mental health in your everyday work.

(2) *Raise your profile*: remember that nurses make up a quarter of the CAMHS workforce and you have most face-to-face contact with children and families. You have a duty to share your knowledge and expertise with others.

(3) *Help make sure that local services meet the needs of local people*: you are in key positions to broker the needs of children and families with com-missioners and service providers. Make sure their voice is heard on planning boards.

(4) *Look for resources to develop your practice*: there are lots of opportunities for nurses to get funding if you know where to look. Spend some time each month on the internet looking for research and travel scholarships, bursaries and awards.

(5) *Celebrate your success in the public domain*: articulate your worth by writing and publishing an article, doing some research or speaking at a conference. This will help raise your professional profile and the status of CAMHS nursing.

(6) *Network widely and get your links right*: you do not have time to do every-thing yourself and someone else in the CAMHS world will be able to help you.

(7) *Listen to the evidence and be creative*: you will never have all the answers and one size does not fit all. Strategies that work today may not work tomorrow.

(8)   *Scan the horizon*: keep up with changes in health, education and social services and youth justice agencies. Remember that CAMHS are in a process of evolution and expect change to be part of your working life.

(9)   *Break down professional boundaries*: these are of no use to the child. Remember that nurses rarely practice in isolation and that CAMHS is a multiagency responsibility.

(10) *Learn from your CAMHS colleagues*: be proud to be a nurse but also remember that you work with a range of other professionals who each have something to contribute to the task of providing comprehensive CAMHS.

Index